Praise for *Your Healthy Pregnancy with Thyroid Disease*

"Dana Tren⋯ ⋯roid advocates. This book ⋯ ⋯r babies."

⋯n, MD, founder, ⋯grative Medicine

Pr⋯ ⋯ooks

"This infor⋯

—*Publishers Weekly*

" . . . inspi⋯ ⋯ions . . . offers solid, pract⋯

—⋯*dicine Magazine*

"Shomon e⋯ ⋯s that a patient has to mak⋯

—*Library Journal*

"At last, a ⋯ ⋯cess weight."

—⋯ames, PhD, RN

"Help and hope for millions who have despaired of ever losing weight and regaining their energy."

—Hyla Cass, MD, author of *Natural Highs*

"Mary Shomon is an outstanding advocate for patient health, and you'll find her book to be outstanding as well!"

—Jacob Teitelbaum, MD, author of *From Fatigued to Fantastic*

"Mary Shomon offers practical and effective solutions that will help millions finally conquer their weight problems."

—Steve Langer, MD, author, *Solved: The Riddle of Illness*

"I can think of few conditions more challenging to patients and the medical profession than fibromyalgia and chronic fatigue syndrome. Once again Mary Shomon has shed an incredible light on what really matters—everything from how to get an accurate diagnosis to finding the best treatment."

—Marie Savard, author of *How to Save Your Own Life*

"If you're one of the millions afflicted with fibromyalgia or chronic fatigue, or think you may be, start changing your life for the better now by reading this crucial book. There are very real answers that will help you even more than you dare to hope, and Mary Shomon has done an absolutely masterful job of providing them to you here."

—Dr. Joseph Mercola, author of *The No-Grain Diet*

"[Mary Shomon] provides a comprehensive service for sufferers of thyroid disease."

—*Time*

"Mary Shomon is 'rattling the cages of the thyroid mandarins.'"

—*Elle*

Your Healthy Pregnancy

with Thyroid Disease

Also by Mary Shomon:

The Thyroid Diet

Living Well with Hypothyroidism

The Thyroid Diet Revolution

Living Well with Autoimmune Disease

The Menopause Thyroid Solution

Living Well with Graves' Disease and Hyperthyroidism

The Thyroid Hormone Breakthrough

Living Well with Chronic Fatigue and Fibromyalgia

Your Healthy Pregnancy

with Thyroid Disease

A Guide to Fertility, Pregnancy,
and Postpartum Wellness

DANA TRENTINI AND MARY SHOMON

Da Capo
LIFE
LONG
A Member of the Perseus Books Group

Designed by Brent Wilcox
Set in 11 point Adobe Garamond Pro by Perseus Books

Cataloging-in-Publication data for this book is available from the Library of Congress.

First Da Capo Press edition 2016
ISBN: 978-0-7382-1867-0 (paperback)
ISBN: 978-0-7382-1868-7 (e-book)

Published by Da Capo Press, an imprint of Perseus Books, a division of PBG Publishing, LLC, a subsidiary of Hachette Book Group, Inc.
www.dacapopress.com

Note: The information in this book is true and complete to the best of our knowledge. This book is intended only as an informative guide for those wishing to know more about health issues. In no way is this book intended to replace, countermand, or conflict with the advice given to you by your own physician. The ultimate decision concerning care should be made between you and your doctor. We strongly recommend you follow his or her advice. Information in this book is general and is offered with no guarantees on the part of the authors or Da Capo Press. The authors and publisher disclaim all liability in connection with the use of this book.

Da Capo Press books are available at special discounts for bulk purchases in the U.S. by corporations, institutions, and other organizations. For more information, please contact the Special Markets Department at 2300 Chestnut Street, Suite 200, Philadelphia, PA, 19103, or call (800) 810-4145, ext. 5000, or e-mail special.markets@perseusbooks.com.

10 9 8 7 6 5 4 3 2 1

This book is written in memory of my lost baby and in dedication to my sons Benjamin and Hudson who beat the odds and made it to the world.

—**DT**

For Julia and Danny—you have all my love—and to my lost little one, I love you, too; you deserved a chance to be in this world.

—**MS**

Contents

Part 3
Your Healthy Pregnancy Plans from Preconception to Postpartum

Part 4
Into the Future

Acknowledgments

How do I thank the woman who helped me get pregnant with my son Hudson when doctors discouraged me from having more children after my miscarriage? You are my thyroid hero, Mary Shomon. I remember the day I met our agent, Carol Mann, in her New York City office, and I knew this woman would change my life. Renée Sedliar, with your sweet manner, you put me at ease throughout the entire process of creating my very first book. Thank you, Lisa Kaufman, for your edit recommendations that made this book flow perfectly. To the Perseus team, you rock! Thank you to all the incredible experts we interviewed. I hope you know that by generously sharing your knowledge for this book, you will save babies around the world. Thank you to the thyroid advocates who work tirelessly to let people know they are not alone—Michelle Bickford, Izabella Wentz, Suzy Cohen, Danna Bowman, Stacey Robbins, Lorraine Cleaver, Denise Fleming, Sarah Downing, Beth Jones, Helle Sydendal, Tiffany Mladinich, Jen Wittman, Karen Fitzpatrick-Dame, Zen Thyroid, Blythe Clifford, Marissa Ravelo, Robert Chapman, Laura Scheunemann, Marc Ryan, Carol Gray, Jill A. Gurfinkel, Maggie Hadleigh-West, and Gena Lee Nolin. To my *Hypothyroid Mom* followers, you are a blessing to me. Thank you to my mom, Ron, Marie, Paul, Jenny, Johann, John, Gloria, Norm, Jennifer, Anthony, John Paul, Elise, Laura, Jennifer, Carmen, Maria, Rina, Leo, Manuel, Milana, Nicholas, Sylvia, Ricky, Lola, John, Sorena, Zackery, Giselle, and my angels (my dad, grandparents, Giulio, and Patrick).

—*Dana Trentini*

I would first like to thank Dana Trentini, my coauthor, for her amazing vision, energy, and advocacy for our fellow thyroid patients. Dana is a pleasure and joy to work with, and I know this is just the first of many books to come from her. Many thanks to literary superagent Carol Mann and her staff, who are

gurus at transforming dreams and passions into amazing books. Much gratitude to our editor, Renée Sedliar, and her top-notch colleagues at Perseus, who
shared our vision of the importance of this book and helped us make it a far
better book at each step in the process. I must also thank all of the amazing
doctors and experts who shared information for the book—your knowledge
and generous spirits are helping more women become mothers, and helping
babies have a healthier start. Many thanks to all the advocates Dana listed—I'm proud to be in the thyroid trenches with you all, helping to spread
the word! Love and thanks to my right-hand go-to person, BFF, and "most
organized person in the world," Jane Frank. I also want to thank Cynthia Wal-
lentine and Julia Schopick for their help and support. I must include my
friends around the United States and the world, whose faith, love, and support
is oxygen. And finally, my family, and in particular, my children who have
given me the immense joy of motherhood, an experience that should never be
denied any woman due to misdiagnosis or mismanagement of her thyroid
problem.

—*Mary Shomon*

Introduction
by Dana Trentini

On a cold, snowy day in New York City in January 2009, I lay on a medical exam table on what would be one of the worst days of my life. I had miscarried a much-wanted child at 12 weeks and was being prepared for a D&C, a surgical procedure to remove the fetus. A technician had just taken an ultrasound and walked out of the room to reconfirm to the medical staff that my baby had no heartbeat. I sprang off my bed and ran to the image on the screen. I felt my body shake and my fists clench as I stared at the image of my unborn child. From a place deep in my soul came a wail.

What Happened to My Child?

When asked my choice of anesthesia, I asked for general anesthesia because there was no way in the world that I wanted to be awake through this procedure. I didn't want to remember a single thing about their removing my child from my body. The anesthesiologist assured me that it would all be over soon and asked me to count backward from 10.

10 . . .

When I was pregnant with my first son, Benjamin, in 2006, I had fantasies of being a supermom. I was going to do it all—career, home, and family—and I was going to do it brilliantly.

Then fatigue came crashing over me.

I was diagnosed with hypothyroidism the year following Benjamin's birth. I was given levothyroxine, the number one drug prescribed by mainstream doctors for hypothyroidism. You'll discover in this book that while some do great on this treatment, many do not. I was one of those who didn't.

Despite my thyroid hormone replacement medication, low-thyroid symptoms overtook my life. I was overwhelmed with a crushing fatigue that no amount of sleep could undo. The weight I'd gained during pregnancy stayed on and kept climbing. My hair was falling out in massive clumps and my scalp itched. My breast milk supply was low. The outer third of my eyebrows were missing. The heels of my feet were cracked and the skin on my body was pale, dry, and itchy. My face was pale, dry, and puffy. My eyes were red and inflamed with dark circles. My eyelids twitched. My legs were numb to the touch. Unusually heavy menstrual bleeding, chronic constipation, persistent headaches, itchy eczema, repeat urinary tract infections, low libido, allergies, anxiety, mood swings, insomnia, brain fog, and constant infections plagued me. Kidney stones landed me in the emergency room. A healthy woman prior to pregnancy, I now had blood levels indicating I had elevated cholesterol and blood sugar levels.

I watched other mothers doing it all and tried to keep up, but every day was a struggle. I felt like a failure.

What had happened to me?

. . . 9 . . .

When I was a girl, my father would sing Frank Sinatra's song "New York, New York." He would sing it at the top of his lungs and I believed that if I could make it in New York City, I really could make it anywhere. In New York City, one of the greatest cities in the world, I expected the best possible medical care. I trusted my Ivy League medical school–trained, award-winning New York City doctors. I never once thought they might not know everything there was to know about hypothyroidism—especially the dangers of thyroid disease in pregnancy. And I continued to trust them when I became pregnant for the second time in late 2008, following my thyroid drug protocol to the letter.

In my first trimester, I was overcome by a sick, tired, weak feeling. I recall the night I said, "I am worried that something is wrong with the baby." But when I shared my anxiety with my doctors, they responded that my thyroid levels were safe and that it was normal in early pregnancy to be tired. I'd been pregnant before, and the way I felt now didn't seem normal to me, but I disregarded my body's warning.

. . . 8 . . .

Why didn't I trust my gut instincts?

Why didn't I put up a better fight with my doctors, and insist that something seemed seriously wrong with me and my baby?

Why did I naively think, "Doctor always knows best"?

I graduated in 1993 with an honors BA in neuroscience from the University of Toronto with high distinction, receiving multiple scholarships and prestigious awards. I worked for several years as a high school science teacher in a specialized school for intellectually gifted students. At Columbia University in 2002, I obtained an MA in organizational psychology and an EdM in counseling psychology. A distinguished Columbia University professor selected me as the team leader for his research team during the course of my studies. I was no stranger to scientific research. So, why hadn't I used my science background and research skills to learn everything I could about my thyroid disease?

Why didn't I get a second medical opinion?

You have no idea how many times I've asked myself these questions and beat myself up over them. I was once interviewed by a large digital media company for a story it wished to include about me online. I was being interviewed on camera in my home and I'll never forget it.

The interviewer asked, "If you knew you weren't feeling well, why didn't you get a second medical opinion?"

I sat silent, thoughts racing through my head, feelings overwhelming me, then said, "I don't know why."

When the interview was over and the camera crew left my apartment, I'll never forget closing the door and dropping down on the ground and crying. I cried like a baby after that interview. That interviewer had no idea how her simple fifteen-word question crushed me.

I'm not even sure how to answer that question. I've asked myself over and over again, going over scenarios of what I should have done but didn't.

. . . 7 . . .

Thyroid-stimulating hormone (TSH) is a measure taken from a blood sample to test thyroid functioning. High TSH levels above the normal reference range are interpreted as indicating an underactive thyroid, known as hypothyroidism. Low TSH levels below the normal reference range are interpreted as indicating an overactive thyroid, called hyperthyroidism.

The Endocrine Society's 2007 clinical guidelines "Management of Thyroid Dysfunction During Pregnancy and Postpartum" includes the following recommendations:

- If hypothyroidism has been diagnosed before pregnancy, thyroid hormone replacement medication dosage should be adjusted to reach a TSH level not higher than 2.5 mIU/L prior to pregnancy.
- If overt hypothyroidism is diagnosed during pregnancy, thyroid function tests should be normalized as rapidly as possible to TSH levels of less than 2.5 mIU/L in the first trimester (or 3 mIU/L in the second and third trimester).

Throughout my first trimester, my TSH remained higher than the above recommended 2.5 mIU/L, soaring close to 10.0 mIU/L. My doctors said that everything was fine and that TSH was only a concern in pregnancy above 10.0 mIU/L.

Wait . . . rewind . . . yes you read that correctly.

My doctors did not realize that my TSH close to 10.0 in pregnancy was a danger to me and my baby, because my doctors clearly had *never read* the guidelines.

And even if they had, while TSH is considered the gold standard in mainstream medicine for the testing of thyroid function, it does not give a complete picture of thyroid health. As you'll learn in this book, there is much more to thyroid testing than TSH.

. . . 6 . . .

Scientific research reveals unequivocally that undiagnosed, untreated, or improperly treated thyroid disease:

- Increases the risk of infertility
- Increases the risk of miscarriage
- Increases the risk of stillbirth
- Increases the risk of maternal anemia
- Increases the risk of preeclampsia
- Increases the risk of placental abruption
- Increases the risk of premature delivery
- Increases the risk of breech birth
- Increases the risk of postpartum hemorrhage

- Increases the risk of low birth weight
- Increases the risk of neonatal respiratory distress
- Increases the risk of admission to neonatal intensive care
- Increases the risk of impaired fetal cognitive development
- Increases the risk of breastfeeding difficulties
- Increases the risk of postpartum depression

Given this knowledge, it would make sense that women would be routinely screened during pregnancy, right? And it would make sense that physicians providing obstetric care and physicians specializing in endocrinology would be especially careful to know and follow the latest treatment guidelines with their patients who have thyroid problems, and who develop thyroid disease during and after pregnancy?

Unfortunately, that is not the case.

In a study published in *Thyroid* in 2010, three waves of mail surveys were distributed to 1,601 Wisconsin health-care providers who were members of the American College of Obstetricians and Gynecologists or the American Academy of Family Physicians and who had a history of providing obstetric care. Of the 575 providers who completed the survey, only 11.5 percent (66/575) had actually read the Endocrine Society's 2007 clinical guidelines.

In another study, a survey was distributed to 260 surgeons attending the 2009 American Association of Endocrine Surgeons' meeting and 109 surgeons returned the survey. Only 23 percent (26/109) had read the Endocrine Society's guidelines. Reading the guidelines was associated with a significantly greater likelihood of the doctors informing patients of the TSH guidelines for pregnancy, but the study didn't indicate how many of the 23 percent who read them didn't follow the guidelines themselves.

The upshot: an army of uninformed health-care providers is treating women with thyroid disease, and most of these practitioners have little understanding of the complexities or standards of care for pregnant thyroid patients and their babies.

. . . 5 . . .

A survey conducted in 2012 asked American Thyroid Association participating physicians—the majority of them endocrinologists—whether they thought all pregnant women should be screened for thyroid dysfunction. The results were reported at the 83rd Annual Meeting of the American Thyroid

Association in 2013: Universal thyroid screening in pregnancy was recommended by 74 percent of the survey respondents. This was not the first time that universal thyroid screening in pregnancy had been recommended; it is likely not the last. Yet despite the fact that abnormal maternal thyroid function can have a detrimental effect on the mother and her fetus, universal screening is still not recommended as a guideline.

In 2014 the Endocrine Society reported that, according to recent World Health Organization (WHO) estimates, thyroid disorders affect 750 million people worldwide, making them even more prevalent than diabetes. Conservative estimates find that at minimum there are 27 million Americans with thyroid disease, but the experts believe that the actual number is closer to 60 million—at least half are undiagnosed.

In 2015, the Endocrine Society reported that, for every 1,000 Americans, up to

- 8 have overt hypothyroidism
- 130 have subclinical hypothyroidism
- 5 have overt hyperthyroidism
- 4 have overt hypothyroidism

Thyroid conditions are five to ten times more common in women compared to men.

Given these statistics, there are pregnant women around the world right now who have thyroid disease. At least half of those women don't even know they have a thyroid problem, and their doctors are not aware they are at risk. Some of these women will experience miscarriage, stillbirth, infertility, maternal anemia, preeclampsia, placental abruption, postpartum hemorrhage, premature delivery, breech birth, low birth weight, and births of babies with impaired cognitive development. These mothers will have no idea their thyroid problems were to blame.

In 2012 the Endocrine Society updated its 2007 guidelines for the management of thyroid dysfunction during pregnancy and postpartum. The committee tasked with creating the new guidelines did not reach agreement with regard to thyroid screening recommendations in pregnancy. Some members recommended screening of all pregnant women by the ninth week or at the time of their first prenatal visit. Other members recommended neither for nor against universal thyroid screening in pregnancy. There was unanimous agreement, however, that targeted screening of high-risk women was recommended.

Women planning pregnancy or who are newly pregnant are high risk if they meet one or more of these criteria:

- Are over age 30
- Have a family history of autoimmune thyroid disease or hypothyroidism
- Have a goiter
- Have thyroid antibodies, primarily thyroid peroxidase antibodies
- Present with symptoms or clinical signs suggestive of low thyroid function
- Have been diagnosed with type 1 diabetes mellitus or other autoimmune disorders
- Have a history of infertility
- Have a prior history of miscarriage or preterm delivery
- Have had prior therapeutic head or neck irradiation or prior thyroid surgery
- Currently receive levothyroxine replacement
- Live in a region with presumed iodine deficiency

However, on page 2560 of its guidelines, the Endocrine Society states:

There is unanimous task force agreement that targeted screening of high-risk women is recommended during the prenatal and perinatal periods. With this approach, the committee acknowledges the important data confirming that such case finding will unfortunately miss 30 percent or more of women with overt or subclinical hypothyroidism.

. . . 4 . . .

My miscarriage was the tipping point for me. After that, my hypothyroidism symptoms raged and I hit rock bottom. To tell you the truth, I don't know how I made it through that dark time in my life. Following my miscarriage, my hypothyroidism symptoms worsened so dramatically that I struggled to stay awake to care for my young son. I knew that something was very wrong. If you've ever reached rock bottom with thyroid disease—where you can't keep your eyes open and function each day—you already know there are no words that will ever come close to describing it.

I am a bookworm. I have been all my life. When I was a little girl, my mother was always telling me to go outside and play, while I hid in my room to read my books. At night when the lights were out, I would read with a flashlight under the covers. So, it figures that, when I reached my lowest point with hypothyroidism and worried I would never get back up, my climb out of that dark hole began with a book.

The day I stumbled upon the book *Living Well with Hypothyroidism: What Your Doctor Doesn't Tell You . . . That You Need to Know* by world-renowned thyroid expert and *New York Times* best-selling author Mary Shomon was a miracle.

This book was my gut-wrenching "Aha!" moment. In reading it I realized that I lost my child all because my doctors did not optimally treat my hypothyroidism. I sobbed for days.

But until you are broken, you have no idea just how strong you really are.

. . . **3** . . .

It is a dream come true that I am joining forces to write this book with the woman that changed my life: Mary Shomon.

For three years after my miscarriage, I had dreams of writing my own book. One day I mentioned this to a friend. When she suggested I create a blog to help build a following for my future book, I asked, "What is a blog?"

This shows you just how little I understood about social media and about writing books.

But, on October 1, 2012, I took a leap of faith and launched my blog, *Hypothyroid Mom*.

October is National Miscarriage Awareness month in the United States, and I'd intentionally timed the launch for October in memory of the baby I lost to hypothyroidism and in dedication to my two boys who beat the odds and made it to the world.

Within two years, *Hypothyroid Mom* had almost 3 million monthly visits from readers in more than two hundred countries around the world. I was voted the winner of two 2014 WEGO Health Activist Awards: Health Activist Hero and Best in Show Twitter. The blog has reached hundreds of thousands. Now, there are so many times that I lay my head down on my desk in gratitude. I am blessed to have connected with readers from around the world.

You may wonder why I created *Hypothyroid Mom* in the first place and why I am now writing this book with Mary. Here's the real reason—pure rage. Mothers and babies are being needlessly harmed from medical lack of awareness about thyroid disease. That is unacceptable!

I lost my child because I failed to be an advocate for myself and my child, and I have to live with that regret for the rest of my life. But I know that I'm not alone.

I know there are women like me, raised to respect authority and not challenge the status quo; women who hate confrontation; who right now are *not* advocating for themselves with their doctors.

I know there are women like me, who believe the "doctor knows best" and expect doctors to have all the answers.

I know there are women like me all around the world being told by their doctors their symptoms are "all in their head"—and who believe it.

I know there are women like me being handed prescriptions for antidepressants, sleeping pills, and/or anxiety medication when they complain of typical thyroid symptoms.

I know there are women like me being told they are hypochondriacs by family members and friends who just don't understand what this illness does to us.

I know there are women like me feeling guilty because they don't have the same energy that others around them do to keep up, to be a supermom.

I know there are women like me hesitant to speak up about their medical concerns for fear of being told they are overreacting.

I know there are women like me who feel that they are all alone.

You aren't alone. You aren't overreacting. You *can* feel better.

After years of intense research and an unstoppable quest to find the top thyroid health professionals, I am now in the best health ever. At the age of forty, I got pregnant naturally with my second son, Hudson, and gave birth to him in 2010. *Yes,* miracle babies are possible for women with thyroid disease.

. . . **2** . . .

What is my hope for this book?

I hope that every woman with thyroid disease, whether they are struggling with hypothyroidism, Hashimoto's disease, hyperthyroidism, Graves' disease, thyroiditis, goiter, nodules, or thyroid cancer, will know there is hope to be well.

I hope that every woman suffering with infertility, due to undiagnosed or improperly treated thyroid problems, will have hope that pregnancy is possible and miracle babies do happen for us.

I hope that every woman who has suffered through a miscarriage or stillbirth due to undiagnosed or improperly treated thyroid problems will know that she is not alone, and that my heart and passion is with her and our lost children. Our babies are precious, and their short lives inspire us to make change.

I hope that every woman who is currently pregnant and has undiagnosed or improperly treated thyroid problems will learn key action steps to help protect her unborn baby.

I hope that every family with a baby born with cognitive and developmental problems due to undiagnosed or improperly treated maternal thyroid problems will know that my heart is with them and that I hope with all hope that these children have blessed lives.

I hope that every woman who wants to breastfeed her newborn but finds herself unable to nurse or provide enough milk due to undiagnosed or improperly treated thyroid problems will know there is an underlying cause that can be resolved.

I hope that every woman experiencing fatigue, depression, and a host of other physical, mental, and emotional symptoms after childbirth due to undiagnosed or improperly treated thyroid problems will know that her symptoms are *not* all in her head. They are very real.

I hope that this book will bring about universal thyroid screening in pregnancy around the world.

I hope that, years from now, I will hear from the babies born to mothers with thyroid disease, thanks to this book, and I will smile.

One thought that has repeatedly struck me is how much easier my journey might have been if somehow, magically, some of the things I know now, I could have known when I was first diagnosed with hypothyroidism, or when my body first whispered a warning to me that something was wrong. Instead, I had to learn those things the hard way. I hope that by my sharing my story, my readers who suffer from this disease, and those who suspect they have it, might benefit from my experiences and what I have learned. If my story saves the life of even one baby, I will have realized my mission.

. . . 1

—Dana Trentini, September 2015

How to Use This Book

We know all too well the fatigue that can overwhelm you with thyroid disease. You may feel that you don't have the energy to read an entire book; that it is just impossible to read about the basics of thyroid disease in fertility, pregnancy, and postpartum, and specifics of testing, medications, and more.

"Just tell me what to do!" you may be saying.

If that describes you, skip right to Part 3. This is the part that we intentionally designed to summarize the key action steps you can take right now, and put you on a successful path from fertility to a healthy baby. This section is also formatted to make it easier for you to use, like a workbook, with checklists and summaries of key information to guide you through key steps.

Parts 1 and 2 provide an in-depth look at the conventional approaches to diagnosis and management of thyroid issues in preconception, pregnancy, and the postpartum phase. Specifically, you'll learn about the Endocrine Society's updated 2012 guidelines "Management of Thyroid Dysfunction During Pregnancy and Postpartum." You'll also learn about the 2011 "Guidelines of the American Thyroid Association for the Diagnosis and Management of Thyroid Disease During Pregnancy and Postpartum"—we refer to these as the "Pregnancy Guidelines"—which are considered the standard of care, and yet are themselves controversial and not widely disseminated to practitioners.

You will also explore cutting-edge medical advice from leading health practitioners, including many nationally and internationally known doctors and experts in thyroid, hormones, autoimmune disease, nutrition, cancer, fertility, and pregnancy.

Also, please keep in mind that there are links and additional resources available at the book's website, http://www.ThyroidPregnancyBook.com, and we invite you to connect with us online.

Your Thyroid and Its Role

How Your Thyroid Works—and What Happens When It Doesn't

Your thyroid, a small, butterfly-shaped gland weighing about an ounce, located below and behind the Adam's apple area of the neck, is the master gland of metabolism. Its function is to produce hormones that deliver oxygen and energy to your cells, tissues, glands, and organs.

Every cell in your body depends on thyroid hormone for energy. Your thyroid has an effect on every physical function, including the function of your muscles and your heart, proper respiration, digestion, sexual development and reproduction, and the growth of your bones, hair, and nails. The thyroid affects the functioning of the brain as well, impacting how clearly you think.

Your thyroid is part of the endocrine system, a system of glands that secrete hormones, which then affect various body functions and organs. The major endocrine glands include the pineal gland, pituitary gland, pancreas, ovaries, testes, thyroid gland, parathyroid gland, hypothalamus, gastrointestinal tract, and adrenal glands.

How the Thyroid Works

The function of the thyroid gland is for its cells to combine dietary iodine—obtained through food, iodized salt, or supplements—with the amino acid tyrosine, converting the iodine and tyrosine into thyroxine and triiodothyronine.

The majority of thyroid hormone produced—around 80 percent—is thyroxine, or T4; the 4 refers to the four atoms of iodine on the molecule. Thyroxine is a prohormone, or storage hormone. In its typical form, it doesn't have any direct action in the body. Instead, it goes through a conversion process in the thyroid and other tissues to become usable in the body. In this conversion process—known as monodeiodination (or more simply, T4-to-T3 conversion)—T4 loses one atom of iodine and becomes triiodothyronine, or

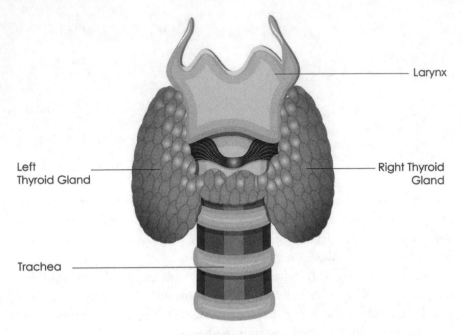

THYROID GLAND

T3. T3 is the active thyroid hormone that transports oxygen and energy into cells throughout the body, regulating your metabolism.

The thyroid operates in a feedback loop with the brain—specifically, with the hypothalamus and the pituitary gland. When low levels of thyroid hormone in the bloodstream are detected, the hypothalamus produces thyrotropin-releasing hormone (TRH). TRH stimulates the pituitary to release thyroid-stimulating hormone (TSH) and prolactin. The TSH acts as a messenger, telling your thyroid gland, "Make more thyroid hormone." When increasing blood levels of thyroid hormones are detected, levels of TSH production drop. This time the message is, "Slow down production of thyroid hormone."

This feedback process operates similarly to your home's thermostat, causing heat or air-conditioning to go on and off to maintain a particular temperature. In the case of your thyroid, the objective is to keep thyroid hormones balanced: not too high and not too low.

The Prevalence of Thyroid Problems

When it comes to statistics about the thyroid, there is one thing we can agree on: there is little agreement! Epidemiologists, endocrinologists, health research organizations, and integrative physicians all offer widely different estimates of the number of people affected by thyroid disease in the United States and other countries.

The American Association of Clinical Endocrinologists has often said that 13 million Americans have thyroid conditions. This is generally thought to be an underestimate.

The American Thyroid Association (ATA) claims that more than 12 percent of the American population will develop a thyroid condition during their lifetime. That would put the total number at around 38 million people. Yet the ATA also says that an estimated 20 million Americans have some form of thyroid disease. According to the ATA, as many as 60 percent of those with thyroid disease are unaware of their condition, and undiagnosed. That would mean that the actual prevalence of thyroid disease in the United States would exceed 60 million.

The American Medical Women's Association and the ATA agree that one in eight women in the United States have a thyroid problem during their lifetime.

The Colorado Thyroid Disease Prevalence Survey found that 8.5 percent of the population has hypothyroidism, specifically. That would translate to more than 27 million Americans with hypothyroidism, and doesn't include those with hyperthyroidism or other thyroid disorders.

In other English-speaking countries, conservative estimates of the number of thyroid sufferers are as follows:

- Canada—around 3 million diagnosed, with 2.5 million undiagnosed
- United Kingdom—around 5 million diagnosed, with an estimated 3 million undiagnosed
- Australia—around 2 million diagnosed, with 1 million undiagnosed

One point of general agreement, however, is that thyroid problems affect women up to ten times more often than men. Medical science has not yet definitively determined why this is the case, but many think one possible reason is that fluctuating hormones in women—in puberty, throughout the menstrual cycle, in pregnancy, in perimenopause—destabilize the endocrine system, affecting the thyroid. Also, women who are pregnant or nursing have a much higher need for iodine—the building block of thyroid hormone—and are more at risk of thyroid disorders due to iodine deficiency. (Iodine deficiency in pregnant mothers is the leading cause of preventable mental retardation in children around the world.)

Another theory is that many thyroid problems are related to autoimmune disease, which women are far more likely than men to develop, for reasons that also are not yet known. Outside of iodine-deficient areas in the developing world, the majority of thyroid problems are autoimmune, primarily Hashimoto's disease.

Whatever the reasons, everyone's statistics show that

- Millions of women have diagnosed thyroid conditions.
- For every woman with a thyroid diagnosis, there is at least one other woman who also has a thyroid problem not yet diagnosed.

Geographic Issues

In the United States, a key geographic factor affecting thyroid risk is the presence of iodine in the soil. Before the introduction of iodized salt, there was a higher prevalence of thyroid problems in what was known as the "Goiter Belt," an area around the Great Lakes that had never been covered by ocean, and whose soil (and produce) were low in iodine. The iodine deficiency in the population put them at higher risk of goiters (enlarged thyroid glands).

With iodized salt, the Goiter Belt has been significantly reduced. However, anywhere there is iodine deficiency—whether due to lack of iodization of salt, or reliance on iodine-poor locally grown produce—there is a great risk of thyroid disease. Lack of iodine is the most significant thyroid risk factor in developing countries in Africa, Asia, and South America, and is particularly problematic in inland mountainous areas, such as the Andes, Alps, and Himalayas. According to the World Health Organization (WHO), the countries at greatest risk are India, Pakistan, Bangladesh, Afghanistan, Angola, Bolivia, China, Egypt, Ethiopia, Ghana, Guatemala, Haiti, Indonesia, Niger, the Philippines, Russia, Senegal, Sudan, Ukraine, and Vietnam.

According to the WHO, in only a few countries do the majority of people achieve an adequate level of iodine intake. These include the United States, Canada, Norway, Sweden, Finland, Switzerland, Austria, Bhutan, Peru, Panama, Macedonia, and Japan.

Another geographic issue related to thyroid disease is exposure to radioactivity. Areas where people have been exposed to nuclear fallout, such as areas downwind of Chernobyl and Fukushima; or have been in the vicinity of nuclear weapons testing, such as in the American West, have higher rates of thyroid problems, including thyroid cancer. The gland is easily damaged by exposure to radioactive materials, especially radioactive iodine I-131. The thyroid glands of unborn children, infants, and children are at the greatest risk from radiation exposure.

Exposure to perchlorate is also linked to various thyroid disorders. Perchlorate is a by-product of the manufacture of rocket fuel, fireworks, and explosives, and is also found in some fertilizers. It also occurs naturally in some soil. In the western United States, perchlorate has gotten into drinking water and irrigation water supplies, and perchlorate-contaminated water is used to irrigate many crops in major agricultural states, such as California, which then raises perchlorate levels in the farmed produce. The United States is also a major importer of produce from Chile, whose soil has significant perchlorate contamination due to fertilizer usage, making Chilean produce a risk factor for exposure as well.

Risk Factors

Outside the United States and other Western nations, the key risk factor for thyroid disease is insufficient iodine. But in the Westernized world, the majority of thyroid conditions are triggered by autoimmune disease. There are numerous risk factors that play a complex role in the development of thyroid disease.

Some key risk factors include:

- Gender: women are at greater risk than men.
- Periods of hormonal change for women: puberty, pregnancy, postpartum, perimenopause, menopause
- Age: women age 50 and above are at the highest risk.
- Family history: a family history of thyroid disease—especially in a mother, sister, daughter, grandmother), or any history of autoimmune disease in the family
- Personal history: previous thyroid issues or autoimmune disease
- Radiation exposure: exposure to nuclear accidents (Chernobyl, Fukushima, living near a nuclear plant), or having had radiation treatment to the head or neck area
- Certain medications: lithium, amiodarone, immunosuppressants, and others
- Smoking: past or current
- Iodine: deficiency or excess
- Diet: overexposure to soy or to raw goitrogenic vegetables (cruciferous vegetables, such as cabbage, cauliflower, broccoli, and Brussels sprouts)

- Celiac disease or gluten intolerance
- History of head or neck trauma
- Toxic exposures: excessive exposure to fluoride, perchlorate, chlorine, or pesticides
- Chronic infections: there is a link between Epstein-Barr virus, candidiasis, chronic Lyme disease, chronic gingivitis, intestinal dysbiosis (bacterial infections in the gut), and other ongoing viral, bacterial, or fungal infections and an increased risk of autoimmune thyroid disease.

Types of Thyroid Conditions

The following thyroid conditions—hypothyroidism, hyperthyroidism, goiter, or nodules—are symptoms of underlying diseases, such as Hashimoto's disease, Graves' disease, thyroiditis, and thyroid cancer. We'll discuss the diseases themselves in the next section.

Hypothyroidism/Underactive Thyroid

Hypothyroidism essentially means there is too little—or no—thyroid hormone. There are a number of causes of hypothyroidism:

- Your gland is damaged due to Hashimoto's disease.
- Your gland has been removed surgically, all or in part.
- Your gland was deformed, missing, or in the wrong place from birth (congenital hypothyroidism).
- Your thyroid has been radioactively ablated.
- Your thyroid is affected by particular drugs that slow the gland.
- Your thyroid is incapable of producing enough hormone due to nodules, inflammation, or infection.
- You are iodine deficient, and your thyroid thus can't produce sufficient thyroid hormone.
- You have been exposed to radiation, excessive amounts of raw goitrogenic foods, fluoride, or perchlorate.

The symptoms of hypothyroidism usually reflect the lack of oxygen and energy that results from insufficient thyroid hormone. The common signs of an underactive thyroid include fatigue, a slowed digestion, hair loss, loss of the outer edge of your eyebrows, fatigue, weight gain, swelling and puffiness, constipation, brain fog, poor memory, slow reflexes, slowed pulse and heart rate, lower blood pressure, muscle aches and pains, and other signs of physical slowdown. A longer, more detailed checklist of hundreds of hypothyroidism symptoms is featured on the website for this book at http://www.Thyroid PregnancyBook.com.

Hyperthyroidism/Overactive Thyroid

Hyperthyroidism means that your gland is producing an excess of thyroid hormone.

There are a number of causes of hyperthyroidism:

- Autoimmune thyroid disease, such as Graves' disease, and the overactive phase of Hashimoto's disease
- Toxic nodules that produce excess thyroid hormone
- Certain medications that cause the thyroid to become overactive
- Overdosage of thyroid hormone replacement drugs
- Ingestion of over-the-counter supplements that contain thyroid hormone

The symptoms of hyperthyroidism usually reflect a speeding-up of your body's processes. They most commonly include a high pulse and heart rate, high blood pressure, anxiety or panic, insomnia, weight loss, an increased appetite with no weight gain, diarrhea or loose stools, tremor or shakiness, weakness in the arms and legs, sensitivity in the eyes, bulging eyes, vision disturbances, fatigue, heart palpitations, and lack of menstrual periods. A longer, more detailed checklist of hundreds of hyperthyroidism symptoms is featured on the book's website at http://www.ThyroidPregnancyBook.com.

Goiter/Enlarged Thyroid

Goiter is an enlarged thyroid gland. There are a number of causes of goiter:

- Iodine deficiency or excess
- Thyroid inflammation
- Infection
- Autoimmune thyroid disease, such as Hashimoto's disease or Graves' disease

In some cases, goiter may have no symptoms. But if it is large enough, it may be visible as a thickening in the neck, or visible bulging in the neck area.

Symptoms of goiter include a swollen, tender or tight feeling in the neck or throat, hoarseness, coughing, and difficulty swallowing or breathing.

A large goiter can be diagnosed by manual examination, but a smaller goiter can be identified with visual tests such as ultrasound, CT scan, MRI, or X-rays.

Nodules/Lumps/Cysts

Nodules are fairly common, and it's estimated that up to 10 percent of the population have thyroid nodules. They become more common as we age.

Nodules are sometimes referred to as lumps. Fluid-filled nodules are referred to as cysts.

A healthy thyroid can have nodules with no symptoms or other signs of disease. But in some cases, nodules are caused by:

- Toxic nodular disease—whereby autoimmune disease causes the gland to produce nodules, which then overproduce thyroid hormone
- Hashimoto's disease
- Infection
- Thyroid cancer

Many nodules cause no symptoms at all, are not visible, and you can't feel them externally. Larger nodules may be visible as a lump in the neck, or may be able to be felt with manual examination. Very large nodules may cause breathing or swallowing difficulties.

Except for toxic nodules, which produce excess thyroid hormone and cause hyperthyroidism symptoms, the symptoms of nodules usually track back to the cause. For example, nodules in Hashimoto's may damage the thyroid's ability to produce hormone, with hypothyroidism symptoms. Large or fast-growing nodules may cause swallowing difficulties, a fullness or pressure in the neck, pain, tenderness, or hoarseness.

A small percentage of nodules are cancerous. In nonpregnant patients, 90 to 95 percent of nodules are benign. In pregnant women, however, as many as one in three nodules are cancerous.

Thyroid Diseases

Several diseases are at the root of the thyroid conditions just discussed.

Hashimoto's Disease

Autoimmune thyroid disease describes a condition in which your immune system mistakenly targets your own thyroid gland. The most common autoimmune disease affecting the thyroid is Hashimoto's disease.

In Hashimoto's, the gland becomes inflamed. An inflammation of the thyroid is referred to as thyroiditis, though the condition is also commonly called Hashimoto's disease. Hashimoto's causes the body to produce antibodies that attack proteins in the gland, which can gradually destroy the gland, cause it to atrophy, and make it incapable of producing enough thyroid hormone. The result is hypothyroidism.

Some patients may have some periods of hyperthyroidism—when the gland goes into overproduction of thyroid hormone—before it slows down permanently. These periods are known as Hashitoxicosis. In most patients, however, periods of normal thyroid function, Hashitoxicosis, and/or slowdown eventually result in a permanent slowdown of the gland.

The cause of Hashimoto's, as with most autoimmune diseases, is unknown. Autoimmune diseases are the subject of extensive study, and there are many theories as to why the immune system malfunctions and attacks itself. In the case of Hashimoto's disease, however, it is known that gluten sensitivity or celiac disease—as well as overexposure to certain toxins, and certain nutritional imbalances—may be contributing factors.

Symptoms of Hashimoto's usually parallel those of the hypothyroidism that results. However, the thyroid can periodically sputter into life during Hashitoxic periods, causing hyperthyroidism symptoms. Hashimoto's can also be accompanied by neck tenderness, hoarseness, or other throat and neck symptoms.

Graves' Disease

In Graves' disease—sometimes referred to as diffuse toxic goiter because patients with Graves' usually develop a goiter—antibodies bind to the gland, causing the thyroid to overproduce hormone, causing hyperthyroidism. In the United States, Graves' disease affects slightly less than 1 percent of the population, or slightly less than 3 million people, but some experts believe that as many as 4 percent of Americans, or 12 million people, may have a mild, subclinical case. These patients may have few or no symptoms, but exhibit blood test evidence of slight hyperthyroidism.

As is the case with Hashimoto's disease, the cause of Graves' disease—also an autoimmune disease—is not clear. But one known trigger or contributing factor appears to be significant physical or emotional stress.

The symptoms of Graves' disease are usually manifestations of hyperthyroidism. Graves' patients may also have various eye-related symptoms, including bulging, dryness, sensitivity, and double vision.

Thyroiditis

Thyroiditis refers to an inflammation of the thyroid. There are a number of forms or categories of thyroiditis, Hashimoto's being the most common, but here are the other key types:

- Painless thyroiditis/silent thyroiditis/lymphocytic thyroiditis—this type of thyroiditis is usually temporary or short term. It may start with mild hyperthyroidism, followed by a period of hypothyroidism, and then the thyroid returns to normal. It's not clear what causes this type of thyroiditis.
- Postpartum thyroiditis—a painless thyroiditis that develops within a year of giving birth is considered postpartum thyroiditis. It's thought to affect as many as 10 percent of women after delivery. It typically starts out with a period of hyperthyroidism, and may shift to hypothyroidism before returning to normal. This type of thyroiditis is triggered by pregnancy or delivery.
- De Quervain's thyroiditis/granulomatous thyroiditis/painful thyroiditis/subacute thyroiditis—these interchangeable terms refer to a form of thyroiditis that is triggered by a viral infection. It is often accompanied by a hyperthyroid phase.
- Acute suppurative thyroiditis—this is the least common form of thyroiditis, and is caused by a bacterial infection in the gland, usually accompanied by an infected abscess in the thyroid gland.

If you have thyroiditis, your symptoms may include any of the hyperthyroid or hypothyroid symptoms discussed earlier. Except for painless thyroiditis, you may also have some degree of pain and/or tenderness in the neck or throat, hoarseness, neck stiffness, and difficulty sleeping.

Thyroid Cancer

Thyroid cancer is one of the least common cancers in the United States, but is one of the nation's fastest-growing types of cancer. There is controversy over the increased rate of thyroid cancer, and some experts believe that it is not an actual increase in the rate but, rather, better detection of smaller nodules via ultrasound, neck or dental X-rays, and other imaging tests.

Oncologist and thyroid cancer expert Scot Remick, MD, believes that the rise in thyroid cancer is not just a result of better or earlier detection. According to Dr. Remick: "If you look at all stages of thyroid cancer, you see an increase in instances, not just the smaller tumors."

According to the American Cancer Society, almost 63,000 cases of thyroid cancer were diagnosed in 2015 (around 47,000 in women, 16,000 in men). Still, the death rate from thyroid cancer has been fairly stable for many years, and remains very low compared with most other cancers.

In the United States, the majority of people diagnosed with thyroid cancer are diagnosed at fifty-five years of age, and a small percentage of thyroid cancers are found in children and teenagers.

There are several risk factors for thyroid cancer:

- Radiation therapy and/or exposure to radiation during childhood
- Family history/genetics—a family history of thyroid cancer, in particular medullary thyroid cancer
- Hashimoto's disease, especially with associated subclinical or overt hypothyroidism

There are several types of thyroid cancer.

- Papillary and follicular thyroid cancer—these make up around 80 to 90 percent of all thyroid cancers. When discovered early, they are usually treatable and survivable.
- Medullary thyroid cancer (MTC)—MTC makes up around 5 to 10 percent of all thyroid cancers. If discovered before it spreads, MTC has a good cure rate. People with a genetic or familial risk of MTC sometimes have the thyroid surgically removed to prevent development of cancer.
- Anaplastic thyroid cancer—this type of cancer is rare, and accounts for around 1 to 2 percent of all thyroid cancers. This is typically a very aggressive cancer, and has a much lower survival rate. There are no known cures.

Some thyroid cancers, especially when the cancer/nodule is very small, have no symptoms at all. Some patients have a visible or palpable lump in the neck, hoarseness or changes in the voice, difficulty breathing or swallowing, swelling or sensitivity in the neck, or swelling of the lymph nodes.

Hypothyroidism: The Common Outcome

It's important to recognize that except for temporary thyroid conditions or remissions, most thyroid conditions, or the treatments for them, result in life-long hypothyroidism—a gland that is unable to produce enough, or any, thyroid hormone. For example:

- Hashimoto's disease usually results in atrophy or destruction of the gland.
- Graves' disease that does not go into remission is typically treated with radioactive iodine (RAI), which permanently disables the gland in most cases.
- Thyroidectomy—thyroid surgery—which is used to treat some cases of Graves' disease or hyperthyroidism, large nodules or goiter, and thyroid cancer, results in lifelong hypothyroidism.

So, whether you have had thyroid cancer and surgical removal of your thyroid in the past, or radioiodine ablation for Graves' disease, or a thyroid atrophied due to Hashimoto's, your current condition is in fact hypothyroidism.

Now that you understand the basic function of the thyroid and the different types of thyroid conditions and disease, we'll discuss how doctors diagnose thyroid dysfunctions, and how to make sure you have all the information you need to understand and address your own situation. If you have already been diagnosed with a thyroid condition or disease, you may want to read the next chapter to make sure your doctor runs all the necessary tests, and interprets the results in a way that will help support your fertility or pregnancy.

Understanding Diagnostic Tests and Test Results

2

One of the most important parts of being an advocate for yourself before, during, and after pregnancy is understanding the different tests doctors use to diagnose thyroid disease. Proper diagnosis involves a number of components, including a thorough history of symptoms, risks and medical history, a clinical evaluation, blood tests, imaging tests, and biopsies.

Symptoms and Medical History

To diagnose a thyroid condition, your doctor should take a complete medical history and thoroughly discuss your risks for and any symptoms of thyroid disease. Chapters 5 and 6 include detailed checklists of risks and symptoms for hypothyroidism/Hashimoto's, and hyperthyroidism/Graves', respectively. These risks and symptoms checklists are also available at the book's website, at http://www.ThyroidPregnancyBook.com. Your doctor should review any family history of thyroid conditions, as well as thyroid autoimmune disease and other diseases. The practitioner should also ask about: radiation and chemical exposures; medications you take or have taken in the past; your use of vitamins, herbs, or supplements; your fertility and pregnancy history; your smoking history; previous surgeries and treatments; and other thyroid risk factors.

The Clinical Evaluation

An important part of thyroid diagnosis is the clinical evaluation by a knowledgeable physician. A thorough clinical examination of your thyroid and related symptoms should include the following steps:

- **Feeling your neck/palpation:** Your practitioner should feel your neck area, to identify any enlargement (goiter) and to look for lumps or masses that can be felt externally.
- **Listening to your thyroid with a stethoscope:** Your practitioner is listening for increased blood flow in the gland, known as bruit.
- **Testing your reflexes:** This is when a rubber mallet is tapped on the knees and on the Achilles area of the feet. An exaggerated response may be a sign of hyperthyroidism, and slowed reflexes may be a sign of hypothyroidism.
- **Checking your heart rate, rhythm, and blood pressure:** Your practitioner is looking for slowed heart rate (bradycardia) or low blood pressure, often associated with hypothyroidism; or high heart rate (tachycardia) or high blood pressure, often suggestive of hyperthyroidism. (Periods of hyperthyroidism, with the associated increased heart rate, may also be associated with Hashimoto's disease.) Your physician may also be listening for heart rhythm changes, as palpitations are associated with both hyperthyroidism and hypothyroidism, and atrial fibrillation—an irregular and rapid heart rate—is associated with hyperthyroidism.
- **Measuring your weight:** Rapid weight gain that is not associated with changes to your diet or exercise can be a sign of hypothyroidism. In addition, inability to lose weight despite a reduction in calories and increase in exercise is also associated with hypothyroidism. Rapid weight loss—or an increased appetite without weight gain—may point to hyperthyroidism.
- **Taking your body temperature:** A low body temperature may be a sign of an underactive thyroid, and a higher-than-normal body temperature, in the absence of infection, may be a sign of an overactive thyroid.
- **Examining your face:** Your doctor will be looking for some characteristic thyroid signs, including loss of hair from the outer edges of your eyebrows—a unique symptom of hypothyroidism—as well as puffiness or swelling in the eyelids or face, another common hypothyroidism symptom. Other signs include unusually smooth, young-looking skin, or blisterlike bumps on the forehead and face (known as milaria bumps), which can be signs of hyperthyroidism.
- **Examining your eyes:** The eyes are often affected in thyroid patients, and common clinical symptoms your physician will be looking for are bulging or protrusion of the eyes, a stare, retraction of your upper eyelids, infrequent blinking, and "lid lag"—your upper eyelids not smoothly following the downward movements of your eyes when you look down. Symptoms such as double vision, dry eyes, blurriness, and eye strain will

also be evaluated. Eye-related symptoms can be seen in both hypothyroidism and Graves' disease, but are more common in Graves' patients. In some cases they are symptoms of the thyroid disease, but they may also exist as a separate autoimmune condition known as thyroid associated ophthalmopathy (TAO) or thyroid eye disease (TED), which is more common in autoimmune thyroid patients.

- **Observing the general quantity and quality of your hair:** Hair loss is seen in both overactive and underactive thyroid conditions. Coarse, brittle, or strawlike hair can point to hypothyroidism. Thinning, finer hair may point to hyperthyroidism.

- **Examining your skin:** Hypothyroidism may manifest as dryness in the skin, especially heels and elbows. Hyperthyroidism can show up in a variety of skin-related symptoms, including a yellowish, jaundiced cast to the skin; hives; and lesions or patches of rough skin on the shins (known as pretibial myxedema or Graves' dermopathy).

- **Examining your nails and hands:** Your practitioner will look for hyperthyroidism-related signs, including onycholysis—a separation of the nail from the underlying nail bed, also called Plummer's nails—and swollen fingertips, also called acropachy.

Your practitioner should also look for some other clinical signs of hyperthyroidism, including tremors—shaky hands—or nervous movements, such as table drumming or tapping feet; and for other signs of hypothyroidism, such as a dull facial expression, slow speech or movement, hoarseness of the voice, and swelling (known as edema) of the hands and/or feet.

Thyroid Blood Tests

Thyroid-Stimulating Hormone/TSH

The most common thyroid test is the blood test that measures the amount of thyroid-stimulating hormone (TSH) in your bloodstream. The test is sometimes called the thyrotropin-stimulating hormone test.

TSH is measured in milli-international units per liter (mIU/L), and values are interpreted using a reference range, sometimes called the "normal" range. The reference range can vary among labs, but for TSH, typically runs from around 0.5 mIU/L to 4.5 mIU/L or so. TSH that is elevated, or above the top cutoff for the reference range, is considered evidence of a thyroid slowdown. (Remember that the pituitary produces more TSH when there is not enough thyroid hormone, to help stimulate production, so the more TSH, the more the pituitary is yelling, "Make more thyroid hormone!") TSH that is below normal is considered evidence of an overactive thyroid. (When the pituitary detects too much thyroid hormone, it produces less TSH, as a message to the gland to slow down or stop production of thyroid hormone.)

Some practitioners rely only on the TSH test to diagnose an underactive or overactive thyroid, and conventional endocrinology considers TSH to be the gold standard for diagnosis and monitoring of many thyroid conditions. It is important to note, however, that even among conventional endocrinologists, there is controversy about the top cutoff of the reference range. Around 2003, the two leading national endocrinology organizations made an unofficial recommendation that the top of the range be lowered from 4.5 to 3.0 mIU/L, in recognition of the fact that levels in this part of the range indicated a possible subclinical, or mild, hypothyroidism. They were also recognizing that the general population samples used to determine the reference range included people who have Hashimoto's disease, and that the normal TSH levels for those without any evidence of autoimmunity tended to be below 3.0 mIU/L.

Some doctors adopted these new recommendations. But laboratory reports continued to use the older ranges, and only flagged those results that were below 0.5 or above 4.5. So, many doctors continued diagnosing and treating using the older, broader range. More recently, the endocrinology organizations backed away from the reference range adjustment they'd suggested in 2003, so now most doctors use the older ranges.

Endocrinologists disagree as to whether levels under 10.0 mIU/L should even be treated. Some doctors believe that these levels warrant treatment with thyroid hormone replacement drugs, while others consider them to indicate subclinical hypothyroidism—and that treatment is only needed after levels exceed 10.0 mIU/L.

Among integrative hormone specialists, a level above 2.0 mIU/L is typically considered possible evidence of a thyroid slowdown, particularly when other blood tests show low or low-normal circulating levels of thyroid hormone, or in the presence of elevated thyroid antibodies.

It is important to note that optimal TSH for fertility differs from the general population's reference range. Some endocrinologists, fertility experts, and integrative hormone specialists believe that TSH should be on the lower end of the reference range, in the 1.0 mIU/L to 2.0 mIU/L range, for optimal fertility. During pregnancy, there are specific target ranges that experts consider ideal for each trimester (this is discussed more fully in Chapter 3), but in general, TSH should not rise about 2.5 mIU/L during pregnancy without additional treatment and evaluation.

Thyroxine/T4—Total and Free

As we discussed in Chapter 1, the majority of hormone produced by the thyroid gland is thyroxine, also known as T4. Thyroxine is considered a "storage" hormone in that, alone, it is not usable by the body to produce energy and deliver oxygen to cells. It must lose an atom of iodine, a process called mono-deiodination (or T4-to-T3 conversion), and become triiodothyronine (T3) to be used by cells. We also discussed how not all of the hormones the thyroid produces are available for use by the body, because some get bound to proteins—as a response to the use of certain medications or drugs, illness, or physical changes such as pregnancy.

The blood test for total thyroxine (Total T4) measures the total amount of T4 circulating in the bloodstream, and the Free T4 test measures the free, available, and unbound levels of thyroxine in the bloodstream.

Total T4 levels can be artificially elevated due to pregnancy and other high-estrogen states, including use of estrogen replacement drugs or birth control pills. In general, and particularly during pregnancy, the free or unbound T4 levels represent the level of hormone available for uptake and use by cells, and are considered more accurate

Total T4 is usually measured in micrograms of lead per deciliter of blood, abbreviated as µg/dL. Free T4 is measured in nanograms per deciliter, or ng/dL. Reference ranges tend to vary more at laboratories around the country, but generally, the range for total T4 is 4.5 to 12.5 µg/dL, and for Free T4, 0.8 to 1.8 ng/dL.

Generally, levels above the top of the reference range suggest that the thyroid is overproducing thyroid hormone—and that the thyroid is overactive, or hyperthyroid. Levels below the bottom of the reference range suggest that the thyroid is underproducing thyroid hormone—and that the thyroid is underactive, or hypothyroid. Levels within the reference range are considered "normal" by conventional physicians.

Again, there are controversies over the reference range. Some integrative physicians and hormone experts believe that if Free T4 is not in the top half of the reference range, it is not optimal.

Triiodothyronine/T3—Total and Free

Triiodothyronine (T3) is the active thyroid hormone that delivers oxygen and energy to cells. The thyroid gland produces some T3. The remainder of T3 is produced by a process by which T4 converts into T3, by losing a molecule of iodine. As with T4, Free T3 measures the free, unbound, and available levels of the hormone, and is considered by some practitioners to be a more accurate picture of the available levels of hormone in the blood.

While ranges can vary among labs, the following are general reference ranges for adults: Total T3: 80 to 200 ng/dL; Free T3: 23 to 61.9 ng/dL. Elevated levels or levels above the reference range may be indicative of hyperthyroidism. Lower levels or levels below the reference range may be indicative of hypothyroidism.

Testing for T3 and Free T3 is even more controversial than T4 testing. This is primarily because many conventional practitioners do not believe that the T3 level affects symptoms and that there is no place for treatment with T3 hormone. Whereas many integrative physicians and hormone experts believe, however, that if Free T3 is not in the top half—or even the top quarter—of the reference range, it is not optimal, and thyroid patients will not feel well.

Reverse T3/RT3

Under normal circumstances, during the process of T4 to T3 conversion, some of the T4 is converted to a substance known as Reverse T3, or RT3. Stress, nutritional deficiencies, and illness, however, can increase the production of Reverse T3. Reverse T3 is inactive and has no function in the body except to, in some cases, block cells' use of actual T3. In some cases, the body seemingly becomes "stuck" in a pattern of high RT3 production.

The test for Reverse T3 is a controversial one. Conventional endocrinology for the most part dismisses the value of RT3 measurement in diagnosing, treating, and managing hypothyroidism—again, because the role of T3 levels, and T3 treatment, is largely ignored.

Integrative physicians and those who focus on optimal hormone balance, however, consider elevated RT3 to be a key sign of an underactive or dysfunctional thyroid.

Their perspective is that by displacing actual T3, RT3 makes blood test results less accurate, and can block the body's ability to properly absorb thyroid hormone. Integrative physician Kent Holtorf calls Reverse T3 the body's "emergency brake," and looks for irregular levels of RT3 to help identify thyroid issues, even when TSH and T4/T3 levels are otherwise within the normal reference range.

The reference range for RT3 is typically 10 to 24 ng/dL. Ideally, Reverse T3 should fall in the lower half of the range.

Thyroid Peroxidase Antibodies (TPOAb)/ Antithyroid Peroxidase Antibodies

Thyroid peroxidase antibodies (TPOAb) are also known as antithyroid per-oxidase antibodies. (In the past, these antibodies were referred to as antithy-roid microsomal antibodies or antimicrosomal antibodies). They work against thyroid peroxidase, an enzyme that plays a role in the conversion of T4 to T3. The presence of TPOAb can be evidence of inflammation of the gland, or tissue destruction such as that caused by Hashimoto's disease. Less commonly, TPOAb are seen in other forms of thyroiditis, such as postpartum thyroiditis.

It's estimated that TPOAb are detectable in approximately 95 percent of patients with Hashimoto's disease, and 50 to 85 percent of Graves' disease patients. The concentrations of antibodies found in patients with Graves' disease are usually lower than in patients with Hashimoto's disease.

Some patients have elevated TPOAb, but are otherwise euthyroid—meaning their T4/T3 and TSH levels fall within the reference range. Some research has shown that preventative treatment with levothyroxine may be warranted in those patients, as it may slow down elevation of antibodies, relieve symptoms, and help prevent progression to overt hypothyroidism.

At many labs, the reference range for TPOAb is 0 to 35 IU/mL.

Thyroid-Stimulating Immunoglobulins (TSI)

Thyroid-stimulating immunoglobulins (TSI), also known as thyroid receptor antibodies (TRAb), stimulate the thyroid gland to enlarge (goiter) and release excessive thyroid hormone, resulting in hyperthyroidism. In this book, we will refer to them as TSI, but understand that some doctors measure TRAb. The test, interpretation, and implications are the same.

The TSI test is typically done:

- To detect Graves' disease and to evaluate toxic multinodular goiter. TSI can be detected in the majority—some estimates say as many as 75 to 90 percent—of Graves' disease patients. The higher the levels, the more active the Graves' disease is thought to be. (The absence of these antibodies does not, however, rule out Graves' disease.)
- To help predict the relapse of Graves' disease. Lowered levels may indicate that Graves' disease treatment is working.

- To determine the cause of hyperthyroidism in patients whose tests are not definitive, or who cannot have any radioactive diagnosing tests (such as when pregnant or breastfeeding)
- To diagnose Graves' disease in patients who have symptoms, but otherwise normal thyroid tests
- To determine whether a pregnant woman has a short-term gestational hyperthyroidism, versus a recurrence of Graves' disease
- To determine whether long-term antithyroid drug treatment has resulted in a remission
- To determine whether Graves' disease has recurred after antithyroid drug treatment
- To determine—in a woman who has active Graves' disease during pregnancy (or a past history of Graves' disease)—whether, during the last months of pregnancy, her fetus is at risk of fetal hyperthyroidism, or of being born with an excess of thyroid hormone, known as neonatal hyperthyroidism
- To determine the risk of hyperthyroidism in a newborn

Thyroglobulin (Tg)

Thyroglobulin (Tg) is a protein produced by the thyroid gland, and its presence in the blood is a sign that a patient still has some active thyroid tissue—whether the entire gland or a remnant left after surgery or radioactive iodine (RAI) treatments.

Thyroglobulin is tested mainly in thyroid cancer patients, for several reasons: to determine whether the cancerous tissue is producing thyroglobulin prior to treatment, to assess whether treatment is working, and to help detect recurrence after treatment.

Since most of the common thyroid cancers—i.e., papillary and follicular—produce thyroglobulin, increased levels of thyroglobulin may be a sign of cancer recurrence.

Thyroglobulin testing may also be done, though less commonly, to evaluate hyperthyroidism and Graves' disease.

A low level of thyroglobulin is normal in people who don't have thyroid disease.

Thyroglobulin levels should be 0 or very low after thyroid surgery or after RAI treatments. If they are still detectable, additional treatment may be required.

If thyroglobulin levels begin to rise after thyroid cancer treatment, that may be a sign that the cancer has recurred.

Thyroglobulin levels that drop may be a sign that Graves' disease and hyperthyroidism treatment is working.

If you have no thyroid gland, thyroglobulin should be less than 0.1 ng/mL. If you still have a gland, it should be less than or equal to 33 ng/mL.

Thyroglobulin Antibodies (TgAb)/Antithyroglobulin Antibodies

Thyroglobulin antibodies—known as TgAb—are also called antithyroglobulin antibodies.

They are found in around 10 percent of people with normal thyroid function, and as many as 15 to 20 percent of people with thyroid cancer. TgAb are positive in about 60 percent of Hashimoto's patients and 30 percent of Graves' patients.

Some patients with Hashimoto's may not have elevated TPOAb, but will have elevated TgAb, and so some doctors use tests for both TPOAb and TgAb in making an initial diagnosis of Hashimoto's.

TgAb can interfere with the thyroglobulin (Tg) results, and so it's important for those with thyroid cancer to have TgAb levels monitored, along with Tg, at regular intervals. When levels are elevated, this can mean that the Tg test levels are not accurate, and that Tg levels may actually be higher than test results show.

The reference range is less than 4.0 IU/mL.

Unconventional Testing

Some other tests that you may encounter are considered unconventional ways to evaluate the thyroid. Many mainstream practitioners are skeptical of these tests and find their use controversial. Some of the tests, however, are well accepted and in use among alternative, integrative, and holistic physicians.

- **Thyroflex:** Thyroflex is a device that measures the reflex response of a tendon located near the elbow. Slow responses are indicative of hypothyroidism; unusually fast ones indicative of hyperthyroidism. Thyroflex manufacturers say the device is more accurate than reflex testing of the Achilles tendon, and claim an accuracy rate of almost 99 percent compared to laboratory testing. There are some limited research studies showing that in terms of general TSH level, Thyroflex tests have some degree of accuracy; however, the test is primarily used by chiropractors and holistic practitioners, and is not generally accepted by conventional medicine as a valid test.

- **Saliva testing:** Saliva testing is growing in popularity with complementary and integrative practitioners. There are a number of companies that provide saliva testing for thyroid function. Saliva tests for thyroid function may have some accuracy, but again, are not considered diagnostic by most physicians.
- **Urinary testing:** Urinary testing for thyroid dysfunction is not in wide use, and is rarely done in the United States. It's primarily performed by physicians in Europe.
- **Basal body temperature testing:** Some practitioners believe that thyroid function—and response to thyroid treatment—can be measured by basal body temperature (BBT) monitoring. According to the late Dr. Broda Barnes, a basal temperature consistently below 97.8°F was a possible indicator of low thyroid function. A small percentage of alternative practitioners rely on basal body temperature results as their primary means of diagnosis. Other alternative practitioners feel that it may be one criterion among several to consider in diagnosis. Most conventional practitioners do not consider the test useful in thyroid diagnosis.
- **Iodine patch test:** with this test, a patch of iodine solution is painted on the skin. Fast evaporation is considered evidence of low iodine status and a thyroid dysfunction. It's generally considered quite controversial, however, and research has found that this test has limited correlation to actual thyroid function.

Thyroid Imaging Tests

A number of imaging tests are performed for diagnosis of various thyroid conditions.

Nuclear Scan/Radioactive Iodine Uptake (RAIU)

A radioactive iodine uptake (RAIU) test can help tell whether you have Graves' disease, toxic multinodular goiter, or thyroiditis. It can also help pinpoint suspicious thyroid nodules. Many doctors like to do the RAIU test, because it's one they may be able to do in their own office.

In this test, a small dose of radioactive iodine 123 is given in pill form. Iodine-123 is considered better and safer for testing because it has a shorter half-life, and gives off a lower level of radiation compared to radioactive iodine

I-131—the type of iodine used for ablation of the thyroid (RAI) and cancer treatment.

Several hours later, the amount of iodine in the bloodstream is measured, often accompanied by an X-ray that views how the iodine concentrates in the thyroid. An overactive thyroid usually absorbs or "takes up" higher amounts of iodine than normal and that uptake is visible in the X-ray. A thyroid that takes up iodine is considered "hot," or overactive, as opposed to a "cold," or underactive, thyroid.

In Graves' disease, RAIU is elevated, and the entire gland shows up as hot. In Hashimoto's disease, the uptake is usually low, but may have small hot spots in the gland.

RAIU can show when thyroid nodules are hot. If you are hyperthyroid due to a hot nodule and not Graves' disease, the nodule will show up as hot, and the rest of your thyroid will be cold. Hot nodules may overproduce thyroid hormone but they are rarely cancerous.

RAIU can also show which thyroid nodules are cold—not taking up iodine. It's estimated that some 10 to 20 percent of cold nodules are cancerous.

Some important notes about the RAIU test:

- If you have high amounts of iodine in your diet, this can interfere with your test results, so your doctor may recommend avoiding iodine for a period prior to the test. Be sure you tell your doctor about any medications or supplements you are taking, particularly those that may contain iodine, such as prenatal vitamins, multivitamins, kelp, bladderwrack, and seaweed. Also, if in recent weeks or the past month you've had any medical tests that use iodine contrast dyes, be sure to let your doctor know.
- This test should *never* be done in a woman who is pregnant, or who might be pregnant. It can be damaging to the thyroid gland of the fetus. The test should also not be done in a woman who is breastfeeding. If this type of imaging is needed in a breastfeeding woman, the physician can substitute technetium 99M instead of iodine. The half-life of technetium is six hours. So, a nursing mother can "pump and dump" breast milk and resume breastfeeding at a point after the test that her physician recommends.

CT Scan

A CT scan, known as computed tomography or "CAT scan," is a specialized type of X-ray that is sometimes used to evaluate the thyroid. A CT scan can't detect smaller nodules, but may help detect and diagnose a goiter or larger thyroid nodules.

CT is considered generally safe during pregnancy as long as it does not include the abdomen or pelvis. Some CT scans require contrast material, and unless necessary, physicians do try to avoid use of contrast materials during pregnancy, as they cross the placenta and may harm the fetus. In particular, iodine-based contrast materials may produce hypothyroidism in a newborn, and are usually avoided. However, if you have had any iodine-based contrast during pregnancy, it's especially important to confirm that required screenings of thyroid function have taken place in your newborn.

It's important to note that some experts recommend that a woman receiving a nonradioactive contrast material—whether iodine-based, or gadolinium—should discontinue breastfeeding for 24 hours, and discard pumped milk. Breastfeeding can be resumed 24 hours after the procedure.

Magnetic Resonance Imaging (MRI)

Magnetic resonance imaging, or MRI, is done when the size and shape of the thyroid needs to be evaluated. MRI can't tell how the thyroid is functioning (i.e., it can't diagnose hyperthyroidism or hypothyroidism), but it can detect enlargement of the gland, and may be able to identify atrophy, irregular shape, and nodules.

In pregnant or nursing women, a thyroid MRI is considered preferable to X-rays or CT scans because it doesn't require any injection of contrast dye, and doesn't involve radiation.

The FDA's current guidelines state that the safety of MRI with respect to the fetus "has not been established." In general, though, most studies have shown no impact of MRI during pregnancy.

Thyroid Ultrasound

Ultrasound of the thyroid is done to evaluate nodules, lumps, and enlargement of your gland.

Ultrasound can tell whether a nodule is a fluid-filled cyst or a mass of solid tissue, but it can't determine whether a nodule or lump is malignant.

Because the thyroid typically enlarges (goiter) in Graves' disease, and the gland typically shrinks when responding to antithyroid drug treatment, some practitioners use ultrasound to monitor the success of antithyroid treatment.

Thyroid ultrasound is considered safe during pregnancy or breastfeeding.

Thyroid Biopsy/Fine-Needle Aspiration (FNA)

A needle biopsy, also known as fine-needle aspiration (FNA), is used to help evaluate "cold," or suspicious, nodules. Large size or rapid growth are some of the characteristics that make a nodule suspicious. Biopsy results can show evidence of Hashimoto's disease, but are primarily used to diagnose or rule out thyroid cancer.

In a needle biopsy, a thin needle is inserted directly into the lump and some cells are withdrawn and evaluated. One or more samples may be needed for thorough testing. Some practitioners use a local anesthetic while doing this procedure, but others do not, believing that better results are obtained without the inflammation caused by the anesthetic injection. Some practitioners use ultrasound—known as an ultrasound-guided biopsy—to ensure that the needle goes into the right position.

Typically, FNAs are done by endocrinologists, cytopathologists, or surgeons. The cells are studied and assessed by a cytopathologist. Many FNAs are performed in a doctor's office, although some might be done as an outpatient procedure in a hospital or surgery center.

It is important that the practitioner performing your FNA have extensive experience, to make sure the procedure produces the best possible samples. A percentage of FNA biopsy results are considered nondiagnostic, meaning they cannot be used at all, and must be redone, an outcome more likely to happen when less experienced practitioners do the sampling. When you are choosing a practitioner to perform your FNA, ask the practitioner to share his or her nondiagnostic FNA rate. More experienced practitioners have very low rates.

The main risk of thyroid FNA is bleeding or hemorrhage. But with an experienced practitioner, that risk is small, and thyroid FNA is generally considered safe, almost never resulting in any complications.

One of the most frustrating challenges you can face is when your FNA results are "inconclusive" or "indeterminate." In this case, the pathology assessment cannot rule out cancer. The conventional next step for this situation is thyroidectomy—a surgery to remove the thyroid, which is then evaluated to conclusively diagnose or rule out thyroid cancer.

When no thyroid cancer is discovered, which happens in the majority of cases, the patient needs to live with lifelong hypothyroidism, after an otherwise unnecessary thyroidectomy.

It's estimated that almost a half-million FNA biopsies are conducted in the United States each year, and up to 30 percent of those come back as indeterminate or inconclusive. Only 20 to 30 percent of inconclusive nodules are found to be malignant.

You should therefore be aware of a test called the Afirma Thyroid FNA Analysis, which, if conducted at the time of the initial biopsy, eliminates almost all inconclusive and indeterminate FNA results. Note that you would need to confirm that your doctor is using this system *before* your FNA is scheduled, or find a doctor who works with this particular testing.

After this overview of the thyroid, thyroid conditions, and the methods and tests used to diagnosis various thyroid problems, we now move on to explore the crucial role that the thyroid plays in your fertility, and your ability to have a healthy pregnancy. The next chapter explains this important relationship, and what it means for you.

The Thyroid's Role in Fertility and Pregnancy

3

Healthy thyroid function is an essential part of your ability to have a healthy reproductive system, and your ability to conceive. The thyroid—along with the reproductive glands—is part of the endocrine system. These glands all interact to affect your fertility in a variety of ways. In addition, the vast majority of thyroid problems in most developed countries is due to Hashimoto's disease. Autoimmunity—including thyroid autoimmunity—is associated with other immune issues and conditions that contribute to or even cause infertility.

Your Reproductive Milestones and Timetable

To understand how thyroid issues can complicate fertility, it's helpful first to review the hormonal milestones of a woman's reproductive life.

As a woman, you're born with all the eggs you will ever have—somewhere from 1 to 2 million eggs. By puberty, the total number of eggs is typically less than 500,000. Around 300 of them are typically released throughout your reproductive years.

The average age for a first menstrual period is from 12 to 13 years. It usually takes several years for your cycle to regulate into a more consistent pattern, and for ovulation to occur during each cycle. For most women, optimal fertility is during their twenties. Some experts say that from ages 19 to 26, you have a 50 percent chance of conceiving during the highest fertility period, typically two days prior to ovulation. This goes down to 40 percent for women ages 27 to 34, and 30 percent for women after the age of 35.

Miscarriage rates track similarly with age as well. The general miscarriage rate is around 8 to 10 percent for women in their twenties, goes to 12 percent for the early thirties, jumps to 18 percent in the mid- to late thirties, and hits

34 percent for women in their early forties. By age 45, the miscarriage rate is more than 50 percent.

Perimenopause is the period of time when the level of your sex hormones fluctuates and eventually declines. It can begin as long as ten years before your actual menopause, which is defined as the point at which it's been a year since your last menstrual period. In the United States, the average age of menopause is around 51, so most women have had their last menstrual periods by age 50.

Given that women begin having periods around age 12 or 13, and stop around age 50, they experience thirty-five or more years of menstrual cycles, and around twenty "childbearing" years.

Your Reproductive/Menstrual Cycle

In looking at the impact of the thyroid on the menstrual cycle and fertility, it's important to first understand how this reproductive and menstrual cycle works each month.

Typically, the first day of your cycle—known as Day 1—is the start of what's known as the follicular phase. During this phase, your pituitary gland releases follicle-stimulating hormone (FSH), to direct some of your eggs to mature and to create fluid-containing follicles around those eggs. During each cycle, a varying number of follicles may develop.

Around Day 10 of your cycle, one follicle typically matures, become dominant, and grows more quickly than the others. (Less commonly, several follicles may become dominant; if they are fertilized, this can lead to multiple births.)

The growth of the follicle causes increasing estrogen to be released, and this causes your uterine lining to thicken over the next few days. Around Day 13 of your cycle, as FSH and estrogen peak, you have a surge of another hormone, called luteinizing hormone (LH). (Your LH surge is what a home ovulation detection kit measures.)

Meanwhile, the fallopian tubes get ready for a fertilized egg. The increased estrogen causes the cervical fluid to become more hospitable to sperm, and it becomes sticky and stringier, and, viewed under a microscope, displays a characteristic fernlike pattern. The cervix also becomes slightly more open, to allow for easier passage of sperm.

Around 28 to 36 hours after the LH surge, and about 12 hours after LH reaches its peak, ovulation occurs. In ovulation, the fully mature egg moves to the surface of the ovary, ruptures, and is released toward the fallopian tube. As the egg is released, some women experience a bit of pain or a pinching feeling in the area of the ovary. You can also have a small discharge, or even light spotting, at ovulation.

Ovulation generally occurs around Day 14 of the cycle. It also signals the end of the follicular phase and the start of the luteal phase of the cycle.

After the egg has left the dominant follicle, the remnants of the follicle become the corpus luteum. This generates the release of progesterone, along with some estrogen. The purpose is to cause the uterus to build up a lining—known as the endometrium—where a fertilized egg would implant.

Toni Weschler, author of the groundbreaking book *Taking Charge of Your Fertility,* shared these thoughts about fertility:

> A woman must have fertile-quality cervical fluid present in order for the sperm to be able to swim through the cervix to reach the short-lived egg in the fallopian tube. Sperm can live up to about two to three days, and occasionally five days in the woman's fertile cervical fluid. The egg can only live about twelve to fourteen hours. You are only fertile on the few days leading up to ovulation, and the day of ovulation itself. So the total time a woman is fertile is less than a week.

After ovulation, FSH drops, and the other follicles are reabsorbed into the ovary.

Once you've ovulated, there are two possible courses for the cycle to take:

- If the egg is fertilized, it will typically take place in the fallopian tube. The fertilized egg will then travel down the tube, and implant in the uterus, and pregnancy has begun.
- If the egg is not fertilized, around 10 days after ovulation (Day 24), the corpus luteum breaks down, and production of estrogen and progesterone slows to a halt. (This time frame, from around Day 24 to Day 28, is typically when premenstrual symptoms are most evident.) The eventual drop in progesterone triggers the endometrium to shed from the uterus—the start of the menstrual period—around Day 28.

Day 28—the start of menstrual bleeding—is also when FSH is released, and the cycle starts again as Day 1. The menstrual phase, when you're bleeding, can last anywhere from one to eight days, but four or five is most common.

Every woman's cycle is different, and can range in length, but the general overview is as follows:

Day 1—Menstrual period starts
Day 1—Follicular phase starts
Days 1–14—Follicular phase
Day 14—Ovulation
Days 14–18—Luteal phase begins
Days 26–28—Premenstrual phase
Day 28/Day 1—Menstrual period starts

Your Thyroid, Your Menstrual Cycle, and Fertility

The ability to get pregnant usually requires a menstrual cycle that functions as nature intended—the process just described. When a woman has an undiagnosed or insufficiently treated thyroid condition, fertility can be affected via a number of menstrual irregularities.

Anovulatory Cycles

An anovulatory cycle is a cycle when no egg is released. There are a number of causes of anovulatory cycles, including but not limited to:

• Puberty
• Breastfeeding
• Perimenopause/age
• Physical/emotional stress
• Adrenal dysfunction
• Anorexia
• Ovarian insufficiency—low ovarian reserve, antiovarian antibodies
• Polycystic ovary syndrome (PCOS)
• Pituitary disorders
• Ovarian cancer

It's important to know that even when you have an anovulatory cycle, you can still have a menstrual period; but since no egg is released, you can't conceive. If you have an undiagnosed or insufficiently treated thyroid condition, you are at a higher risk of having anovulatory cycles than are other women your age. Any cycle when an egg is not released is a cycle during which you will be unable to become pregnant.

Luteal Phase Defects

When a thyroid condition is undiagnosed or untreated, luteal phase defects are also more common.

As discussed earlier, the luteal phase is the second half of the cycle, the time between ovulation and either the fertilization of the egg or the start of menstruation. A healthy luteal phase lasts between 13 and 15 days on average. This allows enough time for hormones to properly prepare the uterine lining, and for the fertilized egg to successfully implant.

If a luteal phase is too short, a fertilized egg doesn't have time to implant before hormones trigger the endometrial lining to shed. If that happens, the fertilized egg ends up expelled as part of the menstrual period. This is essentially a very early miscarriage, but since few women learn they are pregnant this early in the process, they do not recognize it as such.

Luteal phase defects are typically due to low progesterone, or less commonly, an endometrium that is not responding to progesterone. Research has shown that women with undiagnosed or untreated hypothyroidism and hyperthyroidism can have a short luteal phase and insufficient progesterone.

Any cycle during which sufficient progesterone is not produced, resulting in a suboptimal endometrial lining, or a short luteal phase, is a cycle when you will be unable to become pregnant.

In addition to detailed fertility and cycle charting, discussed in Chapter 4, tests that can be helpful in diagnosing a luteal phase defect include:

- Follicle-stimulating hormone (FSH) level
- Luteinizing hormone (LH) level
- Progesterone level

Hyperprolactinemia

As described in Chapter 1, the hypothalamus produces thyroid-releasing hormone (TRH) and prolactin. The TRH's role is to stimulate the pituitary gland to produce TSH. One of prolactin's key roles is in the stimulating production of milk in the breasts. Prolactin also plays a role in metabolism and the immune system, among other functions.

When the thyroid is not functioning properly, excessive amounts of TRH may be produced, and this can cause the pituitary to release too much prolactin, a condition known as hyperprolactinemia. Elevated prolactin can cause a variety of hormonal issues that affect fertility, including:

- Irregular ovulation
- Anovulatory cycles
- Irregular menstruation
- Lack of menstrual periods
- Inhibition of conception/pregnancy

Cycle charting, along with blood tests for prolactin levels, can help to diagnose hyperprolactinemia. If ensuring proper and optimal thyroid functioning does not resolve elevated prolactin levels, the drugs bromocriptine or cabergoline are often used to lower the prolactin levels and restore normal cycles and ovulation.

Early Menopause

The medical literature notes a link between thyroid disorders and a slightly earlier onset of menopause. For some women, perimenopause may begin earlier than is common, thereby shortening their childbearing years and causing reduced fertility at an earlier age.

Pregnenolone Conversion Issues

Thyroid hormone plays a role in converting cholesterol into the hormone pregnenolone. Pregnenolone then ends up being converted into progesterone, estrogen, testosterone, and DHEA. When you don't have enough thyroid hormone, you can end up with deficiencies in these other hormones, which can disrupt the proper functioning of the menstrual cycle and impair fertility.

The Thyroid/Estrogen Relationship

There is a complex relationship between estrogen and thyroid function. Estrogen competes with the thyroid to attach to thyroid receptor sites throughout the body. When there is too much estrogen, it can block the thyroid hormone's ability to be transported into your cells. So, higher estrogen levels, whether due to the introduction of outside hormones or through an imbalance known as estrogen dominance, can disrupt hormonal balance and menstrual cycles as well as impair fertility. High estrogen levels increase a woman's need for thyroid hormone at the cellular level, even when circulating blood levels seem normal.

Sex Hormone Binding Globulin (SHBG) Imbalances

In women with undiagnosed or insufficiently treated hypothyroidism, it's common to see decreased levels of sex hormone binding globulin (SHBG). SHBG is a protein that binds to estrogen. When SHBG is low, estrogen levels can become too high. Excessive estrogen, in addition to creating the imbalance just discussed, can also interfere with growth and development of follicles and get in the way of proper FSH and LH surges associated with ovulation. In hyperthyroidism, SHBG can be elevated, which then lowers progesterone, a situation that can also lead to estrogen dominance.

Menstrual Symptoms and Signs

A number of menstrual symptoms or disorders are common in women with undiagnosed or insufficiently treated thyroid issues.

In women with hypothyroidism, the most common menstrual problems are:

- Metrorrhagia—irregular bleeding and erratic cycles, spotting, midcycle bleeding
- Menorrhagia—extremely heavy or prolonged bleeding
- Oligomenorrhea—cycles that are repeatedly longer than 35 days—or only 4 to 9 periods per year

The most common menstrual disorders in women with hyperthyroidism are:

- Oligomenorrhea
- Amenorrhea—a lack of menstrual periods
- Hypomenorrhea—significantly reduced heaviness of menstrual flow

Oligomenorrhea is associated with greater difficulty getting pregnant, because it can be a symptom of erratic ovulation, anovulatory cycles, and luteal phase defects. Amenorrhea may be a sign of anovulatory cycles, which also prevent pregnancy.

Your Thyroid and Pregnancy

During pregnancy, your thyroid gland needs to expand its function so as to meet the needs of both mother and developing baby. Thyroid hormone is an essential part of the neurological and brain development of the fetus, most significantly during the first trimester. Your baby does not develop a gland capable of producing thyroid hormone until around 12 weeks of gestation, or around the beginning of the second trimester of pregnancy. So, during the first trimester, all the thyroid hormone needed for proper neurological development in the fetus comes from you. This results in an increased demand for thyroid hormone early in your pregnancy.

Once you become pregnant, if you have a healthy thyroid, increased thyroid hormone production begins. During pregnancy, your placenta releases human chorionic gonadotropin (HCG), which additionally stimulates the thyroid gland, especially during the first trimester. Increased estrogen in pregnancy causes an increase in production of T4-binding globulin, known as TBG, a protein that acts as a transporter for thyroid hormone in the bloodstream. This TBG increase sets off a chain of events that affect the overall hormonal picture in pregnancy:

- The TBG actually binds to thyroxine (T4) in the bloodstream, which lowers the Free T4 levels.
- The brain perceives the lowered Free T4 levels as being insufficient (hypothyroidism), and so TSH elevates.
- The elevated TSH triggers the thyroid to produce more thyroid hormone.
- T4 and T3 levels increase.

After the first trimester, your developing baby is getting thyroid hormone from two sources: its own gland, and your thyroid, via transfer across the placenta. The increased demand for thyroid hormones caused by pregnancy continues until your baby is born.

If your iodine intake is not sufficient, or your thyroid gland is compromised (as it is in autoimmune thyroid disease, or due to surgical removal), your body itself can't meet the increased need for thyroid hormone. This results in a drop in thyroid hormone levels, an increase in TSH levels, and hypothyroidism. This condition hinders successful assisted reproduction treatments (ART) and is associated with adverse outcomes, including miscarriage, preterm birth, stillbirth, gestational diabetes, breech delivery, a higher risk of a C-section, and cognitive function deficits—including ADHD, autism, cognitive and learning disabilities, and even mental retardation—in the child.

According to the 2011 "Guidelines of the American Thyroid Association for the Diagnosis and Management of Thyroid Disease During Pregnancy and Postpartum," or Pregnancy Guidelines, a summary of key thyroid changes that take place during pregnancy include the following:

- In women who are not iodine-deficient, the thyroid typically increases around 10 percent in size during pregnancy.
- In women who are iodine-deficient, the gland typically increases from 20 to 40 percent in size during pregnancy.
- Typically, production of thyroxine (T4) and triiodothyronine (T3) increases by 50 percent during pregnancy.
- A pregnant woman has a 50 percent increase in her daily iodine requirement.
- During the first trimester, approximately 10 to 20 percent of pregnant women are thyroid peroxidase antibody (TPOAb) or thyroglobulin antibody (TgAb) positive, with thyroid-stimulating hormone (TSH) in the normal reference range.
- An estimated 16 percent of women who are within the normal reference range but positive for TPOAb or TgAb during the first trimester will go on to have a TSH above 4.0 mIU/L during the third trimester.
- Some 33 to 50 percent of pregnant women who are positive for TPOAb or TgAb in the first trimester will develop postpartum thyroiditis.

The Pregnancy Guidelines authors write: "In essence, pregnancy is a stress test for the thyroid, resulting in hypothyroidism in women with limited thyroidal reserve or iodine deficiency, and postpartum thyroiditis in women with underlying Hashimoto's disease who were euthyroid (had normal thyroid function) prior to conception."

Autoimmune Thyroid Disease, Infertility, and Miscarriage

The relationship between elevated thyroid antibodies indicative of autoimmune thyroid disease, and both infertility and the risk of miscarriage, has been known for several decades.

Infertility is often defined as twelve months of unprotected sexual intercourse without conception, and the general rate in the population is around 10 to 15 percent; however, infertility rates among women with autoimmune thyroid disease can be as high as 50 percent. Miscarriage is defined as the loss of a pregnancy before 24 weeks of gestation, and the general miscarriage rate is around 20 percent, or one in five pregnancies. The risk of miscarriage for a woman who tests positive for thyroid antibodies, however, according to most studies—even when the woman is considered euthyroid, and her blood levels of thyroid hormone are within the reference range—is at least doubled, especially during the first trimester. One study found that thyroid autoantibody-positive women miscarried at a rate of 17 percent, more than double the rate of 8.4 percent for the autoantibody-negative women studied. And a meta-review of research on the subject, published in the *British Medical Journal* in 2011, found more than two dozen studies showing that the risk of miscarriage was increased by 290 percent—almost *tripled*—in pregnant women with thyroid antibodies.

According to the American Thyroid Association, some 10 to 20 percent of all pregnant women test positive for Hashimoto's antibodies (thyroid peroxidase antibodies, or TPOAb) during their first trimester, but otherwise are euthyroid. This means that some 10 to 20 percent of pregnant women face double to triple the risk of miscarriage in the first trimester due to the presence of TPOAb.

In a woman who has had more than one miscarriage, the presence of antibodies also raises the risk of subsequent pregnancy loss, known as recurrent miscarriage, or in medical terminology, recurrent abortion.

Even in women who remain euthyroid but positive for antibodies throughout the pregnancy, there is an increased risk of later miscarriage, stillbirth, and preterm delivery.

Some women with antibodies who start out euthyroid will go on to develop hypothyroidism during the pregnancy. If not detected or sufficiently treated, the hypothyroidism can also increase the risk of miscarriage, preterm delivery, and stillbirth, as well as neurocognitive and developmental problems for the newborn.

Graves' disease is also associated with infertility. A Brazilian study published in 2013 found that infertility is seen in more than half of all Graves' patients. Infertility, due to primary ovarian insufficiency, occurs in around 8 percent of Graves' patients.

Control of TSH levels is also important in women undergoing assisted reproduction who are positive for TPOAb. Unsuccessful procedures and miscarriage rates are higher in women who have a TSH level above 2.8 who also test positive for TPO.

The Thyroid and Assisted Reproduction

Some assisted reproductive technologies, known as ART, can be impacted by thyroid function and thyroid autoimmunity. These include:

- Use of fertility drugs—in particular, Clomid (clomiphene citrate), which helps increase the levels of follicle stimulating hormone (FSH), increasing ovulation rates, and in some cases, the number of follicles released
- Artificial insemination, including intrauterine insemination (IUI) and intracervical insemination (ICI)
- In vitro fertilization (IVF)—in which an egg is fertilized outside the body, and the fertilized embryo is transferred into the uterus

Assisted reproduction puts an additional strain on the thyroid. Studies have shown that the need for increased thyroid hormone typically occurs earlier, and is greater, in women undergoing ART.

Various studies have shown that women with hypothyroidism, even when treated, aren't as responsive to fertility drugs; basically, the ovaries are less likely to respond with ovulation.

Also, the stimulation of the ovaries done in preparation for various ART causes higher estrogen levels, which can impair fertility via blockage of the thyroid receptors. (Note: Some research has shown that thyroid hormone support for these women may improve the success rates of the procedures.)

There is controversy about the thyroid and IVF. Some studies have shown that once fertilized, embryos transferred after IVF have similar success rates in women with treated hypothyroidism; but other studies have shown that even treated hypothyroidism is associated with significantly decreased implantation, pregnancy, and live birth rates compared to women who do not have a thyroid problem and who are not taking thyroid hormone replacement medication. You will find information on these studies in Appendix C.

Now that we've established how thyroid disease can affect fertility and how important healthy thyroid function is to a successful pregnancy, we can begin to directly address how you can assess your own situation, plan, and give yourself the best possible odds for conceiving a child, staying healthy during pregnancy, and giving birth at full term to a healthy baby.

Your Thyroid, from Preconception to Postpartum

Planning Ahead for Pregnancy

4

If you have been diagnosed with a thyroid condition and want to have a baby, you need to plan for pregnancy even before you try to conceive. We all know that when we're trying to get pregnant, we shouldn't smoke and should start taking folic acid, but women with thyroid disease need to think about and do far more than that—even if the condition is "under control" with the help of medication.

As we discussed earlier, thyroid problems are often not being treated properly, which can interfere with your ability to conceive, create health problems during pregnancy, cause pregnancy complications, and threaten the health of your baby. Thyroid patients are more prone to miscarriage. And having an imbalance in a key endocrine gland can destabilize your entire endocrine system, affecting everything from menstrual cycles to your ability to maintain a healthy blood sugar level—all factors that affect fertility and a healthy pregnancy.

When you are ready to have a baby, you are entering one of the most important passages of your life. As a thyroid patient, the experience can also be a challenge. We encourage you to make a preconception plan and consider all of the important factors that can help ensure that you have a healthy pregnancy and baby.

Most physicians recommend that you start planning at least six months before you start trying to conceive. Eggs take several months to mature, and what you start doing today can have an impact on your egg quality months down the road. A six- to twelve-month preconception phase also allows you enough time to ensure that you have achieved optimal and stable thyroid function, have any necessary tests to detect nutritional deficiencies and shore up any missing nutrients, have made dietary and lifestyle changes, reduced inflammation, and taken other important steps. The first step in the process is to find the right doctor to be your partner and guide.

Choosing a Doctor

What type of doctor should you see for your preconception planning? In general, we recommend an integrative physician. Integrative physicians are medical doctors (MDs), naturopathic doctors (NDs), or osteopathic physicians (DOs) who can order tests and prescribe medication, but who also have a thorough understanding of optimal hormone balance and nutrition, and can use both conventional and holistic/alternative approaches to help you achieve optimal health. If you have a history of Graves' disease, hyperthyroidism, thyroid nodules, or thyroid cancer during pregnancy, you will also need to have an endocrinologist as part of your team.

Once you get pregnant, you will also need to see an obstetrician (OB). Keep in mind that very few OBs are considered integrative. Your OB's job will be to monitor the progress of your pregnancy, and ultimately, deliver your baby. Unfortunately, most OBs are not particularly knowledgeable about managing pregnancy in a thyroid patient. A research survey exploring obstetrician-gynecologists' level of knowledge about thyroid disorders and their typical treatment practices found that only 50 percent of the doctors felt that they had received "adequate" training in thyroid disorders during pregnancy.

The same is true of endocrinologists, who, despite specializing in hormonal disorders, are not necessarily knowledgeable about managing thyroid problems in a pregnant patient, or about optimal thyroid health for fertility and pregnancy. You may want to look specifically for a reproductive endocrinologist; they tend to be more knowledgeable because they specialize in fertility and in the hormones that impact fertility and pregnancy.

You really need to make sure that you are working with knowledgeable practitioners from every specialty. Joan and her husband spent several years and a lot of money trying to get pregnant with their first child:

> We finally gave up and focused on my health instead. When I went back to my primary doctor instead of a fertility specialist, he immediately diagnosed Hashimoto's. Six months later I was pregnant—and much better informed! Our second son came quickly and without issue. But when I was pregnant with my third, my new endocrinologist insisted that I lower my Synthroid. When I pointed out that this could cause miscarriage, she asked if I was a religious person and said I should go home and pray. In addition, she told me that it was irresponsible for me to have gotten pregnant knowing that I had a thyroid disorder. Luckily my OB-GYN referred me to a different doctor to deal with my thyroid treatment during pregnancy.

If you don't already have the right doctor, Appendix A of this book includes a list of resources to help you find an integrative physician in your area.

Charting Your Cycle

Charting your menstrual and fertility cycle allows you to identify when you ovulate, pinpoint your fertile days, and discover irregularities in your cycle that may make getting pregnant more difficult. Some women prefer to try to get pregnant without tracking, because doing so makes them feel self-conscious, or risks turning "baby-making" into a pressure-filled "command performance." If you already have a diagnosed thyroid condition, however, you are at greater risk of cycle irregularities that can make it harder to get pregnant. Several months of charting your menstrual and fertility cycle will give you useful information to share with your doctor at your first visit.

Fertility expert and author Toni Weschler recommends that in your charting or tracking, you keep track of three key fertility signs:

- Your cervical fluid, which will go from dry to wet, and at your most fertile—around ovulation—will become clear, slippery, or stretchy. These latter characteristics are fertility signs, and the longer your cervical fluid displays them, the more likely you are to become pregnant.
- Your waking basal body temperature, which will tend to hover in a low range before ovulation (97°–97.5°F), and a higher range after ovulation (97.6°F and higher). The shift in temperature is a good sign of ovulation. Low temperatures after ovulation can indicate higher risk of a miscarriage.
- Your cervix, which you may notice can become softer, higher, more open and wetter right around ovulation

Once you have charted several cycles, you will also be looking to determine whether your luteal phase (from ovulation to menstruation) is at least ten days. A shorter phase can increase your risk of infertility or miscarriage

How to Chart Your Cycles

There are free and fee-based online services and apps that allow you to chart your cycle in great detail. (See Appendix A for some of the sites and apps that can help.) You can also do it manually, using graph paper or a preprinted fertility chart. (You can download a preprinted chart from our website at http://www.ThyroidPregnancyBook.com.)

Toni Weschler offers these instructions on how to chart your cycle:

1. Take your temperature first thing upon awakening, before any other activity, such as drinking, talking on the phone, or getting up to use the bathroom.

2. You should take your temperature about the same time every morning, give or take about an hour.

3. If using a digital thermometer, wait until it beeps, usually about a minute. Some women may prefer to leave it in another minute beyond to be absolutely sure it reflects your correct temperature.

4. Take your temperature orally. (If you find that you don't get a clear temperature pattern, you may want to switch to taking it vaginally. Just be aware that it's important to be consistent and always take it the same way throughout the cycle because vaginal temps tend to be higher than oral temps.)

5. Record your temperatures on a fertility chart.

6. If your temperatures don't reflect a very obvious change in temperature—known as a "thermal shift"—you will need to look for more subtle changes, even small changes of one or two tenths of a degree. If you don't have a thermal shift, this can be a sign that you are not ovulating.

7. Your temperatures before ovulation will probably range from about 97° to 97.5°F. If they tend to remain in the 96s or 98s, it could be an indication of hypo- or hyperthyroidism.

8. Normally, temperatures after ovulation will remain higher for at least 10 days before you get your period. If they don't, you may have a short luteal phase that could indicate that you are at risk for infertility or miscarriages.

Your First Preconception Visit

When you go to your first preconception visit, it's helpful to arrive prepared. Here are some things to bring with you:

- Copies of any blood work, saliva, imaging or nutritional testing you have had done in the past two years. This can help your doctor evaluate your past thyroid, hormonal, and nutritional status.
- A list of all prescription drugs and supplements you are currently taking, with the dosages. Some drugs, and many supplements, are not considered

safe during pregnancy; your doctor can review them with you, and make suggestions for safely tapering off or stopping any potentially harmful substances in advance of your trying to get pregnant.

- A food diary, showing what you eat in a typical week. This can help your practitioner give you recommendations regarding dietary changes you may want to make prior to getting pregnant.
- Your fertility charts

At your first visit, it's important to discuss the following topics, which are explained in greater detail in this chapter:

- Optimizing your thyroid levels for fertility
- Testing for and addressing any other hormonal issues, such as sex hormone and adrenal imbalances
- Testing for and balancing any nutritional deficiencies
- Dietary changes
- Addressing autoimmunity and inflammation
- Lifestyle changes

If you are a smoker, discuss smoking cessation methods with your physician. Smoking can lead to fertility problems, and women who smoke during pregnancy—or are exposed to secondhand smoke—are more likely to give birth to small babies with low birth weight.

Also, be direct with your doctor regarding your consumption of alcohol and caffeine, both of which can cause fertility issues if your intake is too high.

A limited amount of caffeine is considered acceptable, but experts recommend that you limit your total daily intake of caffeine to no more than 200 mg a day through preconception and pregnancy. Some experts recommend that you avoid caffeine entirely during your first trimester, as there is evidence that eliminating caffeine entirely may reduce your risk of miscarriage.

Similarly, while having a glass of wine or a beer once or twice a week may not affect your fertility, studies show that even very modest drinking—five drinks a week or fewer—can still affect fertility. In addition, drinking around the time of ovulation lowers your chances of conception. The best course is to refrain from alcohol use when you are trying to conceive; but in any case, you should not drink during your pregnancy. It is important to note that regular alcohol use by your male partner can lower the motility and concentration of his sperm and decrease the likelihood of fertilization. The odds of conception are greatest when both of you refrain from drinking.

The Basics

As soon as you start thinking about getting pregnant, there are a number of things that you can and should do, and vitamins and supplements you can start taking, to help optimize your health, enhance fertility, and help ensure a healthy pregnancy. These recommendations are all considered safe—from pre-conception through breastfeeding.

Prenatal Vitamin

All of the experts who have contributed to this book recommend that you start taking a good brand of prenatal vitamin as early as possible in your pre-conception planning. According to pharmacist and health educator Suzy Cohen, "Eggs begin their journey of maturing about three months before they are actually released for potential fertilization. You'll want to start a prenatal vitamin at least 3 months before you plan to conceive; preferably 6 months ahead, before the eggs start maturing."

Some prenatal vitamins contain iron and calcium. If they do, you will need to take them at least three to four hours apart from your thyroid medication, to prevent any interaction with your thyroid medication that can reduce your absorption.

Integrative nutritionist Laurie Borenstein recommends you chose a brand that is organic and food-based and that contains DHA—docosahexaenoic acid—an omega-3 fatty acid that supports fetal brain development.

You should consider taking a prenatal vitamin that includes methylfolate, versus traditional folic acid. The rationale for this recommendation is discussed in the next section.

Methylfolate/Methylated Folic Acid

All women who are planning to get pregnant, not just ones with a thyroid condition, should take a supplement called methylfolate.

In the past, we've been told to take 400 mcg of folic acid daily before trying to get pregnant. Folic acid plays a key role in cell and tissue formation and DNA production in your growing baby, and help prevent birth defects such as spina bifida, anencephaly, and other neural tube defects. Neural tube defects typically appear in the growing fetus at four weeks of age—long before many women even know they're pregnant, which is why you need to start taking them before you even try to get pregnant.

But physicians are increasingly aware that at least half of the population has a genetic mutation known as MTHFR that affects the methylation process—the activation of the body's use of folic acid—and makes it less effective. As OB-GYN Thomas Moraczewski explains:

> Methylation is important for the proper production of folate. One of the most important tests preconceptionally to do is the MTHFR. Most OB-GYNs don't do this test because they lack knowledge of its importance. The test looks for mutation in these genes inherited from our parents. Its impact on both thyroid and pregnancy can be significant. The neural tube (primordial brain and CNS) develops within the first few weeks of gestation, before the pregnancy test is even positive. If there is a low active form of folate (B_9), then abnormal brain and spinal cord development may occur. There is even some data showing Trisomy 21 (Down syndrome) may have a folate relationship. Therefore the right type of supplementation is crucial in those with MTHFR mutations. Just giving "extra folic acid" that OBs prescribe or that are found in every prenatal vitamin may actually cause harm because the folic acid isn't being transformed into the "active" methylfolate.

You can be tested for the MTHFR genetic mutation during your preconception planning process. However, if you have not been tested, choose a prenatal vitamin that includes methylfolate, versus traditional folic acid. Brands that incorporate methylfolate include Thorne Prenatal Vitamins and NéevoDHA, as well as Optimal Prenatal vitamin and Optimal Prenatal Powder by Seeking Health. If you are taking a prenatal vitamin that includes regular folic acid, add a methylfolate supplement as well.

Omega-3 Fatty Acids

Omega-3 fatty acids are essential during preconception, as well as throughout pregnancy and during breastfeeding. Findings published in the journal *Applied Physiology, Nutrition and Metabolism* have shown that most women don't get enough of these healthy fats, which are found in such foods as fish, walnuts, and avocados—as well as supplements. One specific concern of a diet too low in omega-3s is an insufficient amount of DHA (docosahexaenoic acid), which is necessary for your baby's brain and nervous system development. During pregnancy, only 27 percent of women were getting enough DHA, and only 25 percent in the months postpartum. Low DHA during your pregnancy is linked to preterm labor, preeclampsia, postpartum depression, stillbirth, early infant death, as well as lower cognitive development, lower IQs, and ADHD in your child. Low DHA while you're breastfeeding increases the risk of asthma and allergies. Omega-3s in general and DHA in particular also help you produce more red blood cells, which allows you to provide nutrients and oxygen to the baby, and aids in healthy placenta development.

The experts recommend that you take 2,000 to 3,000 mg of a combined EPA-DHA supplement. EPA (eicosapentaenoic acid) and DHA (docosahexaenoic acid) are the two key omega-3 fatty acids, and typically found in oily fish and seafood. Choose your brand carefully, as some can contain heavy metals, such as mercury, and if you have a gluten sensitivity, be aware that some supplements have gluten in them. Naturopathic physician Kevin Passero recommends that you choose an algae-based supplement, which is guaranteed to not have pollutants that can be found in fish oil–based supplements. If you use a fish oil–based omega-3 supplement, Dr. Passero recommends a company that ensures purity, such as Nordic Naturals. He cautions: "Be careful about recommendations regarding cod liver oil, because it contains vitamin A, and if you are taking too much, it can be toxic to your developing baby." A number of the other experts we consulted also recommended the Nordic Naturals brand as a pure and safe brand of this supplement.

Selenium

Selenium is a mineral that plays a key role in thyroid health. Integrative physician Richard Shames recommends that "a woman ensure that she is getting enough selenium. Selenium helps with T4/T3 conversion, and lowering of thyroid antibodies," and other integrative experts all agree that thyroid patients planning pregnancy should supplement with selenium from preconception through breastfeeding.

The target dose from supplements and food is around 200 mcg—micrograms, not milligrams—per day. Check your prenatal vitamin to see what level of selenium it provides, then supplement with additional selenium to ensure you are getting 200 mcg a day. More is not better, however, and levels above 400 mcg can be toxic, so be careful to check labels of any selenium supplements you are taking to ensure you don't go over the recommended daily level.

It's hard to get much selenium from food, unless you are a fan of Brazil nuts, which are very high in selenium. If you are supplementing with selenium, it's advisable to avoid Brazil nuts. If you want to get your selenium from Brazil nuts, we recommend you consult with a nutritionist to determine a safe daily intake.

Probiotics

Probiotics are "good" bacteria that help promote a healthy digestive tract and support the immune system. They are found in fermented foods—such as yogurt, kefir, kimchi, miso, and kombucha—but experts recommend that you also supplement with probiotics from preconception through breastfeeding. Research has found that probiotics can help enhance fertility in a number of ways—and make assisted reproduction procedures more effective. For example, probiotic supplementation can reduce the risk of bacterial vaginosis, a common infection that can reduce your fertility, make IVF treatments less effective, and, if present during pregnancy, increase the risk of preterm delivery. Probiotics also lowers inflammation, which can also reduce fertility.

Experts recommend you choose a probiotic supplement with active bacterial cultures that include *Lactobacillus rhamnosus* GG, *Bifidobacterium bifidum*, *Lactococcus lactis*, and *Bifido breve*. Most quality probiotic supplements will require refrigeration to keep the bacteria alive.

Ferritin

Ferritin is a type of blood cell protein that stores iron. Ferritin has an impact on your thyroid and on keeping other hormones in balance. While many prenatal vitamins contain some iron, many of the integrative physicians we consulted, including David Borenstein, recommend that at your first preconception visit, you have your ferritin levels tested. According to Dr. Borenstein:

> Ferritin is important for hormonal function and fertility. Before a patient gets pregnant, I test her ferritin, and if it's not in the top half of the reference range, I have her supplement with iron. I have had patients struggling with infertility who, after optimizing their iron and thyroid function, were able to get pregnant fairly quickly and go on to have a healthy baby.

Once you have the results of your ferritin test back so you know how much more of this mineral you need, you can start supplementation. Ferritin levels should then be rechecked again during the preconception period, to ensure that you maintain the optimal level.

Integrative physician Adrienne Clamp feels that relying only on ferritin can be tricky. "Ferritin may be falsely elevated in any inflammatory condition," she points out, "so in that case, I measure TIBC (total iron-binding capacity) and percent saturation. If iron saturation is less than 20, I think iron supplementation is necessary."

If you have an unplanned pregnancy, it's important to ask for ferritin testing as quickly as possible, and if the results are low, to ask your physician to give you a ferritin injection which will immediately raise your levels.

It's also important to get your ferritin levels checked in the second and third trimesters and in the early months postpartum, to make sure you have optimal levels. Naturopathic physician Kevin Passero recommends that you get ferritin to a level between 45 and 85 (on a lab reference range of 15 to 150). Dr. Passero says:

> I typically recommend the iron glycinate form of iron. It's easier on the stomach, and is less likely to cause constipation—which is already enough of an issue during pregnancy. My general rule for iron, though, is go low, and go slow. So, start at a small dose, and work yourself up slowly to the optimal dosage.

A reminder: any iron supplements must be taken at least three to four hours apart from your thyroid medication, to prevent absorption problems.

Iodine

Supplementation with iodine, a trace mineral that the body needs to synthesize thyroid hormones, is a complicated and sometimes controversial topic.

Around the world, iodine deficiency is the number one cause of preventable retardation. While the majority of women of childbearing age in the United States are not iodine deficient, the number of women who are is on the rise. Data from the National Health and Nutrition Examination Survey (NHANES) has shown that iodine intake has been dropping in recent years, and that around 15 percent of women of childbearing age are currently iodine deficient. Other studies done in particular regions of the United States have found even higher rates of iodine deficiency in women of childbearing age.

Integrative physician David Brownstein, author of the book *Iodine*, believes that iodine is essential during preconception and pregnancy, and that the degree of iodine deficiency is far more prevalent than the studies indicate. According to Dr. Brownstein:

My research has shown that over 96 percent of people are deficient in iodine. Iodized table salt may provide enough iodine to prevent goiter in the
vast majority of people, but it is not sufficient to meet the whole body
need for iodine. Only 10 percent of iodide in refined table salt is bioavailable. In our toxic world, table salt does not provide enough iodine for
whole body iodine sufficiency. . . .

All women of pregnancy age should ensure they have optimal amounts
of iodine. My research has found that the average Japanese [person] ingest[s] approximately 15 mg/day of iodine. I have found this dose safe and
effective for providing enough iodine to meet the fetus's needs. Our toxic
world is replete with bromide and fluoride, which has caused our iodine
requirements to increase over the years. . . .

Most of the experts we consulted agree that the most recent recommendation from a number of sources—that a woman supplement with at least 150
mcg of iodine from preconception through breastfeeding—is a good starting
point. The easiest way to ensure this level of intake is to start taking a prenatal
vitamin that contains iodine early in the preconception phase, and continue
taking it through breastfeeding. Inexplicably, the majority of prescription prenatal vitamins and a substantial percentage of over-the-counter prenatal vitamins do not contain any iodine. So, check labels carefully and make sure that
your prenatal vitamin does.

Dr. Brownstein, on the other hand, recommends taking a combination of
iodine and iodide:

Different tissues of the body preferentially utilize different forms of iodine.
A multivitamin is not the best way to supplement with iodine. Good
sources of iodine include Lugol's solution, Iodozyme HP, Lugol Tablets
and Iodoral. All of these forms supply both iodide and iodine. I suggest
getting tested and working with an iodine-literate health care provider.

A number of the other experts we consulted, including OB-GYN Thomas
Moraczewski, highly recommend that your preconception testing include an
iodine test. "I check iodine levels in every thyroid patient, pregnant or not," Dr.
Moraczewski says. "I prefer to use the ZRT Labs Dried Urine Iodine Test. You
urinate on a small card in the morning and before bed and send it in. About half
of my patients have low iodine levels and it must be replaced appropriately."

Some of the experts do, however, have a concern regarding higher doses of
iodine in Hashimoto's patients, as it can sometimes aggravate the disease.

Thus they want to make sure that the levels are controlled. According to naturopathic physician Fiona McCulloch:

> With respect to Hashimoto's, I always recommend a prenatal vitamin containing 250 mcg of iodine *and* 200 mcg of selenium. I find that this combination is very much needed for Hashimoto's patients. Women with Hashimoto's do need additional iodine in pregnancy like any pregnant woman. 250 mcg of iodine is a very small dose, and is very safe, particularly when combined with selenium. So as far as I've seen, the aggravations in Hashimoto's patients don't occur at all at this level of supplementation.

Vitamin D

We now know that vitamin D is more than a vitamin; it functions as a hormone and has an important effect on our immune system. The experts we consulted recommend that rather than starting to take an arbitrary level of vitamin D during preconception, you first have vitamin D testing to determine your current levels.

Integrative physician David Borenstein prefers that patients have a vitamin D level of at least around 50 to 60 or above on a scale of 32 to 100.

Keep in mind that vitamin D is best absorbed when eaten with your fattiest meal of the day—usually dinner.

Vitamin B$_{12}$

Some of the experts recommend having a test to determine your vitamin B$_{12}$ level during preconception, and supplementing if necessary from preconception through breastfeeding. Integrative physician Adrienne Clamp recommends that B$_{12}$ levels be near the top end of the "normal" range, 800 to 900, and that if supplementation is needed, a sublingual—under-the-tongue—form be used.

Phosphatidylcholine

OB-GYN Thomas Moraczewski recommends that women take the supplement phosphatidylcholine during preconception and pregnancy. According to Dr. Moraczewski, "Phosphatidylcholine helps fetal brain function. But only a minority of pregnant women has adequate levels of choline. If purchased by itself, a good dosage in pregnancy would be between 750 and 1,000 mg. One brand that I recommend is Optimal PC."

Magnesium

According to integrative physician Adrienne Clamp, magnesium plays an important role in over 350 different enzyme reactions in the body. Says Dr. Clamp:

> Among other things, magnesium helps normalize blood pressure, improves neurological function, eases muscle pain, helps sleep, and can reduce constipation. In general, it helps relax muscles, and muscle cramps are common in hypothyroidism, especially in early pregnancy. Also, remember that the uterus is one big muscle, and I think that keeping the magnesium level high enough may help to prevent preterm labor and hopefully preeclampsia as well. I do not have research proof of this but it makes sense to me, considering the importance of magnesium in muscle and neurological function. Magnesium must be measured intracellularly, because it is a predominantly intracellular mineral (meaning that serum magnesium testing is not useful). This is why I order the RBC (red blood cell) magnesium. I usually recommend magnesium glycinate as a first measure, magnesium taurate if glycerinate is not successful in raising the levels to good levels. I try to keep my patients' magnesium levels between 5.5 and 6.5. In a minority of patients who don't respond to the oral supplements, I resort to intramuscular magnesium injections.

Hydration

Staying well hydrated, with water, is a crucial component of your health from preconception through breastfeeding. According to integrative nutritionist Laurie Borenstein, hydration helps detoxification, digestion, and absorption of nutrients, and drinking half your body weight in ounces per day is a good target. This is a time to avoid sodas, sports drinks, energy boosters, juices, and other bottled beverages. These drinks are often loaded with sweeteners, as well as artificial flavors and colors.

Weight Loss

If you are carrying around extra weight, the preconception period is a time to do your best to lose some of it. Being overweight or obese can severely impact your fertility. One study published in 2013 examined the impact on close to one hundred obese women, who had been unable to conceive after two to five years of fertility treatments, of a six-month program of dietary changes and exercise. Among the women who went from a body mass index that characterized them as obese, to one considered just slightly overweight, there was a 42 percent increase in spontaneous conception—they got pregnant without any fertility treatment—and there was a 22 percent increase in conception for those getting fertility treatments.

The dietary and supplement recommendations in this book can help you with weight loss. But losing weight as a thyroid patient can be a challenge. For a detailed approach to weight loss for thyroid patients, we recommend you read Mary Shomon's book *Thyroid Diet Revolution*, which provides a comprehensive program and recommendations to help you lose weight.

Remember that weight-loss supplements or medications can be used in the preconception period but should be discontinued once you are pregnant.

Exercise

Increasing your physical activity during preconception and pregnancy can not only enhance fertility, but improve the outcomes of your pregnancy. Even 15 to 20 minutes a day of brisk walking can have an impact, but if you can aim for 30 to 60 minutes a day of some form of activity, even better: Research has shown a reduced risk of respiratory distress in your newborn, a shorter post-partum hospital stay, and a reduced risk of a C-section. Exercise has also been linked to an easier delivery and faster recovery of muscle tone, strength, and fitness after childbirth.

Thyroid Treatment

One of the most important parts of your preconception planning is to ensure that you are properly diagnosed and receiving optimal thyroid treatment.

If you have not yet been diagnosed with a thyroid condition, but suspect you have one, or have a past history of it, it's crucial to see a knowledgeable practitioner to have the clinical examination, testing of TSH, Free T4, Free T3, Reverse T3, TPOAb, TgAb, and TSI, and ultrasound of any enlargement, lumps or nodules, as detailed in Part 1. Again, remember that many doctors only test TSH, and their conventional view of diagnosis is that if your results are "within the reference range," you don't have a thyroid condition, even if you have autoimmune thyroid disease, nodules, or even goiter. So, you need to know the ideal reference ranges for preconception and pregnancy that you doctor may not know. Be aware that many doctors feel that for optimal thyroid function for pregnancy, TSH should be around 1; Free T4 and Free T3 should be in the higher end of the range; Reverse T3, in the lower end of the range, and antibodies should not be significantly elevated.

If you are already diagnosed with a thyroid condition, then as we've discussed, be aware that most women with thyroid conditions, regardless which condition it is, end up hypothyroid. When you're hypothyroid, you may be concerned that pregnancy is going to be particularly difficult for you. You are right to acknowledge that a healthy pregnancy will require some extra planning and effort on your part, but generally, women who are informed, prepared, have a knowledgeable doctor, and whose thyroid condition is properly managed and treated, should be able to go through pregnancy without any significant difficulties.

One of the most critical things you can do in the preconception period is to ensure that your thyroid levels are optimized. Optimal thyroid function can help your fertility, reduce the risk of miscarriage, minimize complications in pregnancy, and help ensure that your baby is healthy.

Most doctors use the thyroid-stimulating hormone (TSH) level as a gauge. What's the optimal TSH level for getting pregnant and for maintaining a successful pregnancy for both mother and baby? That's a difficult question, because different experts have different answers. Some women may have been told that their TSH level is "normal," and that they shouldn't have any trouble getting pregnant, yet suffer years of "unexplained" infertility or recurrent miscarriages. Others may be told not even to attempt conceiving until their thyroid levels stabilize in the TSH range of 1.0 to 2.0.

While we'll discuss in Chapter 5 the ins and outs of hypothyroidism treatment during pregnancy, during the preconception stage, the 2011 "Guidelines of the American Thyroid Association for the Diagnosis and Management of Thyroid Disease During Pregnancy and Postpartum," or Pregnancy Guidelines, recommend that hypothyroid patients planning pregnancy have their provider adjust their dose of thyroid medication so as to optimize serum TSH values to less than 2.5.

If you have had thyroid cancer, and are on a suppressive dose of thyroid medication with a very low TSH, you should discuss your dosage with your doctor. According to cancer specialist Dr. Jennifer Sipos:

> Sometimes in our cancer patients, we'll actually have to decrease their dose if they're planning to get pregnant, because we don't want them to be hyperthyroid while they're trying to get pregnant, which can increase the likelihood of a miscarriage. When we have cancer patients, we like to plan for pregnancies by getting their TSH in an optimal range so that we then don't have to scramble to adjust the levels once they're already pregnant.

Mary Shomon's Story

When I started my preconception planning, my TSH level was 4.1. At that time, I felt pretty well, and it being almost two decades ago, there was little information about safe TSH levels for conception and pregnancy. I saw an endocrinologist—a woman with more than 20 years of treating women with thyroid problems and thyroid-related infertility. She believed firmly at that time that women needed to be maintained at a TSH level between 1 and 2, which was considered low by some doctors, and that a woman with evidence of thyroid disease needed to be in that same range in order to get pregnant, and maintain the pregnancy. She increased my dosage of thyroid medication, dropping my TSH to a 1.1, and I was able to get pregnant the second month we tried, and go on to have a healthy baby.

The integrative practitioners we consulted recommend that the TSH level of a woman being treated for hypothyroidism be around 1.0, with Free T4 and Free T3 both in the top half of the reference range.

Dr. Richard Shames has this recommendation: "Prior to conception, I recommend that a woman's TSH be on the lower end of the normal range, ideally below 1.0. This helps to lower the autoimmune activity and antibodies, and prepares the body more fully for pregnancy."

Note that if you were previously treated for thyroid cancer, and your doctor recommended suppressive therapy, the 2012 Endocrine Society guidelines on managing thyroid dysfunction in pregnancy recommend that you continue with your suppressive dose, as long as your TSH is not 0, and you have a detectable—even if very low—TSH level.

Jennifer's story illustrates the importance of "being optimized." Jennifer was diagnosed with Hashimoto's, along with goiter and nodules, and started on Synthroid treatment.

My thyroid shrunk considerably pretty quickly. My husband and I were trying to get pregnant for almost 3 years, and the blood work and tests always came back normal, and yet I wasn't getting pregnant. We were going to see an infertility specialist, when a friend suggested I see an endocrinologist first. I said that my thyroid was controlled, and that my doctor had said everything was okay, and my thyroid was not the problem. I thought about it later and figured it couldn't hurt just to get a second opinion. The endocrinologist I went to did blood work that my doctor hadn't done, and it came back irregular. He increased my dose by 50 percent. No joke—I got pregnant about 2 months later. I was fortunate to have my medication increased preventing me from going through infertility before taking another look at thyroid. I had an awesome pregnancy and delivered a healthy baby girl who is now eleven years old.

The Pregnancy Guidelines recommend that a woman with hypothyroidism have her dosage adjusted so that TSH is below 2.5 mIU/L prior to conception. This lowers the risk of the TSH elevating in the first trimester. The issue of whether you should take levothyroxine, levothyroxine plus T3, or natural desiccated thyroid, and considerations specific to each form of medication, are discussed at length in Chapter 5. In any case, if your levels are not optimal, work with your practitioner during the preconception phase to change medications and or dosages to ensure that your levels are optimal. And once optimized, give yourself several months of stability before attempting to get pregnant.

You should also have a plan to confirm your pregnancy as early as possible, since once you are pregnant, it's essential that your dosage of thyroid medication immediately be increased. Don't wait until you've missed your period. We recommend that you start using pregnancy tests as early as seven days after you have possibly conceived, and test daily until you either get a positive result, or start your menstrual period. Different practitioners have different recommendations about the extent of the increase. Some suggest that you add two levothyroxine pills a week as soon as you confirm pregnancy, but if you are on a T4/T3 or NDT drug, your doctor may have another recommendation. In any case, discuss with your doctor before getting pregnant what he or she recommends, so you can be prepared to increase your dose by the agreed-upon amount the very day you confirm your pregnancy.

In 2012, the American Association of Clinical Endocrinologists (AACE) and the American Thyroid Association (ATA) published their "Clinical Practice Guidelines for Hypothyroidism in Adults." These guidelines had some recommendations for women who are planning conception or who are going to receive fertility treatments:

- Treatment should be considered in women of child bearing age with thyroid-stimulating hormone (TSH) levels between 2.5 mIU/L and the upper limit of normal if they are planning an upcoming pregnancy using assisted reproduction techniques.
- Treatment should be considered for women who have normal TSH levels who are planning a pregnancy or assisted reproduction if they have or have in the past tested positive for thyroid peroxidase antibodies

(TPOAb). This is considered particularly important if the woman has a history of miscarriage or a past history of hypothyroidism.

- Women who are pregnant or planning a pregnancy, including assisted reproduction in the immediate future, should be treated if they currently or in the past have had positive levels of TPOAb and their TSH level is greater than 2.5 mIU/L.

Vanessa's experience underscores the importance of having the right doctor, and of confirming your pregnancy early and seeing your doctor right away. At age thirty, Vanessa had hypothyroidism and Hashimoto's, with very high antibodies.

> My then-endocrinologist flatly told me that I would have trouble conceiving and carrying a child to term. I was devastated, both by the news and by this doctor's extremely cold and cavalier attitude. I immediately found another endocrinologist, who was wonderful. He switched me to name-brand Synthroid and began monitoring my levels very carefully. At the time, I had less than 10 percent natural thyroid function left. My new endocrinologist told me I was healthy and fit and that, with careful monitoring, he was confident I could have a successful pregnancy. At age 32, I became pregnant on my second month of trying to conceive. I told both my GP and my endocrinologist immediately. The GP dismissively told me to call back when I was further along but my endocrinologist wanted to see me immediately. I was less than two weeks pregnant and already needed an increased dosage of Synthroid. I was carefully monitored throughout my pregnancy and safely delivered a healthy baby girl.

Planning Ahead If You Have Graves' Disease/Hyperthyroidism

If you have active Graves' disease and hyperthyroidism, the Pregnancy Guidelines and integrative experts all recommend that you wait until your thyroid function is stabilized before getting pregnant.

According to the guidelines, "Women who have Graves' disease should conceive only after they are euthyroid—defined as having normal thyroid levels. The Guidelines strongly recommend contraception until this is achieved, and recommend that physicians offer counseling to women regarding the implications of treatment on conception plans."

Physician and naturopath Jonathan Wright also recommends that a woman with Graves' disease and hyperthyroidism get it under control prior to pregnancy, without using the antithyroid drugs—thionamides—often prescribed for treatment:

> I recommend reducing the overproduction of T4, Free T4, T3 and Free T3 to normal, following the procedure published by the Walter Reed Army Medical Center, Washington, DC, in 1980. At the Walter Reed Army Medical Center, subjects with hyperthyroidism were divided into four treatment groups. One group received lithium. The second group received Lugol's iodine. The third group received lithium first and then three or four days later started iodine. The fourth group received Lugol's iodine first and then three or four days later started lithium. They found that the group that started with Lugol's iodine and finished with lithium did significantly better than all of the other groups. This approach is effective in getting hyperthyroidism rapidly under control, and usually occurs in two weeks or less. This step has been effective in all but one hyperthyroid individual; adding small quantities of another essential element to the Walter Reed protocol completely normalized her thyroid function, too.

Note that this treatment is intended to be a done exclusively during preconception, and is not safe for the fetus during pregnancy or for a breastfeeding baby.

Functional medicine expert Amy Myers, MD, recommends that women with hyperthyroidism start by seeing a functional medicine practitioner to see if natural approaches to reducing autoimmunity and manage hyperthyroidism—which can include supplements, dietary changes, and even such treatments as low-dose naltrexone—can put you into remission without use of radioactive iodine treatment or antithyroid medications. Keep in mind that it can take as long as eighteen months to regulate and control Graves' disease and hyperthyroidism using natural approaches.

If you have active Graves' disease and hyperthyroidism, and natural approaches have failed to help you achieve a remission or treatment, then you have three options:

- **Antithyroid medication:** During preconception, the antithyroid drug methimazole is usually used. The objective is to achieve a remission of your symptoms, normalization of your blood work, and lowering of antibodies. Keep in mind that around 30 percent of patients will achieve remission, and that the process can take a number of months. It is not recommended you attempt to get pregnant while actively taking antithyroid drugs, so if you do go into remission, you will want to alter treatment before conceiving. If you are taking antithyroid medications and do become pregnant, the Pregnancy Guidelines recommend that you confirm your pregnancy as early as possible; that you be switched immediately to another antithyroid drug—propylthiouracil (PTU)—as early as possible in the first trimester to reduce risks of birth defects in your baby; and then switch back to methimazole for the second and third trimester. This is particularly important because if you are hyperthyroid and taking methimazole, and you wait for a missed period to test for pregnancy, it may be weeks before your medication will be switched to the recommended PTU in the first trimester.

- **Radioactive iodine therapy (RAI):** RAI can be performed during the preconception period. You should, however, be sure to have a pregnancy test 48 hours prior to the RAI administration, just to ensure that you are not pregnant. After surgery or RAI, the Pregnancy Guidelines recommend waiting for six months to conceive, to allow you to get on a stable dose of thyroid hormone replacement. Some experts recommend that you wait a year, to protect your developing fetus from any residual radiation. Radioactive iodine may also affect your ovaries, and you may have irregular menstrual cycles for as long as a year after RAI, making your fertility more erratic.

- **Surgery:** The Pregnancy Guidelines recommend surgery for a woman who has high TSI levels and who is planning to get pregnant within two years. The rationale is that antibody levels tend to rise after RAI and may remain elevated. Surgery may also be performed if you are allergic or sensitive to antithyroid drugs, antithyroid drug treatment didn't work, and you prefer not to have RAI. If you have surgery for Graves' disease/hyperthyroidism, experts recommend that you wait at least until you are feeling well and have a history of several sets of blood tests showing optimal thyroid hormone replacement. Usually, this will require at least six months.

Even if you have been treated for Graves' disease with either RAI or surgery, if you are planning to become pregnant, you should know that you may still have a high reading of thyroid antibodies in your bloodstream. You should have TSI testing prior to becoming pregnant, and some doctors recommend a course of antithyroid drugs to bring your level of antibodies down to a normal, manageable level before pregnancy.

Thyroid Cancer

No physicians recommend planning pregnancy while being actively treated for thyroid cancer. If you are pregnant, and are diagnosed with thyroid cancer, see Chapter 7 for information on treatments.

If you have already been diagnosed and treated for thyroid cancer, endocrinologist Roberto Negro, MD, one of the Pregnancy Guidelines authors, confirms the guidelines' recommendations: "After thyroid cancer treatment with surgery and radioiodine, you should wait at least six months to a year before attempting to get pregnant, to stabilize thyroid hormone replacement and confirm remission of your thyroid cancer." Once remission is confirmed, prospects for both a healthy pregnancy and good health generally are good: "Pregnancy is not associated with increased risk of disease recurrence if the patient is cured."

As noted earlier, if you are on suppressive doses of thyroid hormone replacement, it's considered safe to consider suppressive doses during pregnancy, as long as you have a detectable—even if very low—TSH level.

Other Hormonal Imbalances

Before pregnancy, and especially if you have menstrual cycle irregularities, anovulatory cycles, or a short luteal phase, your physician may want to test for estrogen and progesterone levels, and if necessary supplement with prescription drugs or hormones—or in the case of progesterone, an over-the-counter progesterone cream.

Dr. Thomas Moraczewski recommends that you have a 4-point salivary hormone test during your luteal phase, around Day 21 of your cycle, to measure estradiol, progesterone, DHEA, testosterone, and cortisol. Says Dr. Moraczewski: "Low thyroid coincides with low progesterone. Progesterone helps to activate the thyroid receptor in women. Low progesterone can lead to faulty implantation site for the embryo. Supplementation with vaginal progesterone cream or gel can rectify this situation." He also tests for pregnenolone, which he calls the "mother of steroid hormones," and recommends replacement with oral pregnenolone to ensure adequate hormone synthesis in pregnancy.

If you have a history of irregular periods, weight gain, facial hair, and fertility problems, your doctor will also evaluate you for a condition known as polycystic ovary syndrome, or PCOS. The conventional treatment for PCOS is a type 2 diabetes medication, such as metformin (Glucophage), which increases insulin sensitivity. Dietary changes are also recommended, and some women have had success reversing PCOS with dietary changes alone.

Integrative nutritionist Laurie Borenstein was diagnosed with PCOS and told that it would be difficult to get pregnant. After changing her diet, she went on to have two healthy children. According to Borenstein:

> If you have polycystic ovary syndrome, how you eat is especially important. I recommend that you reduce sugar intake in all forms. Eliminate refined sugar, most grains (quinoa and millet can be used sparingly), and dramatically reduce your fruit consumption. Try to choose only low-sugar fruit such as blueberries, blackberries, raspberries, and green apples.

Many physicians feel that in women with thyroid disease, adrenal health should be evaluated, addressed, and balanced during the preconception phase as well. This can best be evaluated by taking a 24-hour saliva cortisol test.

Naturopathic physician Kevin Passero evaluates adrenal function, and addresses it during the preconception phase, to enhance hormonal balance and fertility. Dr. Passero uses a combination of adaptogenic herbs, such as ashwagandha; vitamins such as vitamin C; and adrenal glandular supplements—and suggests nutritional, sleep, and lifestyle changes—to get adrenals back in balance. However Dr. Passero notes that it is important to halt intake of most supplements during a woman's fertile phase if she is trying to and may become pregnant:

> I believe in using the fewest supplements possible during pregnancy, and while some nutrients are necessary, I avoid herbs for the most part. If I'm working with a woman on adrenal support—or any regime of supplements and herb—who is actively trying to get pregnant, I have her stop taking it at ovulation, and resume only when her period starts. This helps protect her fetus from inadvertent exposure during the possible several weeks between conception and confirmation of pregnancy.

Dr. Passero also has some more general recommendations regarding adrenal health and pregnancy for woman with thyroid conditions:

> First, if you're a thyroid patient, give yourself some time, and if possible, don't have your babies too close together. Your body needs time to recover from the adrenal drag caused by pregnancy, delivery, breastfeeding, and sleep disruptions after childbirth. Women do themselves a disservice by

not giving themselves the time to rebuild between pregnancies. If I have a patient on an adrenal protocol and they find out they're unexpectedly pregnant, I tell them to stop everything except vitamin C. But I do tell them to call me as soon as possible after delivery—and we'll start getting things back in balance right away.

Some patients who have very low adrenal function—but who do not have a diagnosis of Addison's disease—may be prescribed a physiologic dose of hydrocortisone to help support the adrenals. It's important to know that synthetic steroids, such as prednisone, are what the Food and Drug Administration (FDA) has termed "Pregnancy Category C," meaning that research in animal studies has shown adverse effects on the fetus, though testing in humans has not been done, but that "potential benefits may warrant use of the drug in pregnant women despite potential risks." Hydrocortisone, however, has no FDA pregnancy category. Some animal studies showed an increased risk of cleft palate in offspring, but anecdotally, scientists have not found evidence that use of hydrocortisone in pregnancy is a risk for birth defects. Still, experts caution that hydrocortisone should be given during pregnancy only when the benefit outweighs risk. If you are on hydrocortisone, you should taper off, and ensure adrenal balance, prior to attempting pregnancy.

Integrative physician and midwife Aviva Romm also feels that managing adrenal stress prior to pregnancy is essential

Make sure you are getting enough B complex and magnesium—things that are calming. Some people benefit from supplements that have 5 HTP or GABA; they help calm the nervous system. I use adaptogens quite a bit. These herbs have been in use for thousands of years as some of the top herbs in Ayurvedic and Chinese medicine. The idea behind adaptogens is that they help to normalize the stress response by regulating the adrenal reaction. In Chinese medicine, for example, ginseng is one of the classics. Ginseng is especially helpful for immune problems and a deeper level of fatigue, but it can be stimulating. One of the main adaptogens in Ayurvedic medicine is ashwagandha. It's considered one of the leading herbs for supporting and restoring the nervous system, and it's one of the leading adaptogens, and is especially helpful for sleep and musculoskeletal tension. Rhodiola is useful for people with general anxiety. Holy basil is just sort of a general, feel-good tonic. Eleutherococcus is particularly helpful for cognitive function issues. *I do not, however, use these treatments during pregnancy.* They are great for women to be on when they are trying to conceive. Discontinue as soon as you know that you are pregnant."

Finally, many of the experts recommend that hemoglobin A1C—blood sugar—be tested at the first preconception visit, along with fasting glucose. Elevated levels of A1C can suggest insulin resistance, which can impair your fertility. According to Dr. Kevin Passero, "Insulin sensitive diets are associated with improved fertility. So, switching to a lower carbohydrate, higher protein diet that includes vegetables—but limits sugar and grains—can lower blood sugar, reduce inflammation, improve your insulin sensitivity, and help reduce your risk of gestational diabetes."

Toxins

One of the most important things you can do is to minimize your exposure to toxins prior to, during, and after pregnancy, and to eliminate certain toxins from your body prior to getting pregnant.

According to integrative and functional medicine specialist Dr. Jill Carnahan:

> We are all swimming in toxic soup! Our food supply is totally adulterated with genetically modified foods, there's an increase in food additives and chemicals, an increase in pesticide use on nonorganic foods, etc. There is only so much our body can handle and once we hit the limit of our detox capacity, we overflow into disease states. Your thyroid is one of the most sensitive organs in the body to environmental toxins and chemicals. Thyroid medication by itself will not help someone feel better if they are still in a state of toxic overload. We must address environmental toxicity, the chemical products we apply to our face and body, the products we use to clean our laundry and household and the food we put into our body.

Dr. Amy Myers recommends that one good way to diminish exposure to toxins in general is to use indoor HEPA air filters in your home:

> If you just think about how toxins get in, they get in through the air that we breathe, they get in through our lungs, they get in through our skin, and they get in through us ingesting them. . . . The indoor air is considered, in some places, 10 to 100 times more toxic than the outdoor air, because our houses are so sealed and all the toxins in the products that we

buy now, the TV's and the computers, and the mattresses, and the particle board, this and that.

Here are some other toxins to recognize and avoid:

Heavy Metals

One of the tests your doctor may order at your preconception visit, especially if you have risk factors, is a test for heavy metals. Lead, for example, is a potent neurotoxin that is stored in the bones and can be passed to a developing baby through the placenta. Mercury can impair your fertility. Arsenic, cadmium, and chromium can also be harmful to women and their babies.

Discuss with your doctor whether heavy metals testing is necessary given your occupation, hobbies, possible exposure, and/or symptoms. If elevated levels of any of these substances are found, your physician can recommend various forms of chelation therapy to help detox and clear these levels from your body.

Food Toxins

There are a number of foods to avoid during preconception, as well as throughout your pregnancy and while breastfeeding. These are foods that contain toxins, heavy metals, or that can be contaminated with bacteria that can put your pregnancy or baby at risk. Some recommendations:

- Choose organic, hormone-free, and pesticide-free foods whenever possible.
- Choose only grass-fed, organic meats and poultry. Nonorganic meat and poultry can contain synthetic hormones, antibiotics, and chemicals that concentrate in animal fat, and that are transferred when we eat the meat.
- Avoid raw meat and poultry, which can be infected with a number of bacteria.
- Avoid deli meats; these can be contaminated with *Listeria* bacteria, which can cause miscarriage.
- Avoid raw seafood, including shellfish and sushi, which can be infected with a number of bacteria and parasites.
- Avoid fish with high mercury levels (e.g., shark, swordfish, king mackerel, and tilefish).
- Avoid smoked seafood, as it can contain *Listeria*.

- Avoid locally caught freshwater fish that may have high levels of polychlorinated biphenyls (PCBs) (e.g., bluefish, striped bass, freshwater salmon, pike, trout, and walleye).
- Avoid raw eggs, due to the risk of *Salmonella*.
- Avoid unpasteurized milk and soft cheeses, such as Brie, Camembert, Roquefort, feta, Gorgonzola, and Mexican queso blanco, unless they are pasteurized. Unpasteurized dairy products can contain *Listeria*.
- Avoid pâté, which can contain *Listeria*.

Fluoride

You may want to have your water tested for heavy metals, bacteria, and fluoride levels. Some physicians recommend that you use only filtered water starting with preconception, and avoid ingesting fluoridated water and fluoride. Dr. Richard Shames says:

> I'm specifically concerned about excessive fluoride exposure, and the link to thyroid problems. I recommend that a woman who is trying to get pregnant, or who is pregnant, should limit her exposure to fluoride. If you can drink unfluoridated water—whether through a reverse osmosis system or a fluoride-free bottled water—that is a good choice. I would also avoid fluoridated products like toothpastes and mouthwashes during that time.

Goitrogens

Goitrogens are naturally occurring substances found in various foods that have the ability to cause a goiter—an enlargement of the thyroid gland. The key goitrogen-rich foods are the vegetables in the cruciferous category, but there are a number of other foods that contain significant amounts of goitrogens as well. In addition to promoting goiter formation, goitrogenic foods can act like antithyroid drugs, slowing down the thyroid and ultimately causing hypothyroidism, an underactive thyroid. Goitrogens are able to disrupt normal thyroid function by inhibiting the body's ability to use iodine, block the process by which iodine becomes the thyroid hormones thyroxine (T4) and triiodothyronine (T3), inhibit the actual secretion of thyroid hormone, and disrupt the peripheral conversion of T4 to T3.

Goitrogens can have two functions in pregnancy. If you consume larger quantities of them, ideally raw, you may be able to slow down an overactive thyroid. However, if you consume too much of these foods, and you're hypothyroid, you may worsen your hypothyroidism. (Note, however, that steaming or cooking can reduce their goitrogenic properties.)

Some of the more common and potent goitrogens include:

- African cassava
- Babassu (a palm-tree coconut fruit found in Brazil and Africa)
- Bok choy
- Broccoli
- Broccolini
- Brussels sprouts
- Cabbage
- Cauliflower
- Chinese broccoli
- Collards
- Daikon
- Kale
- Kohlrabi
- Millet
- Mustard
- Peaches
- Peanuts
- Pine nuts
- Radishes
- Rutabaga
- Spinach
- Strawberries
- Turnips
- Watercress

Be aware that raw juices often includes goitrogenic vegetables, such as cabbage and spinach, and these juices end up providing highly concentrated amounts of goiter-promoting ingredients. Don't drink these juices unless you can be sure what is, and isn't, in them.

Chemicals

One key recommendation is to avoid endocrine-disrupting chemicals. A variety of chemicals, including polychlorinated biphenyls (PCBs) and phthalates, can alter your thyroid levels in pregnancy, and may affect fetal brain development. Starting in preconception, try to avoid excessive exposure to the following:

- Flame-retardant cloth
- Spray-on flame retardants
- Paints and adhesives that contain these ingredients
- Teflon and nonstick coated pans
- Spray-on fabric protectors
- Stain-resistant carpets
- New plastic shower curtains

Note: We know that sometimes it's hard to avoid some of these items, so be as vigilant as you can. If you own a stain-resistant carpet and aren't able to replace it right now, keep in mind green alternatives for when it is time to get new carpets.

Dr. Richard Shames also recommends that you use only nontoxic, chemical-free natural cleaning products in your home and office, starting at preconception.

Integrative and functional medicine specialist Dr. Jill Carnahan recommends that you stop using certain types of plastics, because they are endocrine-disruptors.

Some plastic food and beverage containers are made with endocrine-disrupting chemicals that are suspected of causing harm to developing fetuses. Check water bottles, food packaging, and other plastics, looking for the specific resin code on the bottom, usually located in a triangle of arrows. Avoid those numbered 1, 3, 6, or 7 (PC). Never use plastic in microwave or with hot food, as heat promotes leaching of the chemicals into your food. And discard plastics when they begin to have signs of wear and tear.

She also suggests that you use fewer personal care products—e.g., toothpastes, deodorants, shampoos, soaps, body wash, conditioners, etc.—and check the ones you do use carefully. According to Dr. Carnahan:

Many personal care products contain chemicals that disrupt hormones your baby will rely on for proper development. And others contain carcinogens and neurotoxicants, among other things. Look for products with fewer ingredients—ideally those with the USDA Certified Organic Seal. Avoid products containing parabens, phthalates (DEHP, BBP, DBP, DMP,

DEP), DMDM hydantoin, fragrance, triclosan, sodium lauryl/laureth sulfate, DEA (diethanolamine) and TEA (triethanolamine), formaldehyde, PEGs (polyethylene glycol), and anything with "glycol" or "methyl."

Detoxification

If you have been exposed to toxins, your practitioner may recommend a detoxification regimen. Nutritionist Kim Schuette recommends "gentle therapies that support your liver, kidney and lymphatic function, which are all important during preconception. These therapies can include castor oil packs, dry brushing, dry sauna therapy, coffee enemas (in moderation), rebounding, and regular daily movement." Note that regular use of saunas, coffee enemas, and castor oil packs is not recommended during pregnancy, so if you want to explore a detoxification program, do so before conception.

Fertility-Friendly Nutrition

You can change and improve your diet preconception in many ways to help improve your health, increase your chance of fertility, and help ensure that you have a healthy pregnancy and baby. It's up to you to discuss with your practitioner what changes to make to your diet. But at minimum, some important things you should do include the following:

Avoid Known Food Allergens and Food Triggers

If you are lactose-intolerant, or allergic to a particular food, it's especially important that you avoid them during preconception and all the way through breastfeeding. Ingesting substances that you are sensitive to causes inflammation, which is counterproductive to fertility and a healthy pregnancy.

Eliminate Soy from Your Diet

Most of the integrative experts agree: you should eliminate soy. Soy is a phytoestrogen—a naturally occurring nutrient that acts on the body as estrogen does. It can block absorption of thyroid hormones, and most of the soy available is genetically modified. According to Dr. Richard Shames:

> When trying to conceive, or during pregnancy, some women, in an attempt to increase their protein intake, may be tempted to add more soy to

their diet. I don't recommend this. Don't go overboard with soy while trying to conceive or while pregnant, as it can interfere in some cases with thyroid function.

Eat the Rainbow

Integrative nutritionist and mother of two Laurie Borenstein has a wonderful recommendation that can help you eat well: "Eat the rainbow. A wonderful way to ensure you are consuming a wide array of nutrients necessary for an optimal environment for conceiving and nourishing a fetus once pregnant, is to consume a green, yellow, orange, red, and purple vegetable or fruit every day."

Get Enough Iron from Food

Laurie Borenstein further recommends that you ensure that your diet is heavy in iron-rich foods, such as spinach, Swiss chard, kale, and many other dark leafy greens. A word of caution from Borenstein, however:

> Many of these greens are goitrogenic, meaning that if you consume them raw and in larger quantities, they can slow down your thyroid. So, you will want to cook or steam them, and avoid overconsuming them. There are also many other good sources of iron to be found in whole foods. Some of my favorites are lentils, pumpkin seeds, sesame seeds, chickpeas, eggs, and poultry.

Go Gluten-Free

Some experts recommend that thyroid patients planning to get pregnant go gluten-free, because gluten is a common cause of inflammation in many thyroid patients. Functional medicine expert Amy Myers, MD, says: "You're not missing any nutrients by getting off gluten, so I definitely would recommend that anybody who has a thyroid condition and planning to get pregnant, or is pregnant, absolutely get off of gluten."

Autoimmunity and Gut Health

If you have autoimmune diseases, such as Hashimoto's or Graves', an important part of preconception may be addressing your immune system, to calm inflammation, lower antibodies, and reduce your overall state of autoimmunity. Here are things to consider that can specifically help your immune system and reduce inflammation and antibodies.

Low-Dose Naltrexone (LDN)

During preconception, you may want to discuss with your physician the benefits of taking a prescription medication, low-dose naltrexone (LDN). Used at high doses for addiction problems, very low doses of naltrexone—typically less than 5 mg per day—have been shown to reduce antibodies in a number of autoimmune conditions. In some cases, they balance thyroid function, and can even induce a remission from autoimmune thyroid disease. Interestingly, some physicians are also using LDN to enhance fertility, and a number of fertility specialists are using it as part of fertility treatments.

According to the LDN Research Trust, a charitable group involved in advocacy for LDN treatment, low doses of naltrexone are safe during pregnancy and don't affect fetal development. Julia Schopick, author of *Honest Medicine* and an LDN educator, has this input:

> Since 2003, fertility expert Dr. Phil Boyle has successfully used LDN for many of his patients in Ireland. Over 1,000 women in his practice have taken LDN to treat PMS, endometriosis and polycystic ovary syndrome (PCOS). More than 400 of his patients have safely continued their LDN during pregnancy and breastfeeding, and the outcomes have been positive for both mothers and babies. Dr. Boyle estimates that at least 7 to 10 percent of his fertility patients also have an underactive thyroid. Under his care, they take LDN, along with their thyroid medication, before conception, as well as during pregnancy and breastfeeding.

Julia said that Dr. Boyle has one important caution for pregnant women taking LDN: you should stop taking LDN at 38 weeks gestation in case opiate-based medications are needed for pain relief during or after delivery. Also, if you are taking LDN and go into labor early, be sure to let your delivery team know that you have been taking LDN, as it may affect their choice of pain treatments, if needed.

Selenium Supplementation

We've discussed the importance of selenium to thyroid patients planning pregnancy in general, but it is particularly valuable in reducing antibodies in

Hashimoto's patients. Naturopathic physician Fiona McCulloch recommends taking the selenomethionine form, at 200 mcg per day. (Again, a reminder that you should not take more than 400 mcg of selenium per day, from all sources, including food, supplements, and prenatal vitamins.)

Infections

Identifying and treating infections is an important part of immune system support. If you have chronic autoimmunity with elevated antibodies, your physician may want to run tests, including:

- Viral titers—to identify Epstein-Barr or human herpesvirus 6 (HHV6)
- Fecal stool analysis—to identify intestinal bacterial infections and yeast/ *Candida* overgrowth
- Blood tests for other chronic infections, such as Lyme disease

If elevated titers of chronic viral infections are identified, your doctor may recommend a prescription antiviral medication, such as acyclovir, or a natural antiviral protocol. If you have unhealthy bacteria in your intestinal system, your doctor may recommend a course of antibiotics, as well as supplements, to help resolve the infection. For candidiasis, your doctor may recommend prescription medications, supplements, or dietary changes to restore balance and eliminate yeast overgrowth. Lyme disease is typically treated with antibiotics as well as nutritional support.

Gut Health/Leaky Gut

The issue of an inflamed gut, and the role of gut health in immune function and as an autoimmune disease trigger—sometimes referred to as leaky gut—is controversial in conventional medicine, which recognizes the condition yet doesn't have any specific diagnoses or treatments for it, or for many autoimmune diseases. That said, we do know that your gut is the largest organ in your immune system. From the integrative perspective, ensuring healthy gut function is a critical aspect of immune health and addressing autoimmune disease. Functional medicine expert Amy Myers, MD, feels that ensuring good gut and intestinal health is essential to autoimmune health. According to Dr. Myers:

Eighty percent of the immune system is in our gut, so if you have any type of autoimmune disease, then likely, even if you're not having any digestive issues, there's something going on in the gut—known as leaky gut. I like to think of the gut as like a drawbridge, so it can let all the little teeny, tiny boats in, without having to open up. As we're digesting our food, we then absorb these teeny, tiny little particles naturally through the semipermeable barrier. When our gut gets disrupted with molecules such as gluten, infections, or toxins, stress, or medications, it causes these tight junctions in our gut, that are normally open just a tiny bit, to open up a lot; that big drawbridge opens wide, and then big boats can get through. That's where big molecules, such as gluten, or casein, or even infections can slip through our gut, and into our bloodstream, where they are not supposed to be. Our immune system goes on high alert to go in and attack these different molecules or infections that aren't supposed to be there.

Dr. Myers has patients eliminate gluten, all grains, and legumes to help combat leaky gut.

I have people remove a lot of these foods for 30 days or more to see how they respond, and then gradually add them back in. Of course, a big no-no food is gluten. I really don't want people adding that back in, regardless of whether they feel that they have an intolerance to it or not. With the research out there between autoimmunity and gluten, I would recommend [that] anybody with autoimmune [diagnoses] avoid gluten 100 percent of the time.

Integrative physician Mark Hyman, author of the book *Blood Sugar Solution 10-Day Detox Diet*, believes that patients can start to fine-tune their eating by following an elimination diet, meaning that foods likely to cause inflammation—frequently gluten, dairy, soy, nuts, etc.—are eliminated, and reintroduced one at a time to identify the culprits for each individual:

Most of our inflammation comes from diet. It comes from sugar primarily or refined carbs. It comes from refined oils, like from omega-6 fish oils, all the seed oils, canola, sunflower, safflower, corn oil, soybean oil. It comes from lack of anti-inflammatory foods like phytonutrients in our fruits and vegetables and omega-3 fats. It also comes from certain triggers that can be inflammatory for some people. Most common are gluten and dairy. Leaky gut is a big cause of inflammation. It can be caused by gut flora and food sensitivities like gluten.

Dr. Hyman explains leaky gut in this way:

The intestinal lining is really the size of a tennis court when you lay your small intestine all flat. It's only one cell thick. It's like your skin. When that skin or lining becomes damaged because of stress, because of environmental toxins, because of alterations in your gut flora . . . overuse of antibiotics, the increased use of acid-blocking drugs. . . . This ends up causing what we call damage to this lining of the gut or leaky gut. Then the cells separate and food and proteins and bacterial toxins leak into the bloodstream and interact with the immune system. This ends up leaving a problem with the overall immune system because it's triggering inflammation.

Naturopathic physician Fiona McCulloch also recommends an elimination diet:

Typical sensitivities include gluten/grains, dairy, soy, eggs, sugar, nightshades, and nuts. After a period of elimination, the foods are slowly reintroduced one at a time, and reactions are assessed. Any foods which create reactions should be eliminated from the diet for a certain period of time to allow the immune system to heal and regenerate. There are a variety of diets that may be helpful for autoimmune patients including autoimmune paleo, GAPS, and the Specific Carbohydrate Diet (SCD). For more on these diets, see Appendix A.

Once you've identified trigger foods, eliminating them from your diet may help reduce antibodies and calm autoimmunity.

Lifestyle

There are a number of changes to your lifestyle that you can start making as soon as you consider getting pregnant.

The most obvious? Stop smoking. If you need help, your doctor can recommend medications or programs to help you quit. And if you are a recreational user of drugs, abusing prescription medications, or abusing alcohol, you need to discuss this with your doctor and make a plan to help you stop before you consider getting pregnant.

You also need to ensure that you are getting enough sleep. Lack of sufficient sleep—less than seven hours per night—is associated with risks of lowered fertility, miscarriage, and preterm delivery. If you have difficulty falling asleep, staying asleep, or with early waking, talk to your practitioner about supplements that may help, or even prescription medications during preconception.

One supplement that may help with sleep—and that also has been shown to have some benefits for fertility—is a low-dose time-released form of the hormone melatonin. Dosages of up to 3 mg per night, taken one hour before bedtime at or eleven p.m., whichever is earlier, may help with sleep, and can help improve T4-to-T3 conversion. Melatonin is also known to help stimulate the ovaries to produce follicles.

You also want to make sure that you are getting some sun exposure. Studies have shown that being out in sunny weather increases your chances of getting pregnant. One study found that in women undergoing fertility treatments, daily exposure to sunshine increased the success of pregnancy by as much as one third. Sunshine appears to make a difference as eggs are being prepared— the follicular phase—and the sunnier the climate, and the more sun exposure a woman has in the months prior to conception, the better chance she has of getting pregnant. It's also thought that the light exposure enhances melatonin production in the body. Sunshine also helps you produce and metabolize vitamin D, which supports egg quality. Some fertility experts even suggest that if you want to improve your fertility, you should take a vacation in a sunny climate a month before you start trying to get pregnant!

Practicing active stress management is essential during preconception. It doesn't matter what type of practice you use—you just need to plan on fifteen to thirty minutes a day of a physiologically stress-reducing activity. Chronic stress that is not addressed can contribute to reproductive dysfunction, adrenal imbalances, fertility, and healthy pregnancy. Some stress-reducing activities to consider:

- Meditation
- Guided imagery, relaxation audio CDs
- Breath work—paced breathing or pranayama breathing
- Prayer
- Tai chi
- Qi gong
- Slow, contemplative walking
- Gentle yoga
- Needlework
- Coloring

With careful preconception planning and a good program for taking care of your health and enhancing both your fertility and your preparedness for pregnancy, you give yourself the best possible chance to conceive a child. Good luck!

Now let's talk about how to continue to take care of yourself when you get pregnant, to give both you and your baby the best possible chance to thrive. Different issues arise depending on your particular thyroid condition, so we will focus on how to best manage the different conditions in the chapters that follow.

Hypothyroidism/Hashimoto's During Pregnancy

5

Hypothyroidism refers to the condition of insufficient—or nonexistent—thyroid hormone. Hypothyroidism can develop as a result of iodine deficiency, a defect in your thyroid from birth (congenital hypothyroidism), atrophy and self-destruction as part of Hashimoto's disease, radioactive iodine treatment (RAI), surgical removal, or due to some medications, among other causes. The common denominator in hypothyroidism, however, is the need to take prescription thyroid hormone from an external source.

In women who are not iodine-deficient, hypothyroidism is most commonly caused by Hashimoto's disease. According to the 2011 "Guidelines of the American Thyroid Association for the Diagnosis and Management of Thyroid Disease During Pregnancy and Postpartum," or Pregnancy Guidelines, the thyroid peroxidase antibodies (TPOAb) characteristic of Hashimoto's disease are detected in about half of pregnant women with subclinical hypothyroidism—defined as levels between 2.5 and the top end of the reference range (usually around 5.0), and in more than 80 percent of women with overt hypothyroidism, which is defined as a thyroid-stimulating hormone (TSH) level above 10.

Rapid diagnosis and proper management is essential, because hypothyroidism in pregnancy can cause a variety of complications for both you and your baby. For example:

- Uncontrolled or untreated hypothyroidism, especially in the first trimester of pregnancy, increases your risks of early miscarriage, late miscarriage (during the second trimester or later), pregnancy-induced high blood pressure, postpartum hemorrhage, placental abruption, stillbirth, premature delivery, and breech presentation.

- In addition, hypothyroidism in a pregnant woman can lead to significant neurological and cognitive issues for the child, including a reduction in IQ, learning disabilities, attention-deficit/hyperactivity disorder (ADHD), congenital malformations, and low birth weight. Profound hypothyroidism and iodine deficiency in a woman can lead to severely stunted mental and physical development and mental retardation—a condition known as cretinism—in her child. There is also a link between iodine deficiency, hypothyroidism, and the risk or severity of autism.

Even mild or subclinical hypothyroidism increases pregnancy complications. According to the Pregnancy Guidelines, there is almost double the rate of miscarriage in women with Hashimoto's disease who are subclinically hypothyroid, with TSH levels between 2.5 and 5.0 mIU/L, versus women who have Hashimoto's disease with TSH levels below 2.5 mIU/L.

There is also a link between hypothyroidism and autism. The number of American children who are diagnosed with autism or autism-related disorders is growing at worrisome levels. Back in the 1970s and 1980s, it was estimated that 1 in 2,000 children had autism. Now, the US Centers for Disease Control estimates that 1 in 150 in the United States has autism or an autism spectrum disorder by the age of eight. While some experts believe that the increased levels of diagnosis are due to better detection, the authors of a recent study published in the *Annals of Neurology* believe that the rise in autism is at least in part due to maternal hypothyroidism that results from iodine deficiency, as well as maternal hypothyroidism triggered by autoimmune thyroid disease. The researchers showed that pregnant women who are hypothyroid are nearly four times more likely to have children with autism than are women who have no thyroid problems.

While a direct causal relationship between maternal hypothyroidism and autism hasn't been proven, the researchers were adamant that hypothyroidism must be treated, and ideally, identified before pregnancy, or in early pregnancy. The authors of the study conclude: "If confirmed by future research, this study provides arguments in favor of universal thyroid-function screening in the first trimester of pregnancy and may open the possibility of preventive intervention in autism."

Signs and Symptoms

The signs and symptoms of hypothyroidism are the same in pregnancy as in nonpregnant women. Fatigue, mood changes, brain fog, hair loss, intolerance to cold, dry skin, brittle hair, hair loss, puffiness in the face and around the eyes, memory problems, goiter or neck enlargement, sensitivity in the neck, depression, constipation, swelling of hands and feet, and weight gain are all common symptoms.

The challenge is that many of these common symptoms of hypothyroidism are also common in women during pregnancy who don't have a thyroid condition. So, the challenge is in having your physician recognize that your symptoms may be signs of an undiagnosed thyroid condition, and not just normal side effects of pregnancy.

Ultimately, the best thing for women and babies would be universal thyroid screening in early pregnancy. This would help identify many of the women with undiagnosed hypothyroidism, and help prevent many miscarriages, stillbirths, and preterm deliveries, as well as cognitive problems and even ADHD and autism in children. Until we have universal screening, we believe in erring on the side of caution. If you are having *any* symptoms that could point to a thyroid condition, ask for a complete thyroid panel and evaluation.

Diagnosis During Pregnancy

The reference range—also known as the "normal" range—for the thyroid-stimulating hormone TSH test is different during pregnancy than for the nonpregnant population. According to the Pregnancy Guidelines, the typical (TSH) reference range for women who are not pregnant has an upper range of around 4.0 mIU/L. The guidelines recommend, however, that the upper reference range during pregnancy should be approximately 2.5 to 3.0 mIU/L.

Specifically, the guidelines recommend that if a laboratory has not established its own trimester-specific reference ranges for TSH for pregnant women, the following reference ranges should be used:

- First trimester: 0.1 to 2.5 mIU/L
- Second trimester: 0.2 to 3.0 mIU/L
- Third trimester: 0.3 to 3.0 mIU/L

In pregnancy, overt hypothyroidism is defined as a TSH above 2.5 mIU/L, along with a decreased free thyroxine (Free T4) level. Even if a woman has normal Free T4, if TSH is above 10.0 mIU/L during pregnancy, it is also considered to be overt hypothyroidism. Subclinical hypothyroidism is defined as TSH between 2.5 and 10 mIU/L, with a normal Free T4 level.

The guidelines state that both overt and subclinical hypothyroidism should be treated with thyroid hormone replacement medication in pregnancy.

While the conventional diagnosis of hypothyroidism relies on the TSH test, integrative physicians feel that accurate diagnosis of hypothyroidism during pregnancy requires the additional blood tests for Free T4, Free T3, Reverse T3, and TPOAb that we detailed in Chapter 2.

During pregnancy, integrative physicians like to see TSH around 1.0, and Free T4 and Free T3 in the top half—and in some cases, the top 25th percentile—of the reference range. Reverse T3 should not be significantly elevated. TPOAb is monitored periodically during pregnancy to look for changes in antibody levels that may point to increases or reductions in autoimmunity.

For women who have been treated and optimized prior to pregnancy, the objective is to continue to maintain those optimal levels, ensuring that the TSH does not go above the top end of the guidelines' trimester-specific ranges.

Diagnosis Challenges

One of the most common things many doctors say about hypothyroidism is that it's "easy to diagnose and easy to treat." The reality is, it's far more complicated, especially when you're pregnant, because symptoms can be similar to those of pregnancy.

Kristi was in her first trimester, in her early thirties, when she noticed that she was more tired than she expected. Says Kristi:

> I was so exhausted, more so than any of my friends who had been pregnant. I also was gaining weight very quickly, which is not common in the first trimester. And even though I was eating a very healthy diet, my OB told me not to stop "eating for two" and get more rest. But I had a feeling there was more to it. I saw an integrative doctor, who ran a bunch of tests and told me that I had high antibodies for Hashimoto's and was borderline hypothyroid. That doctor put me on a low dose of thyroid drugs, and within a week, I felt like a new person. I was able to go through the rest of my pregnancy fairly normally. But I did get my thyroid rechecked a few times, and adjusted the dose, to keep things on track. I am happy to say I had a healthy, full-term baby girl.

If you complain to your doctor that you're tired or gaining weight during pregnancy and want your thyroid checked, you may be told that your symptoms are from pregnancy and that you don't need thyroid tests. Whether the refusal to test is due to the doctor's ego, or in the case of an HMO doctor, to try to steer you away from additional tests for cost reasons, it is *not* acceptable. When faced with a doctor who is resistant to testing you—particularly if he or she is unwilling to run anything except the TSH test—time is of the essence. Your best option would be to find another doctor, even if you have to pay out of pocket. If you have no options, here are a few tips:

Quantify your symptoms in a nonemotional way. Don't just complain that you're tired or gaining weight. Explain how many more hours of sleep you need, or how many pounds you are gaining per week, and how many calories you are eating. Doctors are more likely to base decisions on data, not complaints. Bring a checklist of hypothyroidism risks and symptoms, to back up your request.

If your doctor reviews your checklist and refuses to order thyroid tests, ask the doctor to sign and date a copy of your checklist, indicating his or her refusal to test, and to put that in your medical record. Keep a signed copy for yourself. Send a copy to the HMO or insurance company's consumer liaison, along with your request that testing be approved.

If you are unable to get your own physician to order the appropriate tests, then consider having your tests done through a patient-directed, direct-to-consumer laboratory testing service. In most states, these services allow you to select the blood tests you want, pay for them out of pocket, or even with insurance coverage—usually at costs that are close to the wholesale rate and not the marked-up consumer rate—have the blood drawn at nationally certified laboratories, and the results sent back to you directly. Appendix A has recommendations for this service.

If your doctor thinks that a TSH of 4 is fine, even during pregnancy, or refuses to test you for thyroid antibodies—because he or she is clearly unaware of the Pregnancy Guidelines—bring in a copy of the guidelines, showing the trimester-specific reference range. (You'll find a link to the complete guidelines in Appendix A.)

Treatment During Pregnancy

When you are pregnant, your Total T4 concentrations need to increase by 20 to 50 percent to meet the demands of pregnancy. In a woman with healthy thyroid function, the thyroid naturally produces the extra hormone that is needed. However, if you are diagnosed with hypothyroidism, or are already being treated for it when you become pregnant, your thyroid probably is unable to respond normally to the hormonal cues to increase T4 production.

This means that you risk becoming more hypothyroid, endangering the pregnancy, and putting your baby at risk, unless you quickly start or confirm your pregnancy as early as possible and increase your dose of thyroid hormone replacement medication right away. Ultimately, 50 to 80 percent of hypothyroid women need to increase their thyroid medication dosages during pregnancy.

According to the Pregnancy Guidelines, the increased demand begins as early as weeks 4 to 6 of pregnancy, and typically increases until weeks 16 to 20, when it plateaus until delivery. Integrative physicians and thyroid patients, however, have found that TSH levels can rise fairly dramatically as early as two to three weeks postconception in women without thyroid conditions, and therefore that supplementation for women with hypothyroidism should begin earlier.

We make the following recommendations:

- If you are pregnant and newly diagnosed with hypothyroidism, start your treatment immediately.
- If you are already being treated for hypothyroidism and are planning for pregnancy, test for pregnancy as early as 7 days postconception.
- If you are already being treated for hypothyroidism and are planning your pregnancy, have a plan in place with your doctor for how much you should increase your dosage as soon as you confirm your pregnancy. (Note: If you are only taking levothyroxine [versus levothyroxine plus T3, or natural desiccated thyroid], the guidelines have a specific recommendation for you: add two more tablets a week—a 29 percent increase in dosage—as soon as your pregnancy is confirmed. Discuss this plan in advance with your doctor, and if your doctor agrees, once you've confirmed your pregnancy, start taking two more tablets a week, and contact your doctor right away for follow-up testing.
- Once your pregnancy is confirmed, increase your dosage accordingly and inform your doctor that you are pregnant, and start on the new, higher dose. Your practitioner will then recommend your next round of testing, usually in several weeks.

Thyroid Hormone Replacement Medications

A number of different thyroid hormone replacement medications are used to treat hypothyroidism.

Levothyroxine (Synthetic Thyroxine/T4)

The most commonly prescribed hypothyroidism drug—favored particularly by conventional physicians and endocrinologists—is a synthetic form of the thyroxine hormone (T4), known generically as levothyroxine. In 2015 *USA Today* named levothyroxine as America's most prescribed drug, with nearly 120 million prescriptions dispensed in the previous year—3 percent of the US prescription drug market!

The theory behind levothyroxine is that by delivering a synthetic version that is virtually identical to T4, your body will convert the T4 into the active triiodothyronine hormone (T3), for use by the cells.

Brand names for tablet forms of levothyroxine in the United States include Synthroid, Levoxyl, and Levothroid. In Canada, Synthroid, Eltroxin, and PMS-Levothyroxine are popular brand names. An important note about the Synthroid brand: Synthroid contains two ingredients, acacia (derived from tree bark), and lactose, that are known allergens in some patients. A hypoallergenic liquid gelcap brand, designed for people with intestinal problems, absorption issues, and allergies, is called Tirosint.

The conventional medical world—as well as HMOs, medical societies, and insurers—typically follow the official practice guidelines from the endocrinology and thyroid professional groups. In 2012, the American Association of Clinical Endocrinologists (AACE) and the American Thyroid Association (ATA) released their "Clinical Practice Guidelines for Hypothyroidism in Adults." These guidelines indicate that levothyroxine is the only recommended treatment for hypothyroidism.

Some physicians do not recommend use of generic versions of levothyroxine—which are naturally far less expensive than brand names. Some insurers also cover only the generic versions of levothyroxine, and not the brand names, due to cost considerations.

The key issue with generic levothyroxine is that while it is FDA approved, safe, and effective, every time you fill a prescription for generic levothyroxine, you may get a levothyroxine made by a different company. Levothyroxine is required by the FDA to fall within 5 percent of its stated potency. Each company's formulas tend to be consistent, so if one company's product usually runs at 96 percent potency, it will be consistent from refill to refill. However, another drug maker's levothyroxine may typically run at 105 percent of potency. Using the example of a generically prescribed 100 mcg levothyroxine tablet, your unknowingly changing from one drug maker to the other would create a difference of around 65 mcg per week—almost like adding or subtracting an extra pill each week. This could affect your thyroid replacement stability and effectiveness, test results, symptoms, and TSH levels.

This is a special concern for thyroid cancer survivors, many of whom require careful and consistent dosing so as to suppress TSH, to prevent cancer recurrence. It is also a concern for women who are taking thyroid medication before or during pregnancy and need to keep levels stable.

If due to cost considerations or insurance coverage you must use a generic levothyroxine, there are a few things to keep in mind.

- If you are stabilized on a generic levothyroxine, find out who the manufacturer is. While your doctor can't prescribe a particular generic manufacturer's levothyroxine, if you have a relationship with your pharmacist, your pharmacist may be able to ensure that you get levothyroxine from the same generic manufacturer with each refill. This is harder—or impossible—with large chains and mail-order pharmacies, however.
- Get a large supply, such as six months' worth. (Make sure it doesn't expire during your usage time, however.)
- If you can't ensure refills from the same manufacturer, pay close attention to your symptoms, and if you notice them worsening after a refill, ask your doctor to check your levels.

If you have thyroid cancer, generics aren't working to control your hypothyroidism, or you are pregnant, your physician may be able to contact your insurance company to get preapproval to write a prescription for a brand-name drug. That preapproval, along with the special designation "DAW" or "dispense as written" and "no generic substitution" on your prescription—should get a brand name covered. If insurance won't offer approval, you may also have the option of a higher copay to get the brand name medication, rather than a generic.

Liothyronine (Synthetic Triiodothyronine/T3)

As discussed in Chapter 1, the thyroid gland makes both thyroxine (T4) and triiodothyronine (T3).

A synthetic form of T3 known as liothyronine is available in a manufactured form as the brand-name drug Cytomel, and also as a generic. Prescription T3 can also be compounded in time-released/sustained-release forms by compounding pharmacies. A new brand of manufactured, sustained-release synthetic T3, called ThyroMax, has been going through clinical trials and is expected to receive FDA approval and reach the market in the near term.

The use of T3—whether in addition to levothyroxine, or as T3-only therapy, is controversial; however some integrative physicians use T3 therapy in patients who don't respond to T4/T3 or natural thyroid drugs.

The AACE and ATA's 2012 "Clinical Practice Guidelines for Hypothyroidism in Adults" state that "patients with hypothyroidism should be treated only with levothyroxine drugs." They go on to say that "the evidence does not support using levothyroxine-plus-T3 combinations to treat hypothyroidism."

In making this recommendation, the task force chose to ignore a number of studies, including a 2009 Danish study published in the prestigious *European Journal of Endocrinology*, which found that when TSH levels are kept consistent, a T4/T3 combination therapy was superior to levothyroxine-only treatment when evaluating for a number of quality-of-life measurements, depression and anxiety scales, and patient preference. A prominent study published in the *New England Journal of Medicine* in 1999 found that patients benefited from and preferred a T4/T3 combination treatment.

Some other studies have failed to demonstrate a benefit, but some experts have pointed out that low and ineffective doses of T3 were used in those studies, making their results questionable. Still, conventional endocrinology, official guidelines—and therefore, most physicians, HMOs, and insurers—do not prescribe or cover the costs of additional T3 for hypothyroid patients, even when Free T3 levels are subpar, or below the reference range, or Reverse T3 is elevated.

Synthetic Combination T4/T3

In the past, a combination synthetic T4/T3 drug, known generically as liotrix, and by the brand name Thyrolar, was available. This drug has been effectively off the market for a number of years, and is rarely available.

Natural Desiccated Thyroid

Natural desiccated thyroid—known as NDT, "natural thyroid," "thyroid extract," or "porcine thyroid" (called by some, derogatorily, "pig thyroid"), is a prescription drug prepared from the dried thyroid gland of pigs. Much as some people refer to tissues as "Kleenex," NDT drugs are sometimes referred to by the name of one particular brand, "Armour Thyroid," which has been on the market for more than one hundred years. (Note that over-the-counter, nonprescription glandular thyroid supplements made from pig, sheep, or cow thyroid glands are not prescription thyroid medication.)

When Armour was introduced, it was the first medication to treat hypothyroidism, and the only drug available until levothyroxine was introduced in the 1950s. At that point, natural thyroid fell out of favor; the synthetic product was touted as more modern and stable, and the idea that the body converted T4 into all the T3 needed was widely accepted. Since that time, generations of physicians have learned—in medical school, seminars, and from drug company reps—that levothyroxine is the only treatment option available for hypothyroidism. Some physicians even mistakenly believe that NDT is no longer on the market, going off the market, or is a nonprescription, over-the-counter supplement.

To produce NDT, the entire gland is dried, processed, and then batches are checked to make sure they are delivering consistent levels of natural forms of both key hormones, T4 and T3, as well as other components found in a thyroid gland—including calcitonin, T1, and T2. Today, several brands of desiccated thyroid are available by prescription, including Nature-Throid and WP Thyroid (both from RLC Labs), Armour Thyroid, and a Canadian natural thyroid from manufacturer Erfa. A generic form of NDT is also available.

Since NDT was on the market before the creation of the Food and Drug Administration (FDA), it was never required to go through the costly and lengthy new drug application (NDA) process. (Levothyroxine had been "grandfathered" along with NDT, but was eventually required to go through the NDA process a decade ago.) Given its status with the FDA, NDT is considered an FDA-regulated—but not FDA-approved—drug. This is why some insurers, Medicaid, and HMOs refuse to cover the costs. Use of NDT is highly controversial in the medical world, which claims that these drugs are out of date and not "consistent."

This situation has been exacerbated by the AACE/ATA's 2012 hypothyroidism guidelines, which state: "There is no evidence to support using natural desiccated thyroid hormone—i.e., Armour, Nature-Throid—in preference to levothyroxine in treating hypothyroidism." The guidelines conclude that "therefore desiccated thyroid hormone should not be used for the treatment of hypothyroidism."

A recent federally funded study conducted at the Walter Reed Medical Center found that natural desiccated thyroid drugs were a safe and effective alternative to levothyroxine, resulted in greater weight loss, and were preferred by the majority of patients, versus levothyroxine. Still, there are no large, peer-reviewed, double-blind, journal-published studies that compare levothyroxine-only treatment to treatment with natural desiccated thyroid drugs, or demonstrate that one is clinically better than the other.

At the same time, there is significant patient-based evidence that demonstrates that a substantial number of patients have better control of their thyroid levels and symptoms when treated with natural desiccated thyroid, compared to levothyroxine, or with the addition of some NDT to their levothyroxine treatment. An increasing number of integrative and holistic practitioners have found these options to be effective with a subset of their patients. As a result, since the 1990s, NDT has enjoyed a resurgence in use, and several million prescriptions for natural desiccated thyroid are written each year. The number of patients taking these drugs, and practitioners prescribing them, is on the rise.

While there are some mainstream physicians who will prescribe NDT, the majority will not. If you want NDT, you may need to work with an integrative, holistic, or alternative physician.

If you are already taking NDT, be prepared for your OB to want to change you to levothyroxine. This was the situation that Jessika faced, when, after struggling for four years on Synthroid, she switched to Armour Thyroid:

It changed my life for the better. I felt like me again. A few years later, I was happily married and learned I was pregnant. I had my first OB appointment, and when she read my chart and saw that I was hypo, stated, "I see that you are on Armour. We will have to change that." My eyes immediately filled with tears and I explained to her my past with Synthroid. She was adamant that I change and called in a prescription immediately (without even doing blood work). I was a mess. I left that office and called every other doctor I knew. I spent every night researching Armour and pregnancies. At my next appointment the doctor asked had I switched medicines yet; my husband spoke up for me as I was extremely intimidated by this doctor and told her that after a lot of research we decided that my thyroid being regulated by Armour was way better for baby than to allow my body to try to regulate between the Armour to Synthroid switch. She looked me directly in the eye and said, "Do not be surprised when you have a stillborn." I was in total shock. I immediately made an appointment for the next day with a different OB in the practice and got a referral to an endocrinologist. Both of these doctors were totally fine with my being on Armour. We did my blood work every 3 weeks and upped my dose as needed. Mommy and baby (girl!) were both thriving. I went into labor and guess who was on call? The doctor who told me that I would have a stillborn. My baby girl is now 7 months old, and I have been on Armour Thyroid the entire time. The best thing I have ever done was advocate for myself and my child's health. The best thing I have ever done was listen to my gut and not trust this particular doctor.

The T3 Treatment Controversy

Levothyroxine is the recommended treatment for all hypothyroidism, according to various conventional guidelines, as well as the recommended treatment for a pregnant woman with hypothyroidism—whether subclinical or overt. According to both the AACE/ATA's hypothyroidism guidelines and ATA's Pregnancy Guidelines, it is "strongly recommended not to use other thyroid preparations, such as T3 or natural desiccated thyroid drugs."

Researchers and endocrinologists have been going back and forth for more than a decade about the value of treatments that include T3 for hypothyroidism, but based on their own practical experience with patients, and on the growing body of research evidence, holistic and integrative hormone experts are increasingly prescribing T3 as a solution to help optimize thyroid treatment for some patients. They add T3 in one of several ways:

- Adding T3 to levothyroxine treatment, via the addition of the prescription synthetic T3 drug Cytomel, or generic liothyronine (synthetic T3)
- Adding synthetic T3 via prescription compounded time-released/sustained-release T3 in addition to levothyroxine
- Adding a dosage of a natural desiccated thyroid, such as the prescription drugs Nature-Throid, Armour Thyroid, or generic natural thyroid to a levothyroxine treatment
- Switching patients to NDT-only treatment
- Putting a patient on a T3-only therapy (this is less common)

Keep in mind that many endocrinologists are resistant to the idea of T3 treatment. They cite concerns that excessive doses of T3 could cause heart palpitations or other side effects.

And it is important to note that because T3 is the active hormone, in some people, it can have an overstimulatory effect on heart rate and pulse, especially in those with a history of heart disease, the elderly, and those with heart irregularities, such as mitral valve prolapse. T3-savvy physicians evaluate the safety of T3 as compared to the potential benefits on a case-by-case basis.

Even in those patients who do not have any heart- or age-related issues that may make T3 problematic, some patients are simply more sensitive to T3. The heart is very sensitive to thyroid hormone in general, and for some people, even low doses of T3 can cause a rise in pulse, or heart palpitations. For those patients, physicians often recommend the time-released, sustained-release, or slow-release form of T3, available by prescription from compounding pharmacies.

Some integrative physicians, in fact, believe that the slow-release T3 is actually the optimal form for supplemental T3, as it more closely resembles the body's own conversion to and release of T3, and because the slow-release form is less likely to cause any side effects.

T3 Treatments in Pregnancy

Both levothyroxine and liothyronine are designated by the FDA as Category A in pregnancy, meaning that "adequate and well-controlled studies have failed to demonstrate a risk to the fetus in the first trimester of pregnancy (and there is no evidence of risk in later trimesters)."

Still, the Pregnancy Guidelines indicate that liothyronine and NDT (which is a natural combination of T4/T3 hormone) are not to be used in pregnancy. The guidelines do not include any citations or explanation regarding this recommendation, but several studies from more than two decades ago suggested that while T4 can cross the placenta, lower levels of T3 cross the placenta and reach the developing baby. Therefore, experts believe T3-only therapy, a synthetic T4/T3 combination, or desiccated thyroid may not provide enough thyroid hormone to the fetus, and are not recommended for women attempting pregnancy or who are pregnant.

Harvard-educated integrative physician Richard Shames, author of a number of books on thyroid disease, and in practice for decades, has helped many thyroid patients optimize their thyroid function and become pregnant. Dr. Shames does not believe that women should be concerned about using NDT or T3 during pregnancy. He says:

> I think that the warnings regarding using T3 can cause unnecessary fear and concern in women who are stabilized and doing well on natural desiccated thyroid, or T4/T3 combination therapy. Before levothyroxine was on the market, generations of women had successful pregnancies and healthy babies using natural desiccated thyroid.

I am especially concerned about the possibility that some physicians might recommend that a patient stop treatment that includes T3, and change to levothyroxine-only therapy early in pregnancy. Maintaining strong thyroid function in early pregnancy is crucial to maintaining the pregnancy, and for the healthy development of the baby. For a woman who is optimized on a treatment that includes T3, the slight concern about T3 not crossing the placenta seems to be much less of a risk than changing medications at this delicate time, which creates the very real risk of hypothyroidism in the mother. Destabilizing thyroid function can endanger the pregnancy, as well as the cognitive development of her fetus.

Manhattan-based integrative physician David Borenstein also feels that a T4/T3 combination therapy, as well as NDT, can be safe in pregnancy. According to Dr. Borenstein:

> The way you best treat a thyroid patient—before, during and after pregnancy—is to make sure that her numbers are optimal. Any patient who is hypothyroid, and who finds out that she is pregnant, should get immediate thyroid blood work. If all the thyroid levels are not optimal for pregnancy, then it should be corrected with the appropriate dosage change. And she should be frequently tested through that critical first trimester, and regularly throughout the pregnancy. As long as the blood work meets the standards set by the Pregnancy Guidelines, I see no problem with a woman maintaining her existing thyroid treatment. I would not, however, recommend T3-only therapy during pregnancy, as we need more understanding of how T3 is metabolized in a pregnant woman.

Naturopathic physician Kevin Passero raises some good points about the use of T3 treatments in pregnancy.

> I am comfortable with my patients continuing on T4/T3 treatment, or natural desiccated thyroid, while pregnant. Both levothyroxine (synthetic T4) and liothyronine (synthetic T3) are FDA Category A, meaning that they are . . . among the safest drugs for women to use during pregnancy. From a scientific perspective, we don't have studies and clear evidence that T4/T3 combination treatment, or NDT, are at all harmful during pregnancy, nor is there clinical data in human studies showing that levothyoxine-only is better than T4/T3 or NDT. We simply don't have the studies on pregnancy outcomes.

My experience is that I have had many patients who were having recurrent miscarriages, while being treated with levothyroxine. After I optimized their thyroid on a T4/T3 or NDT treatment, they were able to get pregnant easily, and carry the pregnancy to term, and deliver a healthy baby. From a clinical perspective, if symptoms are managed and levels are balanced well, there is no reason to switch to levothyroxine-only treatment.

At such a critical time as early pregnancy, why would you switch someone back to the therapy that wasn't working for them before pregnancy? It could be problematic, because those patients that rely on a therapy that includes T3 to safely manage their levels and symptoms may have genetic variations, or conversion problems, and need T3 as part of their treatment in order to have a healthy pregnancy.

My advice is if you're feeling well, and doing well, and confident in your practitioner, there's no evidence to suggest that T4/T3 or NDT aren't safe during pregnancy.

Reproductive endocrinologist and fertility expert Dr. Hugh McInick believes that levothyroxine-only therapy can be problematic for some patients, and prefers NDT during pregnancy:

What concerns me about treatment with a synthetic T4 compound such as Synthroid is the rather high percentage of patients who are not able to convert T4 into T3, which is the active thyroid hormone that enters into every cell in the body and ultimately is responsible for normal cellular function. If there is inadequate T4 to T3 conversion in the mother, her developing fetus may not receive sufficient T3 to promote normal growth and neurological development. That is why I only prescribe a natural desiccated thyroid (NDT) compound, which already contains T3 and does not depend on the conversion of T4 into T3 in the body. A woman taking Synthroid and monitored with TSH levels only could be thought to be on an optimal dose of medicine, yet if her Total and Free T3 levels were measured and found to be low, her therapy would actually be inadequate, since the T4 prescribed was not being converted into T3.

What Is the "Best" Thyroid Drug?

The answer to the question of "what is the best thyroid drug" will vary wildly, depending on who you are asking. If you are asking us, as patient advocates, our answer will always the same: The best thyroid drug to treat your hypothyroidism is the one that safely, consistently, and best resolves your symptoms and maintains you at optimal levels.

If you ask conventional endocrinologists, or read their official "guidelines" (which are funded, not surprisingly, by levothyroxine manufacturers), they unequivocally recommend only levothyroxine, and deliberately exclude other options. Some of them even go so far as to tout one particular brand.

A small subset of integrative practitioners favor only NDT to the exclusion of synthetic drugs, but the majority tend to use whichever combination works best for each patient.

But in the end, one size does not fit all, and the drug or combination of drugs that safely works best to optimize your thyroid function and relieve your symptoms is unique to you—and that, truly, is the "best" drug . . . for you.

Thyroid Medication: Practical Tips

Here are some guidelines regarding how to take your thyroid hormone replacement medications.

First, always double-check your prescription to make sure that you have the prescribed drug, at the correct dosage, and that you've been give the full amount of the prescription. Also verify that generics have not been substituted for brand names when your physician has specified "no substitution."

For best absorption of levothyroxine, T3, or NDT, most doctors recommend taking it on an empty stomach, first thing in the morning.

Ideally, you should wait at least an hour before eating and before drinking coffee (including decaf). Both food and coffee can interfere with proper absorption. According to one study, drinking coffee within an hour of taking levothyroxine impairs absorption by at least 25 percent to as much as 57 percent. (Note: The gelcap Tirosint seems to be immune to coffee's effects.)

When you're pregnant, you may have indigestion and reach for the antacids. Be careful, because such antacids as Tums or Mylanta contain calcium, which can block the absorption of your thyroid medication. If you need an antacid or you're taking calcium supplements, take them at least three to four hours apart from your thyroid medication. The same is true for iron supplements, which many women take during pregnancy. Take them at least three to four hours apart from thyroid medication. Watch out for unexpected places where you might find calcium or iron—such as your prenatal vitamin and calcium-fortified drinks (e.g., orange juice or nondairy milks).

Sometimes during pregnancy, you are so nauseated that you have to eat as soon as you get up. If that's the case, it's best to wait at least an hour after you eat before you take your medication. But if there is no way to avoid eating around the time you take your thyroid hormone, the key is then *consistency.* Take it the same way every day.

While most instructions recommend taking thyroid medication in the morning, there is also the option of taking thyroid medication—specifically levothyroxine—at bedtime. Two important studies—a 2007 study published in the journal *Clinical Endocrinology*, and a follow-up larger randomized trial reported in the December 2010 issue of the *Archives of Internal Medicine*—found that taking the same dose of levothyroxine at bedtime, as compared to first thing in the morning, resulted in greater absorption and lower TSH levels. One benefit of taking it at nighttime is that you don't have to wait for breakfast or coffee, or be concerned about calcium or iron interference.

The studies were conducted with levothyroxine; T3 and NDT were not studied. However, some integrative practitioners recommend taking some T3 or NDT at nighttime, as it may help improve absorption and reduce symptoms. A warning: Some thyroid patients find that if they take a medication with T3 later in the day or in the evening, the slight stimulatory effect of the T3 medication can make it difficult to sleep. So, keep in mind that while it's very possible that if a similar study were conducted with T3 drugs, the results would be similar: there is some chance that it would negatively impact sleep quality in some patients.

Optimally, some doctors have suggested that patients who take medications use a time-released or sustained release formulation of T3, or split their T3 doses. This approach seems to minimize sleep interference.

Again, if you do make a change to how you take your thyroid medication, you'll want to have a reevaluation of blood levels and symptoms after several weeks to determine whether you need to adjust the dosage or timing of your medication.

Storing Your Thyroid Medication

It's important to store your thyroid medication properly. Thyroid medication should be stored in a cool area, away from humidity and moisture. This means that your bathroom is *not* the best place to store medication. Also, keep in mind that the potency of thyroid medication—as well as many other medications—can be dramatically affected by heat. If you take any prescription drug, you need to be aware that transport or storage at high temperatures can quickly degrade the potency and stability of many medications. Be careful then, of some situations that can expose your medications to heat and degrade their potency:

- Your medication is stored in your home, and you are in an area of 90-degree plus heat and you do not have air-conditioning.
- Your medication traveled in an airline's luggage compartment during hot weather (where it could sit on the tarmac and in luggage-handling areas that are not air-conditioned).
- Your medication was sitting in a hot car or trunk for an extended period, including while traveling.
- You have experienced an extended power outage at your home.
- Your pharmacy lost power for an extended period during a storm or power failure, and medications were in an area without air-conditioning.
- Your pharmacy turns off air-conditioning when the store is closed evenings and/or weekends.
- You get your medications from a mail-order pharmacy and your drugs spend time in overheated delivery trucks or shipping areas, and in your mailbox.

One important tip: Always carry your medications with you on an airplane, instead of storing them in your checked luggage. Note that the Transportation Safety Administration (TSA) recommends, but does not require, that your prescription medications be labeled to assist with the screening process. International travelers should travel with medicines in their original containers with pharmacy labels, so you can more easily pass through Customs checkpoints.

Monitoring Your Thyroid During Pregnancy

Women who are hypothyroid and become pregnant, or who are diagnosed during pregnancy, should have thyroid tests run every four weeks at minimum during the first half of pregnancy, to allow for dosage adjustments. The TSH should again be checked between weeks 26 and 32 of pregnancy, at minimum.

Some practitioners suggest multiple checks during the first trimester, and then blood work during the second and third trimesters, to ensure that thyroid function remains optimized during pregnancy.

Our recommendation is that you get regular checks, but any time that your symptoms get worse, or you feel especially nauseated (except for a

> Make sure that, whatever thyroid hormone replacement medication you are taking, you bring several days' worth with you to the hospital during childbirth. Even if you are on levothyroxine, the hospital may not be able to supply the same brand or generic that you're taking. And if you are on additional T3 or NDT, it could be difficult or impossible to get it in the hospital during and after delivery.

normal bout of morning sickness), that's a sign that it's time to get rechecked again, right away.

Hashimoto's Disease

If you go into pregnancy with Hashimoto's disease—typically evidenced by elevated thyroid peroxidase antibodies (TPOAb)—but you have otherwise normal thyroid levels and are not on thyroid hormone replacement medication, you will need careful and frequent monitoring.

According to endocrinologist Roberto Negro, MD:

Women who are positive for thyroid antibodies . . . are prone to develop hypothyroidism during pregnancy. From a clinical point of view, although before pregnancy the thyroid gland works well (euthyroidism), these patients should be strictly monitored, especially at the beginning of pregnancy, to be able to start replacement treatment, if necessary.

The Pregnancy Guidelines recommend that women with elevated antibodies who are not receiving thyroid treatment be monitored every 4 to 6 weeks during pregnancy until midpregnancy, and any subclinical or full hypothyroidism—per the trimester-specific ranges—be treated. You should again be tested at least once between weeks 26 and 32 of pregnancy, and treated if there is evidence of subclinical or overt hypothyroidism.

As discussed earlier in this chapter, some integrative physicians also have found that use of a drug known as naltrexone at low doses may reduce inflammation and [thyroid peroxidase] antibodies, and also help achieve a remission in some autoimmune diseases, including Hashimoto's.

Autologous stem cell transplants—using your own fat cells harvested in a mini-liposuction procedure—are also being studied as therapy for autoimmune thyroid disease, and may result in lowering of antibodies, and even disease remission in some recipients.

Melanie was diagnosed with Hashimoto's and hypothyroidism at age thirty-four. Says Melanie:

> My antibodies numbers were in the thousands, and my endocrinologist said I shouldn't try to conceive because it would either end up as a miscarriage or a baby with neurological issues. I was devastated and was depressed for weeks. I took his prescription for Synthroid but I also researched online before my next visit. He laughed at all my research and the idea of going gluten free. I tried it anyway. While my antibodies didn't reduce as much as I had hoped, they did go down. And then I got pregnant with twins right away. Both babies are extremely bright and could sing their ABCs by their first birthday. I changed doctors, but I'd love to take the babies to his office to show him that he needs to do some more research of his own before he tells women not to try to conceive.

Can Hashimoto's and Hypothyroidism Be Treated Naturally?

Many thyroid patients ask if there are ways to treat hypothyroidism "naturally." To answer the question, the first step needs to be defining what we mean by "natural."

For some patients and practitioners, treating hypothyroidism naturally means using NDT versus levothyroxine. Others view the idea of "natural treatment" as meaning that the treatment does *not* include any prescription drugs.

In our combined three decades as patient advocates, we both have had the unique opportunity to interview hundreds of practitioners. Many of them might be characterized as "alternative" or holistic, including naturopaths, herbalists, chiropractors, acupuncturists, Traditional Chinese Medicine doctors, holistic MDs, homeopaths, and many other types of experts. We have asked them the key question: Can you treat or even "cure" thyroid problems naturally? Most of the ethical practitioners offer the same answer: no.

But that said, there are some cases where they are able to resolve—or essentially cure—thyroid issues, help patients lower the dose of medications needed, and most important, resolve symptoms not relieved by medications.

Some practitioners test for an iodine deficiency, and have found that if there is a significant deficiency that is at the root of the hypothyroidism, proper iodine supplementation may shift levels back to normal and resolve symptoms in some of those patients.

Another subset of patients have developed autoimmune thyroid disease—Hashimoto's disease or Graves' disease—as an inflammatory response to celiac disease or gluten intolerance. For some of those patients, following a gluten-free diet may lower thyroid antibodies and result in a full remission from the autoimmune thyroid disease, and even relief of symptoms, eliminating a need for medication and treatment.

Pharmacist and author Izabella Wentz is one of many practitioners who recommends that Hashimoto's patients consider a gluten-free diet:

> A strong connection between reactions to gluten and Hashimoto's has been emerging in the last decade. While celiac disease has been the most commonly studied condition in how it related to Hashimoto's, in a survey of my readers, 88 percent of the people with Hashimoto's felt better on a gluten-free diet, while only 3.5 percent of them had diagnosed celiac disease.

We have also heard from some Traditional Chinese Medicine practitioners who have said that some of their patients with Graves' and Hashimoto's have responded to longer-term treatment with acupuncture and Chinese herbal medicine.

Natural health experts have cautioned, however, that hypothyroid patients need to be followed and regularly tested by a practitioner who can prescribe, as many of their patients need to take "traditional" drug therapy. Some—not all—of the patients may be able to be gradually weaned off their traditional drug treatments, as thyroid balance is restored by the natural approaches.

But the practitioners caution that it's not a sure thing. Rather, it's a complex process; it almost always takes quite a long time to see results; and some patients find it difficult to follow the detailed and sometimes costly vitamin/supplement/herbal regimen, mind-body practices, lifestyle changes, and dietary restrictions necessary to achieve success.

So, does this mean there's no hope? Never say never! If you have a mild or borderline thyroid problem, you may want to investigate going for a remission or natural cure of your condition, under the direction of a knowledgeable alternative practitioner.

And even if your thyroid problem is not mild, alternative practitioners may be able to recommend approaches to support your thyroid, immune, and hormonal systems, which will allow you to take less medication, get better relief of symptoms, and deal with persistent symptoms that may not be relieved by medication.

One caution: While some ethical chiropractors may be able to help support your immune system and thyroid function with nutritional and supplement testing and recommendations, and can work alongside your prescribing physician as part of your health-care team, chiropractors cannot legally prescribe thyroid medication. This does not stop some chiropractors from marketing costly payment-up-front chiropractic thyroid programs to patients, and in some cases, making fairly dramatic and unsubstantiated claims about their success and results.

Self-Treatment

Can you head on down to the local health food store, pick up some supplements, make a few dietary changes, and fix your thyroid problem yourself, without a doctor?

Probably not, and it's especially risky when you're pregnant. It's challenging even for experienced practitioners to sort out the complexity of a thyroid imbalance and treat it naturally. It's even more of a challenge for the average person. There is also the risk that your condition will get worse. For example, if you load up on high doses of iodine and you aren't deficient, you can actually aggravate your thyroid problem and make it far worse, and endanger your pregnancy.

Or if you take over-the-counter thyroid support supplements, you may be taking one that illegally contains some actual thyroid hormone in it—but in undisclosed amounts. These supplements can cause hyperthyroidism, along with atrial fibrillation. This puts you, your pregnancy, and your unborn baby in danger.

Be especially wary about costly supplements marketed on the Internet or at health food stores that tout themselves as thyroid cures, or suggest that they are alternatives to prescription thyroid medications. Not only do these supplements usually lack the missing thyroid hormone that the body requires, but there are often ingredients—such as iodine—that may worsen thyroid conditions in a subset of people.

Also be careful about self-medicating with prescription drugs obtained without a prescription. While some patients take this controversial course, it can end up doing more harm than good for some patients, and is never recommended during pregnancy.

Hyperthyroidism/Graves' Disease During Pregnancy

6

Hyperthyroidism describes the condition in which you have an overactive thyroid and your own gland is producing an excess of thyroid hormones. In hyperthyroidism, the excess of hormones is not due to overmedication on thyroid hormone replacement. *Thyrotoxicosis* refers to the state of hyperthyroidism that affects the body—whether the excess comes from the gland itself or is due to taking too much thyroid hormone. Graves' disease is an autoimmune disease whereby antibodies attack the gland, causing it to produce excessive amounts of thyroid hormone.

Physicians recommend that you *never* plan to get pregnant while you are hyperthyroid or thyrotoxic due to any cause, because treating these conditions during pregnancy can be complicated and poses increased risks to both you and your baby. However, some women still become pregnant while hyperthyroid or thyrotoxic during pregnancy, or develop problems during the pregnancy.

Hyperthyroidism shows up in pregnancy for a number of reasons:

- Graves' disease—around 1 in 500 women develop Graves' disease during pregnancy, and Graves' is the cause of 80 to 85 percent of the cases of overt hyperthyroidism in pregnancy.
- Toxic adenoma and toxic multinodular goiter—the second most prevalent cause of hyperthyroidism in pregnancy.
- Transient hyperthyroidism of hyperemesis gravidarum (THHG)—affects only 0.3 percent to 1.0 percent of pregnancies.
- First trimester HCG elevation—affects 1 in 5 women
- Being in the hyperthyroid phase of Hashimoto's disease—statistics on this aren't readily available, but given the number of women who have Hashimoto's, it's likely that it may be one of the more common—but overlooked—reasons for hyperthyroidism in pregnancy.

- Other types of thyroiditis—again, statistics aren't readily available, but is probably uncommon.
- Gestational transient thyrotoxicosis (GTT)—affects around 2 to 3 of every 100 pregnancies
- Factitious hyperthyroidism—this is hyperthyroidism resulting from taking too high a dosage of thyroid medication. Levothyroxine is the number one prescribed medication in the United States, and even though statistics about prevalence aren't available, some doctors may overmedicate hypothyroid patients during pregnancy; in that case, the factitious hyperthyroidism is termed iatrogenic, meaning "caused by the doctor." In other cases, patients may deliberately take too much medication, either because they think it will help them lose weight or feel better, or because they suffer from a psychiatric disorder.
- There is also an extreme, life-threatening form of hyperthyroidism, called thyroid storm, which can result from undiagnosed or untreated hyperthyroidism, and in some cases develops after thyroid surgery. In thyroid storm, heart rate and blood pressure become uncontrollably high. This can be triggered by labor and delivery in a woman with untreated hyperthyroidism.

Determining the cause of your hyperthyroidism and getting a specific diagnosis and treatment during pregnancy are crucial, because early diagnosis and treatment can prevent serious consequences for you, complications in your pregnancy, and dangers to your baby.

If you are experiencing uncontrolled or untreated hyperthyroidism, you are at risk of a number of complications, including:

- Pregnancy-induced high blood pressure
- Extreme morning sickness
- Congestive heart failure
- Preeclampsia
- Placental abruption
- Thyroid storm

The risks to your baby are significant, as well. They include:

- Miscarriage
- Intrauterine growth retardation
- Premature delivery

- Low birth weight
- Stillbirth
- Fetal hyperthyroidism
- Neonatal hyperthyroidism

If you are diagnosed with Graves' disease or have uncontrolled or severe hyperthyroidism during pregnancy, it is important to consult with a perinatologist—an obstetrician who specializes in high-risk pregnancy. These doctors are sometimes called "maternal-fetal medicine" or "high-risk pregnancy" specialists.

Signs and Symptoms

The symptoms of hyperthyroidism and thyrotoxicosis reflect a speeding-up of your body's processes. They include:

- Fatigue
- High blood pressure
- Heart palpitations
- Anxiety, panic attacks, restlessness, nervousness
- Insomnia
- Diarrhea or loose stools
- Tremor or shakiness
- Weakness in your arms and legs
- Difficulty climbing stairs
- Difficulty concentrating
- Intolerance to heat, excessive sweating

As you can see, many of the common hyperthyroidism symptoms are also similar to pregnancy symptoms. This means you or your doctor may not instantly suspect that the cause is hyperthyroidism.

However, a few hyperthyroidism symptoms are not typical pregnancy symptoms, but *are* clear symptoms of Graves' disease and hyperthyroidism. They include:

- Neck enlargement (goiter)—this is noticeable in almost all pregnant women with Graves' disease and hyperthyroidism, as the gland usually is enlarged from two to four times its normal size. Enlargement is also common in toxic multinodular goiter.

- Sensitivity or a feeling of fullness in the throat or neck—due to goiter
- Difficulty breathing or swallowing—due to goiter
- Irregular heart rates (arrhythmias) including atrial fibrillation
- A high pulse and heart rate, typically over 100
- A high heart rate in the baby, typically of more than 160 beats per minute
- Vision problems: e.g., sensitivity, protrusion of the eyes, blurred vision, double vision, etc.—also known as ophthalmopathy
- Failure to gain weight during pregnancy, or weight loss, despite increased or normal appetite
- Excessive nausea and vomiting—more common in THHG

The Diagnostic Starting Point

If you are experiencing symptoms at any point in your pregnancy, you should insist on a thorough evaluation of your thyroid. This should include a clinical examination in which the doctor will look for enlargement of your thyroid; eye symptoms, such as bulging of the eyeball; weight loss; rapid pulse; or higher blood pressure. Your baby's fetal heart rate should also be measured.

Blood tests are also necessary. According to the 2011 "Guidelines of the American Thyroid Association for the Diagnosis and Management of Thyroid Disease During Pregnancy and Postpartum," or Pregnancy Guidelines, the diagnosis of hyperthyroidism or thyrotoxicosis in pregnant women should be based primarily on the following two blood test results:

- A thyroid-stimulating hormone (TSH) blood test value of less than 0.01 mIU/L, and
- An elevated Free T4 value. (Note: Free T4 and not Total T4 should be measured, because pregnancy makes Total T4 less accurate.)

If the TSH is low, but the Free T4 is normal or only slightly elevated, Free T3 may also be measured, as elevations in Free T3 can help clarify the diagnosis.

Once clinical hyperthyroidism or thyrotoxicosis—whether mild or subclinical, or more severe—is established, a key diagnostic challenge for your doctor is to determine the cause. The underlying cause helps determine additional testing and monitoring needed, the treatment you may receive, as well as potential risks to your baby.

Note: In nonpregnant patients, a common test—radioactive iodine uptake (RAIU)—is used to evaluate the cause of hyperthyroidism. A small, tracer dose of radioactive iodine is given, and several hours later, a special scanner is used to assess the absorption—or "uptake"—of the iodine by your thyroid. High uptake suggests Graves' disease, and unevenness in the uptake suggests the presence of a nodule or nodules. But the RAIU is never done during pregnancy, due to the risks posed to the fetus by exposure to radiation. This makes diagnosing the cause of hyperthyroidism in pregnancy more difficult.

Treatments

If you are pregnant, and have mild or subclinical hyperthyroidism and few symptoms, your physician will probably not prescribe treatment during your pregnancy. If you have moderate to severe hyperthyroidism, with more significant or debilitating symptoms, treatment is almost always required to protect your health and the health of your unborn baby.

Radioactive Iodine

For American thyroid patients who are not pregnant, the conventional treatment for Graves' disease focuses on disabling the thyroid permanently, by administering radioactive iodine (RAI) treatment. In RAI, you ingest (via a drink or pill) a radioactive form of iodine, which goes directly to the thyroid gland. Unlike conventional radiation treatment, which can damage organs around the target area, RAI targets its action only on thyroid cells, making them incapable of producing thyroid hormone. In some cases, RAI causes the gland to atrophy and shrink. Most patients after RAI end up hypothyroid for life, although some will get a dose that leaves them with some thyroid function and hormone levels in the reference range. Some patients require additional RAI treatment later after a recurrence of hyperthyroidism.

Again, however, RAI is never performed on pregnant women. And women of childbearing age are cautioned to wait from six months to a year after RAI, and only after thyroid levels are stabilized, before attempting to conceive.

There is controversy over the use of RAI for hyperthyroidism, in particular for women of childbearing age. When members of the American Thyroid Association, the European Thyroid Association, and the Japan Thyroid Association were surveyed on their management of Graves' hyperthyroidism in women of childbearing age, RAI was the therapy of choice by American physicians, while the majority of European and Japanese physicians preferred to use antithyroid drugs.

During pregnancy then, antithyroid drugs and surgery are key treatment options for women who are hyperthyroid during pregnancy.

Antithyroid Drugs

Antithyroid drugs are almost always the first course of treatment for a pregnant woman whose hyperthyroidism requires treatment.

The key antithyroid drugs propylthiouracil (PTU), methimazole (MMI), and carbimazole are effective in pregnant women. Babies of mothers taking antithyroid drugs do have a higher risk of goiter and fetal hypothyroidism, however. Still, these drugs are recommended because the risk of hyperthyroidism in a mother and fetus is greater than the risk of taking a low dose of the antithyroid medication.

Among the drugs, PTU is typically recommended during the first trimester, because it is less effective at crossing the placenta, and doesn't pose the rare risk of causing scalp defects, as do the other drugs. The Pregnancy Guidelines recommend the discontinuation of PTU after the first trimester and switching to methimazole, to decrease the risk of liver disease associated with PTU. Taking methimazole during the first trimester, or taking PTU during the second and third trimesters, is only recommended for women who have allergies, sensitivities, or side effects from the other antithyroid drug.

If you are diagnosed during the first trimester, experts recommend that you be started on the lowest possible dose of PTU, and then retested every two weeks until thyroid hormone levels are normalized. In women being treated with antithyroid drugs during pregnancy, the guidelines state that the goal is a Free T4 at the top—or slightly above—the reference range, and TSH in the low-normal range. Physicians typically avoid higher doses (for example, more than 200 mg a day of PTU, or 30 mg of methimazole), because it can cause goiter and hypothyroidism in your developing baby.

> Make sure that whatever antithyroid drug you are taking, that you bring several days' worth with you to the hospital during childbirth. And be sure that you let your doctors and nurses know about your condition and your medication, and that both are noted in your chart.

Once levels normalize, testing should continue every 2 to 4 weeks. This regular monitoring is not just to ensure that thyroid levels are stabilized, but to determine whether the antithyroid drug dosage needs to be reduced or even eliminated entirely.

At the end of your first trimester, around 13 weeks, your doctor will likely switch you from PTU to methimazole. You should be rechecked again in 2 weeks to ensure that the transition to the new medication is keeping thyroid levels in control.

If you are taking antithyroid drugs and develop any of the following symptoms, you should contact your doctor immediately, as they may be signs of adverse reactions to the medication:

- Fatigue
- Weakness
- Abdominal pain
- Loss of appetite
- A skin rash or itching
- Easy bruising
- Yellowing of the skin or whites of the eyes, called jaundice
- Persistent sore throat
- Fever

For women with Graves' disease who are on antithyroid medication, it is particularly important to confirm pregnancy as early as possible, and to take a pregnancy test after any missed periods. Angela shares her story:

> After being diagnosed with Graves' disease and put on antithyroid drugs, I was told I probably wouldn't be able to have children—which seems ridiculous now to hear that. My symptoms were controlled using carbimazole. I'd just turned 30 and even with medication I felt lethargic and I hadn't had a period in over six months, so went to the GP to get checked. He took routine blood tests and found I was 13 weeks pregnant. Immediately my medication was changed and I worried constantly about the baby. He was growing well but always on the lowest percentile. After a difficult labor he was born by emergency C-section at 42 weeks with what looked like open wounds on his scalp. It took three years to get a diagnosis of aplasia cutis but no explanation why. After research I've found being on carbimazole while pregnant can be a cause. He's nine years old now, and besides having large scars on his scalp and allergies to nuts, he's a really healthy, intelligent kid.

Beta-Blockers

If you have moderate to severe hyperthyroidism and an elevated heart rate, elevated blood pressure, or palpitations, beta-blockers may be prescribed. Keep in mind, however, that they are not considered safe to use for more than two weeks. For example, some doctors might treat you with beta-blockers for the two weeks after your diagnosis, while waiting for antithyroid drugs to take effect. Beta-blockers are not prescribed during the end of pregnancy, because they can be linked to growth problems, breathing difficulties, and slow heart rate in newborns.

Surgery

In the United States, surgical removal of the thyroid—known as thyroidectomy—is used to treat hyperthyroidism in nonpregnant patients only if antithyroid drugs can't be tolerated or RAI is unable to control the overactive thyroid. Occasionally, women who want to get pregnant choose to have surgery prior to conception, so that they can avoid the recommended six to twelve month wait after RAI to get pregnant.

Because RAI is not an option in pregnancy, there are some situations where you doctor may recommend surgery to remove your thyroid as a treatment for Graves' disease or hyperthyroidism during your pregnancy. The reasons surgery may be recommended include:

- You have an allergy or experience undesirable side effects from antithyroid drugs. From 3 to 5 percent of patients have drug-related side effects, such as allergic reactions, rashes, or low white cell counts.
- You are on extremely high doses of antithyroid drugs to manage your condition (e.g., more than 30 mg of methimazole or 300 mg of PTU).
- Your condition is not responding to the antithyroid drugs, and you remain hyperthyroid and symptomatic.
- Your fetus is showing evidence of hypothyroidism due to the antithyroid drugs (typically, a slow fetal heart rate and/or slowed bone development).

Surgery is typically performed in the second trimester, when the greatest risk of miscarriage has passed. Second-trimester thyroid surgery is considered safe. Surgery is not typically performed in the third trimester, as this may pose a risk of preterm labor and delivery.

The Pregnancy Guidelines recommend that, at the time of surgery, your antibody levels be measured to assess the potential risk of hyperthyroidism in the fetus. They further recommend that doctors prescribe patients a short course of potassium iodide solution in advance of the surgery.

After thyroid surgery, you will need frequent monitoring of your thyroid levels, because at some point, as soon as the excess thyroid hormone is out of your system, you will become hypothyroid and need to start thyroid hormone replacement. If you have underlying Graves' disease, you will also need antibody monitoring during the later stages of pregnancy, as the Graves' antibodies can remain in your bloodstream long after surgery, and can potentially affect your baby before or after birth.

Chapter 7 has some detailed tips on finding a good thyroid surgeon, and what to expect from thyroid surgery and the recuperation process.

Iodine Therapy

An alternative hyperthyroidism treatment option that some integrative and naturopathic doctors may offer is iodine therapy. Naturopathic physician John Robinson recommends that you consider iodine therapy for treatment of hyperthyroidism in lieu of antithyroid drugs. According to Dr. Robinson:

> This is by far one of the most safe and effective treatments for the hyperthyroid state. There is a long history with the use of iodine for hyperthyroidism. Doses would range from 6.25 mg up to 180 mg daily to keep the thyroid function normal. Historically, reports would show up to a 90 percent effective rate with using 90 mg of iodine daily to control the hyperthyroid state. In my practice, I find that these are the approximate doses that are effective and over time can often be lowered to a general maintenance dose of as low as 12.5 mg daily. For the subclinical hyperthyroid patient with only a low TSH value, iodine therapy, in its proper clinical context, is extremely simple and effective.
>
> Always take 200 mcg of selenium with iodine. Selenium deficiency is associated with autoimmune thyroiditis, such as Graves' disease, and is one of the most important nutrients for thyroid function. It is also important to note that if iodine is used as a therapy for hyperthyroidism, it should be used with a complete nutritional protocol and close clinical monitoring by a competent physician.
>
> Iodine therapy for the pregnant mother, in doses between 6 to 40 mg, have been shown *not* to cause issues with the fetus such as hypothyroidism, but this treatment is not conventionally accepted. Of course, it is extremely important to be monitored by a competent physician who has experience in the use of iodine therapy and thyroid disease.

Dr. Robinson's recommendation is backed up by some new research. A recent Japanese study found that among patients in an iodine-sufficient area switched from methimazole to potassium iodine in the first trimester of pregnancy, versus staying on methimazole, there was a substantial difference of anomalies in the newborns—with 1.5 percent in the potassium iodide group, versus 4.1 percent in the methimazole group. None of the newborns whose mothers were taking potassium iodide had thyroid dysfunction or a goiter. While the researchers felt that more study is needed, substituting potassium iodide for methimazole as a way to treat hyperthyroidism in Graves' disease patients, during the first trimester, may be an effective treatment that also reduces the incidence of congenital anomalies.

Low-Dose Naltrexone (LDN)

Some integrative physicians are using low doses of the addiction drug naltrexone in a therapy that can in some cases lower antibodies and help achieve remission. Practitioners consider low-dose naltrexone (LDN) generally safe during pregnancy.

Hyperthyroid Conditions

We've reviewed how hyperthyroidism/thyrotoxicosis is generally defined, and the treatments—antithyroid drugs, beta-blockers, and surgery—that are commonly available during pregnancy. But diagnosis and treatments depend on the cause of your hyperthyroidism. In this section, we look at the different hyperthyroidism and thyrotoxicosis in pregnancy, as well as how they are typically handled.

Graves' Disease

Graves' disease is an autoimmune condition in which the body produces antibodies that overstimulate the thyroid and cause it to produce too much thyroid hormone.

If you were not pregnant, doctors would frequently do the radioactive iodine uptake (RAIU) test to make a diagnosis of Graves' disease. This test is not used during pregnancy, however, because of the danger the radioactivity poses to a developing baby.

To diagnose Graves' disease in pregnancy, your doctor should take your family and personal medical history, discuss your symptoms, and do a clinical examination, looking particularly for classic clinical signs of Graves', such as goiter, a high pulse rate, and eye-related symptoms.

In Graves', you will not only have a low thyroid-stimulating hormone (TSH) level and elevated Free T4, but you will likely also have an elevated level of thyroid-stimulating immunoglobulins (TSI). These antibodies are positive in as many as 90 percent of patients with Graves' disease, so this blood test can be used to confirm a diagnosis of Graves' disease during pregnancy.

During pregnancy, the treatment is antithyroid drugs, with a goal of keeping Free T4 and TSH within the reference range. If you do not respond to antithyroid drugs, or you have adverse reactions to the drugs, and you are significantly hyperthyroid and symptomatic, surgery will be recommended. Ideally, it should be conducted in the second trimester, the safest time for your baby. In unresponsive hyperthyroidism, however, if there is a risk of thyroid storm, or potential danger to your baby, your doctor may recommend surgery at other points during the pregnancy.

Once you are taking antithyroid drugs, you should be monitored every 2 to 6 weeks. In addition to thyroid testing, at health-care visits, your pulse will be monitored, along with weight gain and thyroid size. Pulse should remain below 100 beats per minute. You should strive to keep your weight gain within the normal ranges for pregnancy, so speak with your doctor about proper nutrition and what types of physical activity are appropriate for your current condition. Fetal growth and pulse rate should also be monitored regularly, and periodic ultrasounds of your fetus should look for any signs of an enlarged thyroid, growth problems, or other evidence of irregularities that may result from your hyperthyroidism.

Once you reach target levels (Free T4 at the top end or just slightly above the top end of the reference range), testing should continue every 2 to 6 weeks. This regular monitoring is not just to ensure that thyroid levels are stabilized, but to determine whether the antithyroid drug dosage needs to be reduced.

At the end of your first trimester, around 13 weeks, your doctor will likely switch you from PTU to methimazole. You should be rechecked again in 2 weeks to ensure that the transition to the new medication is keeping thyroid levels in control.

A complete thyroid panel, including thyroid-stimulating immunoglobulin (TSI) levels, should be checked around the midpoint of pregnancy, from between 20 and 24 weeks gestation. According to endocrinologist Roberto Negro, MD, "In most cases, antithyroid drugs may be discontinued during the second-third trimester as Graves' disease often spontaneously improves, but thyroid function should be checked."

If your TSI levels have dropped, your doctor may start tapering down your dosage, because as many as a third of women can stop taking the medication and the thyroid will normalize before childbirth. Most doctors will not discontinue antithyroid drug treatment until after the thirty-second week of pregnancy, however, because before that time, the risk of relapse is higher.

If you have elevated levels of TSI at this point, it can signal that your baby is at risk of developing fetal or neonatal hyperthyroidism, discussed later in this chapter.

Toxic Adenoma/Toxic Multinodular Goiter

Most thyroid nodules don't impact hormone production, but a toxic adenoma is a benign thyroid nodule that produces excessive amounts of thyroid hormone, and causes hyperthyroidism. Toxic multinodular goiter is a situation where the thyroid gland enlarges due to the growth of numerous benign nodules that produce excessive amounts of thyroid hormone and cause hyperthyroidism. Neither of these conditions is autoimmune in nature.

In a nonpregnant patient, these conditions are typically diagnosed with radioactive iodine uptake (RAIU). Since this test is not done in pregnancy, the diagnosis is typically made with several criteria:

- Blood work that shows hyperthyroidism, but does not show thyroid antibodies
- Your symptoms
- Visible nodules or visible enlargement of your thyroid
- Palpation of your neck, and ability to feel a nodule or nodules
- Ultrasound imaging that shows a nodule or nodules

During pregnancy, the primary treatment is antithyroid drugs. If the hyperthyroidism can't be controlled, and poses a danger to you or your baby, or the nodule(s) are threatening your ability to breathe or swallow, surgery may be recommended.

Following childbirth, and after you conclude breastfeeding, if your nodule(s) continue to cause hyperthyroidism, or significant symptoms, your doctor may recommend radioactive iodine (RAI) treatment or surgery.

Transient Hyperthyroidism of Hyperemesis Gravidarum (THHG)

During the first trimester of pregnancy, a small percentage of women develop a form of hyperthyroidism that is triggered by a severe form of morning sickness known as hyperemesis gravidarum. Hyperemesis gravidarum is characterized by severe nausea, excessive vomiting, electrolyte disturbances, and weight loss. Other symptoms can include fatigue, weakness, excessive salivation, lightheadedness, fainting, and infrequent urination.

The Pregnancy Guidelines recommend that all pregnant women with hyperemesis gravidarum have their thyroid function evaluated, because in some cases, the syndrome is also associated with a short-term hyperthyroidism known as transient hyperthyroidism of hyperemesis gravidarum, or THHG.

There are some factors that distinguish THHG from other types of hyperthyroidism in pregnant women:

- The presence of severe vomiting—not a typical characteristic of hyperthyroidism
- Significant weight loss—not characteristic during pregnancy
- The lack of typical Graves' disease symptoms, including goiter (enlarged thyroid) and eye-related symptoms
- The lack of other "classic" hyperthyroidism symptoms, such as tachycardia (a heart rate greater than 100 beats/minute), diarrhea, muscle weakness, or tremor

Blood test results can also help pinpoint a diagnosis of THHG because free T4 is usually only slightly elevated, and the T3 level will typically be normal in a woman with THHG. According to the Endocrine Society, TSI should also be measured in patients with hyperemesis gravidarum to identify the possibility of Graves' disease.

Some cases of THHG require no thyroid-specific treatment, and the thyroid abnormalities will spontaneously resolve by the end of the second trimester. When symptoms are severe, however, thyroid treatment may take place, usually during the first trimester, and may consist of a short course of antithyroid drugs, usually PTU. Women with hyperemesis gravidarum who are also diagnosed with Graves' disease should be treated with antithyroid drugs as clinically necessary.

For THHG patients without Graves' disease, as pregnancy hormones normalize after the first trimester, by the middle of the pregnancy, most women notice that the hyperthyroid symptoms subside. TSH may remain low or suppressed, however. Usually, any thyroid treatment being given is discontinued and the thyroid function returns to normal before delivery.

In dealing with THHG that involves milder nausea and vomiting, treatment usually involves dietary changes, rest, and antacids. On the alternative front, some women have had success managing THHG with acupressure;

herbal remedies, such as peppermint and ginger; and hypnosis. When nausea and vomiting are severe, dehydration and malnutrition in the mother
and poor weight gain in the developing baby can occur. Severe symptoms,
therefore, may require hospitalization so that the woman can receive intravenous fluids and nutrition. In some severe cases, medications, including
metoclopramide (Reglan), antihistamines, and antireflux drugs, may also be
prescribed.

HCG Elevation

Towards the end of your first trimester, at around 13 weeks, increases in the
pregnancy hormone HCG can in some cases cause your Free T4 to increase,
which can push your TSH levels down to hyperthyroid levels. As many as one
in five pregnant women may have this small, temporary period of hyperthyroidism. Hyperthyroidism due to HCG elevation is almost always asymptom-
atic, with no clinical signs of hyperthyroidism. If at this point in pregnancy
your thyroid blood test levels suggest hyperthyroidism, but you have no symptoms and no thyroid antibodies, you should not automatically be diagnosed
with hyperthyroidism, and treatment is not necessary. Your thyroid will usually return to normal during the second and third trimester of your pregnancy.
If you have HCG-elevated hyperthyroidism, you should however have your
thyroid levels monitored monthly through your pregnancy until levels return
to normal.

Hashimoto's Disease/Hyperthyroid Phase

Hashimoto's disease—as evidenced by elevated thyroid peroxidase antibodies (TPOAb)—usually is characterized by self-destruction of the thyroid
gland and hypothyroidism. But in its earlier stages, some patients have oc-
casional periods of hyperthyroidism as the thyroid sputters into short bursts
of overactivity.

   If you have been diagnosed with Hashimoto's disease prior to pregnancy
and develop hyperthyroidism symptoms during your pregnancy, it's important to have TSH, Free T4, Free T3, TPOAb, and TSI checked. Depending on
how elevated your thyroid levels are, and the severity of your symptoms, if you
are being treated with thyroid hormone replacement medication, your doctor
will reduce your dose. You should be rechecked every two weeks to monitor
your progress, since it's possible that, within weeks, your thyroid may shift
back into hypothyroidism, and your dose will again need to be increased.

If you are not being treated with thyroid hormone replacement medication, depending on how elevated your thyroid levels are, and the severity of your symptoms, your doctor may recommend a short course of antithyroid drugs. Again, you should be rechecked every two weeks to monitor your progress in case the dosage of your antithyroid drugs needs to be reduced or use of them terminated altogether.

Painless Thyroiditis

Painless thyroiditis is usually characterized by a low TSH, elevated Free T4, and the absence of thyroid antibodies. Because painless thyroiditis is a short-term, transient condition and usually doesn't cause severe hyperthyroidism, you will most likely not need treatment.

Gestational Transient Thyrotoxicosis (GTT)

A small number of women develop gestational transient thyrotoxicosis (GTT), especially during early pregnancy. This is a nonautoimmune type of hyperthyroidism that occurs in pregnant women, and is sometimes linked to hyperemesis gravidarum (excessive nausea and vomiting during pregnancy). Diagnosis of GTT is made when you have no history of previous hyperthyroidism, no goiter, and no evidence of thyroid antibodies, but you do have low TSH and elevated Free T4 and Free T3 levels. In the rare case of severe GTT—defined by the Pregnancy Guidelines as having a Free T4 level that is above the reference range and a TSH less than 0.1—you may need treatment with antithyroid drugs. But typically, gestational transient thyrotoxicosis is not treated with any type of thyroid-related medication.

Factitious Hyperthyroidism

Factitious hyperthyroidism refers to hyperthyroidism due to taking too much thyroid medication. If you are hypothyroid prior to pregnancy and taking thyroid hormone replacement medication, it is possible that your doctor's adjustments to your dosage may leave you overmedicated, with blood tests and symptoms that point to hyperthyroidism. There are also pharmacy errors where patients end up taking too high a dosage. Less commonly, some people choose to take too much medication.

If you develop factitious hyperthyroidism, your doctor will lower your dose of thyroid hormone replacement medication. You should be retested within several weeks, and should continue adjusting your dosage and re-checking until the hyperthyroidism resolves, and blood test levels return to normal.

Thyroid Storm

Some people with Graves' disease or uncontrolled hyperthyroidism develop a condition known as thyroid storm. It's not common however; only 1 to 2 percent of patients with any form of hyperthyroidism ever develop thyroid storm. During thyroid storm, your heart rate, blood pressure, and body temperature can become uncontrollably high. If thyroid storm is suspected, call your doctor and go immediately to a hospital emergency room, as this is a life-threatening condition that can develop and worsen quickly, and requires treatment within hours to avoid fatal complications, such as stroke or heart attack.

Untreated Graves' disease and/or hyperthyroidism are specific risk factors, as are being female and pregnant. Even when the Graves' disease is identified and being treated, however, certain other factors raise the risk of thyroid storm:

- Infection—lung infection, throat infection, or pneumonia
- Blood sugar changes—diabetic ketoacidosis, insulin-induced hypoglycemia
- Recent surgery to the thyroid
- Abrupt withdrawal of antithyroid medications
- Radioactive iodine (RAI) treatment of the thyroid
- Excessive palpation (handling/manipulation) of the thyroid
- Severe emotional stress
- An overdose of thyroid hormone
- Toxemia of pregnancy and labor

The symptoms of thyroid storm include:

- Fever of 100 to as high as 106
- A high heart rate that can be as high as 200 beats per minute
- Palpitations, chest pain, shortness of breath
- High blood pressure
- Confusion, delirium, and even psychosis
- Extreme weakness and fatigue
- Extreme restlessness, nervousness, mood swings

- Exaggerated reflexes
- Difficulty breathing
- Nausea, vomiting, diarrhea
- Recent dramatic weight loss may have taken place recently
- Profuse sweating, dehydration
- Stupor or coma

Thyroid storm is treated on an emergency basis with a combination of antithyroid drugs, blockade iodine drug, beta-blockers, and treatment for any underlying nonthyroidal illness or infection that may be contributing to the thyroid storm.

AN IMPORTANT WARNING: If you suspect that you are going into thyroid storm, go to an emergency room immediately!

Natural Approaches

There is one key reason why it's problematic to rely on natural and holistic approaches to managing newly diagnosed or worsening hyperthyroidism—and Graves' disease in particular—during pregnancy: *Natural approaches take time to work.*

Some holistic practitioners tell their Graves' and hyperthyroid patients that it can take as long as a year to get Graves' and hyperthyroidism into remission, if at all. And when you are pregnant and hyperthyroid, you don't have that time. You can't wait weeks or months to see whether different herbs, vitamins, foods, and lifestyle changes will work. To protect your own health, and the health of your baby, you need to start treatment right away. Also, most holistic practitioners are reluctant to use herbal remedies during pregnancy, because they haven't been tested in pregnant women, and we just don't know what potential effects they may have on the unborn baby.

That said, there are some holistic approaches to enhancing your health that you can consider—working with your physician—if you are diagnosed with Graves' disease and hyperthyroidism during pregnancy:

- Eat more goitrogenic foods—some integrative and holistic physicians recommend supplementing antithyroid drug approaches with natural antithyroid foods (goitrogens). This may allow you to take a lower dose of antithyroid medications—which then poses less risk to you and your baby. We provide a list of some common goitrogenic foods on page 69.

- Take l-carnitine—which can slow the thyroid and allow you to take a lower dose of antithyroid medications.
- Take lemon balm—also known as *Melissa* or *Melissa officinalis*—supplements. This herb may block the action of the TSI found in Graves' disease from further stimulating the thyroid gland.
- As discussed in Chapter 6, you may also want to consider following an anti-inflammatory, autoimmune diet, and eliminate gluten, as a way to help reduce or even eliminate antibodies.

> Note: Taking any supplements during pregnancy should only be done under the guidance of a medical professional.

Naturopathic physician John Robinson also recommends that if you're hyperthyroid, you adopt a regular stress-reduction practice:

The hyperthyroid (high thyroid) patient is often extremely stressed emotionally. This stress is often one of the key triggers for the hyperthyroidism in the first place. I suggest that my patients meditate regularly and remove as many stressful situations as possible to provide the space to heal and recover and to avoid additional overstimulation to the nervous system.

Fetal and Neonatal Hyperthyroidism

When you have Graves' hyperthyroidism during pregnancy, there is a small risk—approximately 1 to 5 percent—that your baby will develop hyperthyroidism before birth—a condition known as fetal thyrotoxicosis. There is also a risk that your baby will be born with hyperthyroidism, known as neonatal hyperthyroidism.

Your baby is at risk if:

- You had Graves' disease in the past and had RAI or surgery to treat it.
- You developed Graves' disease during the pregnancy and are being treated with antithyroid drugs.

- You developed Graves' disease during the pregnancy and had surgery to treat it.

It may be surprising to learn that if you had Graves' disease and were treated with RAI or surgery prior to your pregnancy, there is still a risk that your baby will have fetal thyrotoxicosis or neonatal hyperthyroidism. This is due to antibodies in your bloodstream that remain long after RAI or surgery, cross the placenta, and cause an overactive thyroid in your baby before or after birth. No matter how long it has been since you had RAI or a thyroidectomy, antibodies can be present. In fact, according to the Pregnancy Guidelines, more than 95 percent of women with Graves' disease have evidence of thyroid antibodies, including after RAI.

The risk to your baby is higher if your TSI levels, which must be measured between 22 and 26 weeks gestation, are elevated.

If you have a past or current history of Graves' disease, one important first step to take is to make sure that you enlist the help of a pediatric endocrinologist—or a maternal-fetal medicine specialist, perinatologist, or high-risk OB with expertise in fetal and neonatal thyroid issues—to ensure that your baby is properly monitored and treated before and after birth.

Another important recommendation is to advise everyone on your health team of your condition. While your OB or endocrinologist may know that you are hyperthyroid, or have a history of Graves' disease, the attending physicians, pediatricians, and nurses at the hospital may not. Or the information may get overlooked. So, even though the chance that your baby will develop fetal or neonatal hyperthyroidism is very small, it's absolutely essential that you remind every health-care provider who comes in contact with you about your thyroid condition or history.

Monitoring During Pregnancy

If you have Graves' disease or hyperthyroidism during pregnancy, or have a history of Graves' disease, regular fetal monitoring during your pregnancy is essential.

- Your baby's heart rate should be monitored, and fetal thyrotoxicosis is suggested when the baby's heart rate is more than 160 beats per minute. You should also have regular ultrasounds to evaluate the size of your baby's thyroid and whether it's becoming enlarged.

- During ultrasounds, your doctor should also be looking for other possible symptoms of fetal hyperthyroidism, including growth retardation and changes to bones.

Testing During Pregnancy

Whether you were treated for Graves' disease prior to pregnancy, or developed hyperthyroidism or Graves' disease during pregnancy, during the third trimester of your pregnancy doctors should measure your TSI levels. Elevated levels are associated with an increased risk that your baby will be affected.

Fetal Hyperthyroidism

If your unborn baby is determined to be hyperthyroid, your doctor is likely to prescribe the antithyroid drug methimazole for you—whether or not you yourself are hyperthyroid—to help normalize your baby's thyroid function before birth.

Neonatal Hyperthyroidism

If you had elevated antibodies during your third trimester, or your newborn is suspected to be hyperthyroid, your pediatric endocrinologist or specialist should test the newborn's TSH and Free T4 levels right after birth. In those babies born with hyperthyroidism, those tests can confirm it immediately.

In some cases, however, if you are receiving antithyroid drug treatment during your pregnancy, your baby may be born with normal thyroid levels and no hyperthyroidism symptoms, and be sent home, but then several days and up to around three weeks later, start showing symptoms of hyperthyroidism. The hyperthyroidism develops as the antithyroid drug you were taking—which was passing through the placenta to your baby—wears off after birth.

The signs and symptoms of hyperthyroidism in a newborn include the following:

- An unusually small head circumference
- An unusually prominent forehead
- A dangerous accumulation of fluid in the baby's belly and/or organs, including the liver, spleen, heart, or lungs (known as fetal hydrops)
- Enlarged liver and/or spleen

- Low birth weight
- Premature birth
- Warm, moist skin
- High blood pressure
- Fast heartbeat
- Irregular heart rhythms
- Irritability, hyperactivity, restlessness, poor sleep
- An enlarged thyroid (goiter)
- Difficulty breathing due to goiter pressing on the windpipe
- Excessive or normal appetite, with poor weight gain
- Bulging eyes, stare
- Vomiting
- Diarrhea

If you see any of these symptoms in your baby, your baby should be tested immediately.

Treatment for neonatal hyperthyroidism should be started as soon as it's diagnosed. Typically, an antithyroid drug is used, along with a beta-blocker, such as propranolol, to help control muscular and heart overactivity. In some cases, iodine in the form of Lugol's solution or potassium iodide may be given to help inhibit the release of thyroid hormones. If your baby is extremely hyperthyroid, your doctor may prescribe glucocorticoid drugs. These drugs reduce inflammation, can slow your baby's secretion of thyroid hormones, and can lower the conversion of T4 to T3.

Your baby should have weekly thyroid function tests to monitor progress. Once the condition starts to improve, the dosages of medications can be gradually decreased, and ultimately discontinued. This usually takes place between 3 and 12 weeks, as your antibodies disappear from your baby's circulation. There are some rare cases, however, where neonatal hyperthyroidism has continued for as long as six months or more in an infant.

Fetal and Neonatal Hypothyroidism

If you are being treated with antithyroid drugs during pregnancy, your baby is at a slight risk of developing fetal or neonatal hypothyroidism.

There are two key risk factors that can increase the risk:

- Poor control of your hyperthyroidism throughout your pregnancy, which can cause transient central hypothyroidism in the fetus or newborn

- High doses of antithyroid drugs, which can cause hypothyroidism in your fetus or newborn

If your specialist confirms fetal hypothyroidism as a complication of your treatment, he or she will likely reduce your dosage of antithyroid medications.

As part of the postbirth "heel-stick test," babies born in the United States are automatically tested for hypothyroidism at birth. However, if you have any risk factors, or if your newborn shows any of the following symptoms of neonatal hypothyroidism, you should ensure that not only this test, but also a more detailed panel of thyroid tests, be done:

- A dull expression
- Puffiness in the face
- A thickened tongue
- A tongue that sticks out of the baby's mouth
- Episodes of choking
- Constipation
- Jaundice
- Poor feeding
- Excessive sleepiness or lethargy
- Lack of muscle tone
- Unusually short height
- Decreased muscle tone
- Failure to grow
- A hoarse cry
- Large soft spots on the skull

If neonatal hypothyroidism is diagnosed, your baby should start thyroid hormone replacement treatment immediately. Regular follow-up is necessary, because if the hypothyroidism is transient, the baby will eventually be able to stop taking the thyroid medication. But if the thyroid gland has been permanently damaged, then thyroid hormone replacement treatment will need to continue indefinitely.

Thyroiditis, Goiter, Nodules, and Thyroid Cancer in Pregnancy

In addition to hyperthyroidism and hypothyroidism, a number of other thyroid conditions and diseases can affect you while you are pregnant. In this chapter we look at how thyroiditis, goiter, nodules, and thyroid cancer are diagnosed and treated in pregnancy.

Thyroiditis

Thyroiditis refers to any condition that inflames the thyroid. We've talked about the most common type of thyroiditis, Hashimoto's disease. But there are a number of different types of thyroiditis, and all of them can strike during pregnancy. There are few statistics about the number of pregnant women who develop the different types of thyroiditis, but the good news is that thyroiditis is not very common. Still, it's important to know how thyroiditis is diagnosed and treated.

An important note: In nonpregnant patients, a radioiodine uptake (RIU) is often used to identify the type of thyroiditis. But this radioactive test is not done in pregnancy, as it poses a risk to your baby's thyroid, so diagnosis will need to be made by symptoms, clinical examination, blood tests, imaging tests, or in some cases, fine-needle aspiration biopsy.

Painless Thyroiditis/Silent Thyroiditis/Lymphocytic Thyroiditis

Painless thyroiditis is considered a variant form of chronic autoimmune thyroiditis (Hashimoto's), suggesting that it is part of the spectrum of thyroid autoimmune disease.

If you have painless thyroiditis, you are considered to have a form of autoimmune thyroid disease, like Hashimoto's, except that it usually resolves itself and the thyroid function returns to normal. This type of thyroiditis doesn't typically cause any symptoms, and your thyroid usually does not become enlarged (goiter).

It's thought that painless thyroiditis may be responsible for as much as 10 percent of hyperthyroidism, because the typical course of painless thyroiditis is a temporary period of hyperthyroidism, which is then sometimes followed by a period of hypothyroidism, and then a return to normal thyroid function.

There are some medications that can trigger painless thyroiditis. If you are on any of the following medications, your doctor may consider prescribing alternatives:

- Interferon-alfa—a medication used to treat some viral infections and cancers
- Interleukin-2—a medication used as a cancer treatment
- Amiodarone—a medication used to treat an irregular heartbeat
- Lithium—a mood-stabilizing drug used to treat bipolar disorder

Painless thyroiditis is usually characterized by a low TSH and elevated Free T4. Because painless thyroiditis is a short-term, transient condition, and usually doesn't cause severe thyroid dysfunction, you most likely will not need treatment.

De Quervain's Thyroiditis/Granulomatous Thyroiditis/Painful Thyroiditis/Subacute Thyroiditis

The main symptom of De Quervain's thyroiditis—also known as subacute nonsuppurative thyroiditis—is neck pain and tenderness. Some patients experience difficulty swallowing, or even fever. The cause of this particular type of thyroiditis is thought to be a virus.

Diagnosis is done by clinical examination, symptoms, and TSH, Free T4, and Free T3 tests. Typically, this type of thyroiditis starts out with a period of hyperthyroidism that may last from four to six weeks. Thyroid hormone levels then start to drop, becoming normal for about four weeks, and then they continue to decline toward a hypothyroid phase, lasting around four to six weeks.

For treatment in nonpregnant patients, if the primary complaint is pain or swelling, a nonsteroidal anti-inflammatory drug, such as aspirin or ibuprofen, may be recommended. These drugs are not recommended when you are pregnant, however, so you might need to look for non-medication-based treatments, such as hot or cold compresses. If you are experiencing significant hyperthyroid symptoms, a beta-blocker drug may be prescribed—but only for a short time in pregnancy, during the hyperthyroid phase of the condition. If your blood tests show that you are in a hypothyroid phase during pregnancy, most physicians will prescribe thyroid hormone replacement medications to ensure that you are within the TSH range appropriate for your trimester.

Eventually, in most patients, the thyroid gland and hormone production returns to normal.

Very few patients have a recurrence of this type of thyroiditis. One study, however, found that around 15 percent of patients with this type of thyroiditis will eventually develop permanent hypothyroidism that requires treatment. So, if you are diagnosed with De Quervain's thyroiditis, make sure it's noted in your medical records, and pay attention to possible thyroid symptoms down the road. You also should consider making a comprehensive thyroid blood panel a regular part of your annual checkup.

Acute Suppurative Thyroiditis

Acute suppurative thyroiditis is also known as acute infectious thyroiditis. It falls into the category of a "painful" thyroiditis, and symptoms can include neck pain, tenderness, difficulty swallowing, and fever. This type of thyroiditis is usually caused by a bacterial infection—often with staph or strep bacteria. The infection subsequently causes an abscess in the thyroid gland.

If your doctor suspects acute infectious thyroiditis, a number of steps will be taken, including:

- Ultrasound of the thyroid, to determine whether there are any abscesses to be treated. Ultrasound is safe during pregnancy.
- Fine-needle aspiration (FNA) of the mass in your thyroid, and the fluid or material will be cultured to identify infection. FNA is considered safe in pregnancy.
- Blood tests (TSH, Free T4, and Free T3), to evaluate thyroid function and look for signs of infection
- Prescription of an antibiotic medicine that will treat the particular type of infection. (There are antibiotics that are considered safe to take during pregnancy.)
- Drainage of the mass or lump

While most patients respond to drainage and antibiotic treatment, in rare cases, surgical drainage or removal of the gland may be needed, which results in lifelong hypothyroidism. If surgery is needed, it would most likely be performed during the second trimester of pregnancy, or your physician may recommend waiting until after delivery to have the surgery, unless it is an emergency situation.

Postpartum Thyroiditis

Postpartum thyroiditis is one of the more common types of thyroiditis affecting women after pregnancy. The diagnosis and treatment are discussed at length in Chapter 8.

Goiter/Enlarged Thyroid

A slight enlargement of the thyroid is normal during pregnancy. But when the thyroid becomes more significantly enlarged, it's known as goiter. Goiter may not cause any symptoms, and may not even be visible, except on imaging tests. But when goiter is accompanied by symptoms, you may have problems with swallowing, shortness of breath, a hoarse voice, tightness in your throat, coughing, or wheezing. The most obvious symptom of a goiter is a visible swelling, located at the base of your neck.

If a goiter is externally visible or palpable, it can be diagnosed in a clinical examination. But goiter is considered a condition, and not a disease on its own, and is usually the result of another issue that affects the thyroid, including:

- Iodine deficiency
- Hashimoto's disease
- Graves' disease
- Multinodular goiter—where numerous nodules end up causing your gland to enlarge
- A large nodule—that causes the gland to enlarge
- Thyroid cancer
- Thyroiditis

After diagnosing a goiter, the next step for your physician is to determine what is causing the goiter, whether your thyroid levels are within safe ranges for pregnancy, and if there are any other underlying issues that need to be addressed.

Further exploration of goiter can include:

- Blood tests—TSH, Free T4, Free T3, TPOAb, and TSI—to identify whether you are hypothyroid, hyperthyroid, or have Hashimoto's or Graves' disease
- A urinary iodine test—to determine whether you are iodine deficient
- Ultrasound—which can give the doctor a sense of how enlarged the thyroid is, if it contains any nodules, and if it is in a location that could affect breathing or swallowing
- A fine-needle aspiration (FNA) biopsy—which will get a tissue or fluid sample for testing, to identify infection, or other potential causes of goiter

In nonpregnant patients, a radioactive scan is sometimes done to evaluate the thyroid, but these are not done during pregnancy.

The treatment for goiter depends on its underlying cause. A small goiter without any other thyroid hormone imbalances or underlying issues doesn't require treatment. It will typically be monitored during your pregnancy, with regular blood tests and one or more ultrasound tests.

If goiter is the result of an iodine deficiency, the treatment is sufficient iodine in the diet. If the cause of the goiter is autoimmune thyroid disease, such as Hashimoto's, Graves', or other types of thyroiditis, or if any hypothyroidism or hyperthyroidism is found, it will be treated as we explained in previous chapters.

Hoda was in her midtwenties, and being treated for hypothyroidism as a result of Hashimoto's, when she had her first pregnancy. Says Hoda:

> I was noticing some discomfort in my neck, my collars felt tight, and I almost felt like I had a lump in my throat. My doctor was adjusting my dosage of Levoxyl, but at a visit when I was 16 weeks pregnant, I mentioned this neck thing, and the doctor felt my neck, and confirmed that I had developed a goiter. She raised my dose a bit, and also had me get an ultrasound, just to make sure there wasn't anything else going on, and it was fine. It didn't get any bigger the rest of the pregnancy, and I had a healthy baby boy. A few months after I had my son, I noticed that the goiter seemed to go away on its own.

If a goiter is not responding to any of these treatments, is causing pain or movement problems, impairing breathing or swallowing, or is cosmetically unsightly, doctors may recommend surgery to remove all or part of the gland. Even then, unless it's an emergency, surgery to remove the gland would typically be scheduled only in the second trimester, or after delivery. If you have your thyroid surgically removed, you will become hypothyroid and require lifelong thyroid hormone replacement medication.

Nodules/Lumps/Cysts

Thyroid nodules are lumps or cysts located in the gland. They can be fluid-filled or solid.

Most thyroid nodules don't cause any signs or symptoms. Occasionally, if a nodule is very large, you may be able to feel the lump, feel pressure in your neck, or experience shortness of breath or difficulty swallowing.

Nodules can be caused by autoimmune thyroid disease, and when those conditions are present, they are often accompanied by the symptoms of hypothyroidism or hyperthyroidism.

Evaluation and treatment of thyroid nodules depends on the size, characteristics, cause, and symptoms they may be causing. If you have thyroid nodules, it is important to see an endocrinologist with expertise in thyroid disease and thyroid nodules. This is not something that your GP or OB should typically be handling.

For nodules that are not causing physical symptoms, have no suspicious characteristics or cause no concern about the possibility of cancer, and/or have been shown to be benign after biopsy, most doctors recommend monitoring them periodically with ultrasound. If they remain the same size, periodic monitoring continues.

In patients with normal thyroid function or hypothyroidism, there is limited evidence that for some patients, use of higher doses of thyroid hormone medication to suppress thyroid-stimulating hormone (TSH) to the low end of the reference range may shrink nodules, or prevent their growth. This is controversial, however, and experts do not agree on the effectiveness of this approach. It is also not typically recommended during pregnancy.

For a benign cystic (fluid-filled) nodule, one treatment is percutaneous ethanol injection (PEI). In PEI, the nodule is injected with ethanol—sometimes guided by ultrasound. PEI is considered to be effective for these cystic nodules, and some practitioners feel comfortable performing this procedure during pregnancy.

If a benign nodule is affecting breathing or swallowing, or affecting blood vessels, surgical removal of all or part of the thyroid gland may be recommended. Again, in a pregnant woman, this would typically be done in the second trimester, or after delivery.

If a benign thyroid nodule is actually producing thyroid hormones, it is known as a "toxic" nodule, and can cause or worsen a situation of thyrotoxicosis. Radioactive iodine (RAI) treatment is given to nonpregnant patients who have this condition to potentially shrink the gland and nodules. This treatment is not given during pregnancy or breastfeeding, however. (Some good news: several research studies have shown that inadvertent use of RAI prior to 12 weeks of gestation did not appear to damage the fetal thyroid.)

The 2011 "Guidelines of the American Thyroid Association for the Diagnosis and Management of Thyroid Disease During Pregnancy and Postpartum," or Pregnancy Guidelines, suggest that nodules larger than 1 cm should be biopsied, and nodules from 5 mm to 1 cm in size should be biopsied if you have any hereditary thyroid cancer risk or anything suspicious shows up in the ultrasound.

In pregnancy, any hyperthyroidism resulting from your nodules would be treated as described in Chapter 6.

Ablation techniques are used for solid, as opposed to fluid-filled, nodules, and may also be an option for those patients who are not good candidates for surgery. In radiofrequency thermal ablation, a small incision is made after numbing the area, and an electrode is inserted near the nodule, which releases radio waves, creating heat that destroys or shrinks the nodule. In percutaneous laser ablation, after numbing the area and making a small incision, a laser is inserted to directly target the thyroid nodule. We are not aware of any studies that have determined whether this is a safe procedure in pregnancy. You should talk to your endocrinologist about this potential treatment.

The Cancer Risk

Most thyroid nodules are benign, but typically, a small percentage can be cancerous. Thyroid nodules are more common after multiple pregnancies, and thyroid nodules are more likely to increase in size during pregnancy.

While the general risk of a thyroid nodule being malignant is 5 percent, some studies have found that from one in four to one in three nodules found in pregnant women are cancerous. Some experts speculate that pregnancy may speed up the growth of previously cancerous nodules.

Any nodules with suspicious characteristics will typically be biopsied. But given the higher risk of cancer in nodules during pregnancy, we recommend that *any* nodules found during pregnancy be fully evaluated. Evaluation includes thyroid blood work, ultrasound, and if there are any suspicious characteristics or family history of thyroid cancer, a fine-needle aspiration (FNA) biopsy.

In this recommendation we depart from the Pregnancy Guidelines. The guidelines recommend that if nodules are discovered, you should be asked about your family history of benign or malignant thyroid disease and endocrine disorders, previous disease or treatment involving the neck (in particular, any radiation treatments to the head or neck during childhood), as well as when the nodule was detected, and how quickly it is growing. The guidelines further recommend that all women with a thyroid nodule have their TSH and Free T4 measured; that if a woman has a family history of medullary thyroid carcinoma or multiple endocrine neoplasia (MEN) 2, calcitonin levels should also be measured; and that ultrasound be used to determine the features of the nodule, and monitor their growth. They say that if a nodule is less than 10 mm in size, a fine-needle aspiration (FNA) biopsy of the thyroid is not required unless there are suspicious characteristics. We think there are good reasons to be more proactive in evaluating all nodules during pregnancy.

The guidelines do go on to say that, if after you've been given the "all clear" on your nodules, they are growing rapidly, or you have a persistent cough or vocal problems, or a family history of thyroid cancer, FNA should be performed to rule out once again the small possibility of cancer.

Thyroid Cancer

Thyroid cancer, while one of the few cancers whose rates are growing, is still fairly rare, and accounts for only 1.2 percent of all new cancers in the United States annually. According to the American Cancer Society, in 2015 there were around 62,450 new cases of thyroid cancer (47,230 in women, and 15,220 in men), and about 1,950 deaths from thyroid cancer (1,080 women and 870 men). Thyroid cancer is commonly diagnosed at a younger age than most other adult cancers, and around two out of three cases are found in people younger than age fifty-five. Only 2 percent of thyroid cancers occur in children and teens.

Thyroid cancer requires treatment and lifelong monitoring and can have debilitating effects on patients. The survival rates are high, however, with 95 percent of all thyroid cancer patients achieving what would be considered a cure, or long-term survival without reoccurrence.

If your FNA shows thyroid cancer, one of the first steps is to ensure that your practitioner is a thyroid specialist—not just an endocrinologist, but one who has expertise in diagnosing and treating different types of thyroid cancer.

Thyroid Cancer Risk Factors

There are a number of risk factors for thyroid cancer. They include:

- Gender—women are about three times more at risk than men
- A diet low in iodine—in geographic areas of iodine deficiency, follicular thyroid cancers are more common.
- Radiation exposure—whether through early radiation treatments to the head and neck, or exposure to radioactive fallout from nuclear weapons or power plant accidents in childhood or young adulthood
- Heredity—thyroid cancer, and in particular, medullary thyroid cancer, in your family has a genetic component that increases your risk
- A history of Hashimoto's disease, especially untreated

Integrative physician David Brownstein agrees that iodine deficiency is a risk factor for thyroid cancer. According to Dr. Brownstein:

Iodine deficiency is associated with goiter and endocrine cancers such as cancer of the thyroid, ovaries, uterus, breast, prostate and pancreas. I feel the iodine deficiency epidemic we are seeing is, in large part, responsible for the endocrine cancer epidemic we are currently facing. The most common cause of goiter is iodine deficiency, by far. Iodine should be the first item researched for any person having abnormal growths in any endocrine tissues including the thyroid and the breasts.

Thyroid Cancer Signs and Symptoms

Thyroid cancer, especially early in its development, may not cause any symptoms at all. But as a thyroid cancer grows and develops, it is more likely to cause symptoms. Some of the signs and symptoms that may point to thyroid cancer include the following:

- A lump or nodule in the neck—especially in the front of the neck, in the area of the Adam's apple. Sometimes this lump or nodule will grow quickly.
- Enlargement of the neck
- Enlarged lymph nodes in the neck
- Hoarseness, difficulty speaking normally, voice changes

- Difficulty swallowing, or a choking feeling
- Difficulty breathing
- Pain in the neck or throat, including pain from the neck to the ears
- Sensitivity in the neck—discomfort with neckties, turtlenecks, scarves, necklaces
- Persistent or chronic cough not due to allergies or illness
- Asymmetry in the thyroid (big nodule on one side, nothing on the other)

The Thyroid Neck Check

To underscore the importance of early detection, the American Association of Clinical Endocrinologists (AACE) encourages Americans to perform a simple self-exam it calls the "Thyroid Neck Check." Examining your neck can in some cases help you find lumps or enlargements that may point to thyroid conditions, including nodules, goiter, and thyroid cancer.

To detect a thyroid abnormality early, or identify lumps that may indicate potential thyroid cancer, follow these steps to perform your own "Thyroid Neck Check":

1. Stand in front of a mirror
2. Stretch your neck back
3. Swallow water
4. Look for an enlargement in your neck (below the Adam's apple, above the collarbone)
5. Feel the area to confirm enlargement or a bump
6. If any problem is detected, see a doctor.

Note: The "Thyroid Neck Check" is not conclusive. A thorough examination by a physician is needed to diagnose or rule out thyroid cancer.

Testing

As discussed earlier, testing for thyroid cancer during pregnancy typically involves an FNA biopsy, as well as some thyroid blood work, including TSH, Free T4, Free T3, and Tg levels. The radioactive uptake test that is usually done to identify whether nodules are cold, warm, or hot is not done during pregnancy, as it poses a risk to the fetus.

If you have a family history of medullary thyroid carcinoma or multiple endocrine neoplasia (MEN) 2, your calcitonin levels should also be measured.

Papillary and Follicular Cancer

About 80 percent of thyroid cancer is what's known as differentiated thyroid cancer. Most papillary and follicular cancers are differentiated. This means that the cells have not undergone significant changes.

Papillary and follicular cancers are usually the most effectively treated types of thyroid cancer. Treatment for papillary and follicular thyroid cancer depends on the staging of the cancer. For small microcarcinomas that are barely detectable, some doctors are taking a watch and wait approach, with periodic monitoring. But for the most part, when a tumor is smaller, and in the thyroid, and may have spread to the lymph nodes or right outside the thyroid, but no further, the treatment is typically a lobectomy (to remove the affected lobe) or more often a full thyroidectomy to remove the thyroid. If cancer is present in lymph nodes, they will also be surgically removed.

In pregnant women, depending on the size and stage of the cancer, your physician may recommend that you wait until after delivery to have surgery and further treatment. This is considered safe, as these cancers are typically very slow-growing. In this case, your physician will likely prescribe an increased, suppressive dose of thyroid hormone medication to prevent spread of the cancer. You should also have thyroid ultrasounds at least once a trimester to assess for rapid tumor growth, which may indicate a more immediate need for surgery.

Some patients need to follow a low-iodine diet and stay off all thyroid hormone replacement medications for several weeks, and then receive radioactive iodine, which eliminates any remnants of thyroid tissue that could stimulate cancer growth. According to oncologist and thyroid cancer expert, Jochen Lorch, MD:

> RAI after thyroid cancer surgery takes advantage of the fact that these cancer cells are very much like thyroid gland cells that pick up iodine in order to make thyroid hormone. While these tumors usually don't produce any hormone, they still retain their ability to pick up iodine. RAI delivers a targeted form of radiation to the gland, to destroy remaining cells. For RAI treatment to be most effective, your TSH must be well above the normal range, typically above 30. You'll be made significantly hypothyroid in order to allow the TSH to rise, which typically takes from six weeks to two months. At the same time, you follow a low-iodine diet, and take no thyroid hormone replacement medication. For some patients with differentiated cancer, we can avoid putting them through eight weeks of misery off

their thyroid medication, by using recombinant TSH—known as Thyrogen—as an injection prior to their radioiodine treatment. This raises TSH rapidly, and prevents development of hypothyroidism symptoms. The issue is that it can be expensive and frequently is in short supply.

This is followed by thyroid hormone replacement medication treatment, often at "suppressive levels"—designed to keep the TSH low, and prevent any growth or recurrent cancer activity in any remnant thyroid gland.

It is important to note, however, that radioactive iodine treatment is never done in pregnant or breastfeeding women, due to the risks the radiation poses to fetal or infant thyroid health.

There is little research looking at treating metastatic or late-stage papillary and follicular thyroid cancer during pregnancy, so treatment will require careful consultation with your thyroid cancer expert. In the nonpregnant population, for cancers that have spread and are at later stages, or for thyroid cancers that will not take up iodine and are not responsive to RAI, external beam radiation therapy may be done. This therapy uses high-energy beams of radiation, delivered by a machine outside the body, to help treat recurrence or spread.

While most papillary and follicular cancers respond to surgery and RAI, if these treatments are not effective, some drugs, called kinase inhibitors, may block tumor growth and destroy growth-promoting proteins. Oral medications, such as sorafenib (Nexavar) and lenvatinib (Lenvima), are being used in these cases. Other drugs, such as sunitinib (Sutent), pazopanib (Votrient), and vandetanib (Caprelsa), are being studied for possible use.

Chemotherapy is not commonly used, except in advanced thyroid cancers that are unresponsive to hormone therapy and RAI.

Medullary Thyroid Cancer

The treatment for medullary cancer is typically to remove the thyroid and lymph nodes if affected. RAI is not used, as this type of cancer does not take up iodine. For a pregnant woman, the surgery would typically be performed during the second trimester, but based on the staging and aggressiveness of the cancer, the need for immediate surgery may outweigh the risks, and surgery may be recommended and performed any time during the pregnancy. Follow-up with thyroid hormone replacement is necessary.

While there is little research on treating advanced medullary thyroid cancer in pregnancy, in the nonpregnant population, doctors may prescribe vandetanib (Caprelsa) or cabozantinib (Cometriq), oral medications that may help slow the growth of the cancer. The drugs sorafenib (Nexavar) and sunitinib (Sutent) may be tried if vandetanib and cabozantinib are not effective. In rare cases of metastatic medullary thyroid cancer, chemotherapy may also be used.

Anaplastic Thyroid Cancer

Treatment for anaplastic thyroid cancer typically includes a full thyroidectomy. Because this is an aggressive and invasive cancer that may affect the trachea (windpipe), patients may also need a tracheostomy.

External beam radiation therapy, chemotherapy, and clinical trials of new treatment protocols are often recommended, due to the aggressiveness and high mortality rate of this rare type of cancer.

Follow-up

Regular, lifelong follow-up is necessary after thyroid cancer. The entire thyroid is removed as treatment for most thyroid cancers, so almost all thyroid cancer survivors end up hypothyroid, and need to take thyroid replacement hormone for life.

All thyroid cancer patients undergo regular monitoring of thyroid levels via blood test, to make sure that thyroid hormone replacement dose is optimal and that TSH levels are suppressed if necessary. Depending on the type, staging, and progression of the thyroid cancer, follow-up also can include:

- Physical examinations to feel for enlargement or changes in the thyroid area
- Neck ultrasound, to look for any tissue regrowth or cancer recurrence
- RAI scan—this scan is looking for a recurrence of papillary or follicular cancer. In nonpregnant patients, after thyroid surgery, thyroid hormone is withdrawn for around three to six weeks prior to the radioactive iodine scan, to allow for an accurate result. (Or patients are given a one-time shot of Thyrogen, a medication that relieves hypothyroidism symptoms but allows for an accurate scan.) During this period, most patients are also asked to follow a low-iodine diet. (The Thyroid Cancer Survivors' Association [ThyCa] has a free online booklet that describes the diet, with recipes.) After the radioactive iodine scan results are evaluated for any signs of recurrence, patients typically resume their thyroid hormone replacement medication. Note that these scans are never done during pregnancy or while breastfeeding.

- Thyroglobulin (Tg) blood tests—because thyroid cells produce Tg, after surgery, Tg should be low or undetectable. Evidence of Tg cells means that there are still thyroid cells present, and levels that increase may suggest a recurrence of cancer.
- Antithyroglobulin antibodies (TgAb) test—for those cancer patients having Tg testing, TgAb also need to be tested, because they can impair the results—and therefore the validity—of the Tg testing.
- MRI—of the head/neck/chest area—note that gadolinium (not iodine) is typically used for contrast PET/CT scan. A PET scan or CT scan may be done if cancer is suspected but is not showing up on RAI scan or ultrasound. Again, these are not typically done during pregnancy or while breastfeeding.

An excellent resource for information on thyroid cancer treatment and follow-up is the Thyroid Cancer Survivors' Association (ThyCa) (see Appendix A).

Surgery

If thyroid cancer is found, the type of thyroid cancer determines the treatment. For well-differentiated thyroid cancer found during pregnancy, the Pregnancy Guidelines suggest that surgery—known as thyroidectomy—generally be deferred until after delivery. For medullary thyroid cancer, surgery is recommended during pregnancy if there is a large primary tumor, or extensive spread to the lymph nodes. The impact of thyroid surgery during pregnancy has been studied, and generally, if the thyroid surgery is performed during the second trimester, it has not been associated with increased maternal or fetal risk.

Jill S. was diagnosed with papillary cancer when she was in her early thirties and six months pregnant, and her doctor told her she could decide whether to have surgery or wait until after her baby was born:

> I chose surgery. I did not want to have the cancer in my body any longer. To say I was scared was an understatement. I was not only making a decision for my life but for my unborn child as well. I had a total thyroidectomy and some lymph nodes removed. They also found a second cancerous nodule. All went well and my baby was perfectly fine and healthy and so was I. My daughter is now 3 1/2 and she is smart, beautiful and very healthy. I could not be more proud of her.

The guidelines recommend that if surgery for well-differentiated thyroid cancer is being deferred until after delivery, an ultrasound should be performed during each trimester to watch for rapid tumor growth. When there is rapid growth, or there is spread to the lymph nodes, surgery is recommended.

In you have early stage papillary or follicular thyroid cancer and your doctor classifies it as "well-differentiated," you may be offered the opportunity to wait for treatment and surgery until after delivery. These types of cancers are typically very slow-growing, and it's considered safe to wait. However, your doctor will likely recommend that your dosage of thyroid hormone be increased so that you are taking a suppressive dose of medication, keeping your TSH from 0.1 to 1.5 mIU/L at the highest to help prevent spread of the cancer.

Treating Hypothyroidism in Pregnant Thyroid Cancer Survivors

According to the Pregnancy Guidelines, in women who have persistent thyroid cancer, TSH can be maintained below 0.1 mIU/L during pregnancy. In women who are free of thyroid cancer but who had a high risk tumor in the past, suppression should be maintained at TSH levels between 0.1 mIU/L and 0.5 mIU/L. In low-risk patients with no signs of thyroid cancer, TSH can be kept at the lower end of the reference range (0.3–1.5 mIU/L).

Typically, pregnant women who are on thyroid hormone replacement after thyroid cancer require a smaller dose increase compared to women who are hypothyroid due to other disorders. The guidelines recommend that in these women, TSH be monitored every 4 weeks during pregnancy, until 16 to 20 weeks of gestation, and again at least once between 26 and 32 weeks of gestation.

RAI Treatment for Cancer and the Effect on Subsequent Pregnancy

Researchers have not found an increase in infertility, miscarriage, stillbirth, neonatal mortality, congenital malformations, preterm birth, low birth weight, or death during the first year of life after radioactive iodine (RAI) treatment for thyroid cancer in women in their twenties and thirties. There is, however, an increased risk of miscarriage in the months following RAI that can result from insufficient control of thyroid hormones. The Pregnancy Guidelines recommend waiting at least six months after RAI to ensure optimal thyroid management prior to conception.

For some perimenopausal women, RAI can also destabilize hormones, and trigger the onset of menopause.

Pregnancy does not appear to increase the risk for thyroid cancer recurrence in women who have no disease present prior to pregnancy. In women who have any remnant of thyroid cancer, however, either in terms of visible thyroid tissues or elevated thyroglobulin (Tg) levels, pregnancy may stimulate thyroid cancer growth.

If you have had a previously treated differentiated thyroid cancer and undetectable thyroglobulin (Tg) levels, no special monitoring is needed during pregnancy. However, the guidelines recommend an ultrasound during each trimester if you were previously treated for differentiated thyroid cancer and have elevated Tg levels or any evidence of persistent disease.

Postpartum Thyroid Problems

8

Even if you have no history of thyroid problems, the period after childbirth is a time when thyroid problems can start.

Thyroid diagnosis is often associated with periods of hormonal flux, changes to the immune and endocrine system, or periods of physical stress. Pregnancy puts a great strain on your thyroid and adrenal glands. Your immune system also has to make profound changes during pregnancy, to allow a "foreign body"—your baby—to coexist in your body, without attacking or rejecting it. Right after childbirth, you also experience a huge drop in estrogen and progesterone levels. And the sleep deprivation and erratic sleep cycles that affect many new mothers can be especially stressful to your adrenal function and hormones. All of these factors mean that new thyroid conditions may appear during your postpartum period.

If you were diagnosed with a thyroid condition before pregnancy, the many changes that take place during and after pregnancy can destabilize your thyroid function, and fluctuations may occur that change how you feel or the treatment you need.

In this chapter, you'll learn about hypothyroidism/Hashimoto's, hyperthyroidism/Graves', and postpartum thyroiditis that is newly diagnosed after your pregnancy, as well as what to expect in the postpartum period if you are being treated for a thyroid problem during your pregnancy. You will also learn about several postpartum issues—low milk supply, postpartum depression, hair loss, and an inability to lose weight—that can be symptoms of an undiagnosed or insufficiently treated thyroid condition after childbirth.

Hypothyroidism/Hashimoto's

If you were hypothyroid during your pregnancy, in almost all cases, you will continue to be hypothyroid and require treatment after pregnancy. The 2011 "Guidelines of the American Thyroid Association for the Diagnosis

139

and Management of Thyroid Disease During Pregnancy and Postpartum," or Pregnancy Guidelines, recommend that following delivery, your dosage of thyroid hormone replacement be reduced to your prepregnancy dose and rechecked at six weeks postpartum. The guidelines do note, however, that some studies show that more than half the women who have Hashimoto's disease and are on thyroid hormone replacement actually have ended up needing an increased dosage postpartum over the prepregnancy dose, most likely due to worsening of autoimmune thyroid dysfunction after pregnancy. Be aware, therefore, that the guidelines are contradictory. If you are hypothyroid due to Hashimoto's disease, immediately reducing your thyroid dosage after delivery as the guidelines suggest creates a fifty-fifty chance that your thyroid hormone levels will drop, your TSH will increase, and you will become more hypothyroid and symptomatic. Being undertreated after childbirth also puts you at greater risk of hypothyroid-related postpartum symptoms, such as low milk supply, postpartum depression, hair loss, and difficulty losing weight. These issues are discussed at greater length in this chapter.

Integrative physicians recommend having your TSH, Free T4, and Free T3 checked no more than two weeks after delivery, and that any dosage adjustments be made at that time to keep your thyroid levels optimized. Then, get rechecked again no more than eight weeks later, and readjust your thyroid hormone replacement dosage as needed. You should continue to have levels rechecked, and your dosage adjusted, every eight weeks until you are stabilized at optimum thyroid levels.

Integrative physician Richard Shames recommends that after pregnancy, a woman who is hypothyroid due to Hashimoto's disease should have her TSH kept in the lower end of the reference range, around 1.0. According to Dr. Shames: "After years of practice, I saw many women who had a surge of antibodies in the months after childbirth, triggering a variety of postpartum issues, including postpartum depression. Keeping the TSH lower appears to help avoid the risk of this antibody flare-up."

In some cases, you may go through a phase of mild hypothyroidism, with milder symptoms. This is typically associated with postpartum thyroiditis. Postpartum thyroiditis typically resolves on its own over time, and usually does not require treatment, unless you are trying to conceive again. Postpartum thyroiditis is discussed at greater length later in this chapter.

If you had elevated thyroid peroxidase antibodies (TPOAb) before or during your pregnancy, even if your TSH, Free T4, and Free T3 remained within recommended ranges, you are at greater risk of becoming hypothyroid after pregnancy. If you go into the pregnancy with these elevated antibodies, or they are detected during pregnancy, pay close attention to any signs or symptoms of an underactive thyroid after you've given birth.

If you experience any of the following symptoms: fatigue, weight gain (or failure to lose baby weight), depression, constipation, hair loss, or other hypothyroidism symptoms, see your doctor right away to have TSH, Free T4, Free T3, and TPOAb tested. Keep in mind that it is easy for you and even your doctor to assume that these symptoms are "normal" after having a baby. But if you have elevated TPOAb, and you develop symptoms after childbirth, it is essential that you have a comprehensive thyroid workup to look for possible hypothyroidism.

Hyperthyroidism/Graves'

Hyperthyroidism can also appear after childbirth. Most commonly, hyperthyroidism after pregnancy represents the overactive phase of postpartum thyroiditis, a condition discussed in the next section. If that is the case, the hyperthyroidism often resolves itself without treatment, and the thyroid returns to normal. In some cases, this phase can be followed by a period of hypothyroidism, and then again, a return to normal thyroid function.

Women who have had Graves' disease and were treated with antithyroid drugs prior to pregnancy—as well as those who became hyperthyroid after a previous pregnancy—are at greater risk of developing postpartum hyperthyroidism. Statistically, women with Graves' disease who were previously in remission have a higher overall relapse rate—84 percent—after pregnancy, compared to a 56 percent relapse rate in women who have not become pregnant.

If you have preeclampsia during your pregnancy, you should also be aware that this may be a sign that you are at risk of postpartum hyperthyroidism. During Mariah's first pregnancy, she developed preeclampsia and spent seven months on bedrest:

> I was not the same person after I had my son. Five months after I had him I had this huge bulge in my neck. My eyes started to bulge. We made a doctor's appointment, and I was never so scared in my life. I was diagnosed with Graves' disease and hyperthyroidism. I had finally found a great thyroid doctor! We tried antithyroid drugs to try and get my thyroid levels

down, but it wasn't working. Finally almost a year later, I had RAI, and it worked! Now my levels are normal.

Evaluating Postpartum Hyperthyroidism

According to the Pregnancy Guidelines, the challenge of hyperthyroidism that appears after pregnancy is determining whether the overactive thyroid is due to postpartum thyroiditis or to Graves' disease. The two conditions require different treatments and have different outcomes.

To differentiate between the two conditions, the guidelines suggest measuring thyroid-stimulating immunoglobins (TSI), because most women with Graves' disease will test positive for them, but the majority of women with postpartum thyroiditis will not. Doctors will also look for clinical signs of Graves' disease—such as goiter, or thyroid eye symptoms, also called Graves' orbitopathy or Graves' ophthalmopathy. In some cases, doctors may examine radioiodine uptake (RAIU) levels; RAIU will typically be low in postpartum thyroiditis, and higher in Graves' disease.

Radiation can cross over into breast milk, so in women who are breastfeeding, the guidelines recommend that if an RAIU scan is needed, iodine-123 or technetium be used. These two isotopes have short half-lives—versus the longer half-life of iodine-131—and a nursing mother can pump and discard the milk for several days, and then resume breastfeeding.

Treating Hyperthyroidism

The Pregnancy Guidelines recommend that postpartum hyperthyroidism be treated, and that the first choice of treatment should be the antithyroid drug known as methimazole (Tapazole). If you are breastfeeding, doses up to 20 to 30 milligrams a day—taken as divided doses after breastfeeding—are considered safe for you and your baby. The second choice for antithyroid medication after pregnancy is propylthiouracil (known as PTU), at doses up to 300 mg a day. PTU is typically only recommended if you are allergic to methimazole, because PTU is associated with increased risks of liver toxicity.

If you are allergic or sensitive to antithyroid drugs, or your hyperthyroidism does not respond to the medications, your doctor will likely recommend RAI treatment—and less commonly, surgical removal of your thyroid, to permanently slow down your thyroid. The treatment of hyperthyroidism is discussed at greater length in Chapter 6.

Postpartum Thyroiditis

It's common for a new mother to feel tired, experience mood swings, and have a variety of other symptoms in the months after childbirth. But for some women, those symptoms—usually attributed to being a new mother—are actually a sign of a condition known as postpartum thyroiditis. Postpartum thyroiditis is an inflammation of the thyroid that initially occurs in the first year after childbirth, miscarriage, or induced abortion. It's considered a variation of Hashimoto's disease.

Who Is at Risk of Postpartum Thyroiditis?

Any woman who has been pregnant can have postpartum thyroiditis, and the condition is fairly common—approximately 7 percent of women develop it. The risks of developing postpartum thyroiditis are higher for women with the following conditions and thyroid markers:

- Women with type 1 diabetes—up to 25 percent develop postpartum thyroiditis
- Women with elevated antithyroid antibodies, but normal thyroid hormone levels—up to 25 percent
- Women with elevated antithyroid peroxidase antibodies (anti-TPOAb)—up to 50 percent

Postpartum thyroiditis is also far more common in a woman who has had a previous episode of the condition.

The Typical Course of Postpartum Thyroiditis

The most common course for postpartum thyroiditis is mild hypothyroidism, which typically starts around two to six months after delivery. Over time, the thyroid normalizes, and thyroid levels return to normal.

The next most common course starts with mild hyperthyroidism, beginning from around one to four months after delivery. Again, over time, the thyroid normalizes, and levels return to normal.

The least common course starts with mild hyperthyroidism, beginning one to four months after delivery but lasting only around two to eight weeks, which then shifts into mild hypothyroidism, which can last for weeks or months; the thyroid then normalizes over time.

Although some cases of postpartum thyroiditis resolve over time, there is also a strong risk that the postpartum thyroiditis will become chronic thyroid disease. It's estimated that as many as half the patients who experience postpartum thyroiditis will, within four to eight years, develop persistent hypothyroidism, a goiter, or both.

Can Postpartum Thyroiditis Be Prevented?

Some studies have shown that selenium supplementation may help prevent postpartum thyroiditis in women who are positive for TPOAb. One study found specifically that postpartum thyroiditis occurred in 49 percent of a group of TPOAb-positive women who were not supplementing with selenium, versus 29 percent of women who supplemented with 200 mcg daily of selenium. This is a significant difference, and suggests that selenium supplementation started during preconception and continued through pregnancy should be extended throughout the first year after pregnancy.

Symptoms of Postpartum Thyroiditis

A number of symptoms of postpartum thyroiditis can appear during both the hypothyroid and hyperthyroid phases of the condition. These include:

- Decreased milk volume in breastfeeding women
- Hair loss
- Fatigue
- Goiter (an enlarged thyroid gland) that is painless
- Depression, moodiness

The symptoms during the hypothyroid phase of postpartum thyroiditis are milder versions of general hypothyroidism symptoms, including sluggishness, dry skin, difficulty losing weight (or weight gain), constipation, low body temperature, and puffiness in the eyes, face, and hands, among others.

Symptoms during the hyperthyroid phase of postpartum thyroiditis are typically milder versions of general hyperthyroidism symptoms, including anxiety, muscle weakness, irritability, heart palpitations, fast heartbeat, tremor, weight loss, and loose stools or diarrhea.

Diagnosis

Postpartum thyroiditis is usually diagnosed by blood tests. In the hypothyroid phase, TSH is elevated, and T4 is low or low-normal. Antithyroid peroxidase antibody concentrations are likely to be elevated in the majority of postpartum thyroiditis sufferers, especially during the hypothyroid phase. In the hyperthyroid phase, blood tests typically show low TSH and high-normal or elevated T4 and T3. In some cases of postpartum thyroiditis, an ultrasound is performed, and typically will show enlargement of the thyroid gland.

Postpartum thyroiditis and Graves' disease can both cause hyperthyroidism after childbirth. While postpartum thyroiditis is a far more common cause of hyperthyroidism, it is still important that your physician not fail to diagnose Graves' disease if it is present. The main difference is that if you have postpartum thyroiditis, your symptoms will tend to be mild, you are not likely to have much enlargement of your thyroid, and you won't have any of the eye symptoms—such as bulging, stare, or double vision—that are more common in Graves'.

In some cases, a radioiodine uptake test is done to differentiate postpartum thyroiditis from Graves' disease. (Note, however, that this test is not done if you are breastfeeding, to avoid exposing your infant to radiation, which can damage the baby's thyroid gland.)

Treatment

For some women, no treatment is necessary for postpartum thyroiditis, as the hypothyroidism or hyperthyroidism is mild, symptoms are not debilitating, and the condition resolves on its own.

According to the Pregnancy Guidelines, antithyroid drugs are not typically recommended for the hyperthyroid period of postpartum thyroiditis. If you have significant hyperthyroidism symptoms, however, your doctor may prescribe a beta-blocker. The guidelines recommend propranolol, at the lowest possible dose to relieve symptoms. Propranolol is also considered to be safe while breastfeeding, because only low levels are found in breast milk, and it doesn't appear to cause any negative effects in breastfed infants. The guidelines recommend that after the hyperthyroid phase, TSH should be monitored every two months until one year postpartum, to screen for hypothyroidism.

If you are in the hypothyroid phase of postpartum thyroiditis and have severe symptoms, or if you are planning to try to get pregnant again, the guidelines recommend that you be treated with thyroid hormone replacement medication. If you have no symptoms, but are in the hypothyroid phase of postpartum thyroiditis, the guidelines recommend that you have your TSH rechecked every four to eight weeks until the thyroid normalizes. The integrative thyroid experts disagree, however, and recommend that you should have a more complete thyroid panel—including TSH, Free T4, and Free T3—rechecked every four to eight weeks, and that if your thyroid levels are not optimal and you are symptomatic, treatment should be considered.

Common Challenges

The time after pregnancy is a time when some women first develop signs and symptoms of a thyroid problem. Postpartum depression, breastfeeding difficulties and issues, hair loss after childbirth, and weight loss challenges after childbirth can all be signs that a new mother has an undiagnosed thyroid condition.

If you are already being treated for hypothyroidism, you still may experience these same challenges after pregnancy, and they are more likely if your treatment is not optimal.

Postpartum Depression

Depression after childbirth—called perinatal depression, or postpartum depression, abbreviated as PPD—is far more common than most people realize. It's estimated that from 15 to 17 percent of women experience some significant PPD. Women who have tested positive previously for thyroid peroxidase antibodies (TPOAb) face a higher risk of PPD.

The symptoms of PPD include:

- A lack of interest in your baby
- A lack of maternal feelings toward your baby
- Not feeling that "bonded" connection that everyone else seems to have
- Changes in your appetite—either eating more or less than usual, with associated weight gain/loss
- Difficulty sleeping; insomnia

- Sleeping more than usual
- Feelings of anger and irritability
- Feeling easily frustrated, especially about minor issues
- Feeling out-of-control rage, including over small, insignificant things
- Crying frequently
- Feelings of intense sadness
- Feelings of hopelessness and guilt
- Feeling guilty every time your baby cries
- Wondering what the point is of having a baby
- Thinking perhaps it was not a good idea to become a mother
- Thoughts of harming yourself or your baby
- A fear of being alone with the baby
- Thinking, "It would be better if this baby had not been born."
- Loss of interest or pleasure in things that you used to enjoy, such as reading, cooking, or hobbies
- Lack of interest in family time or family outings
- Excessive worries about your baby's health
- Constant fears that your baby isn't breathing
- Obsessive thinking—such as "Is the oven off?" or "Is the door locked?"—that interferes with your daily life

These symptoms can start as early as immediately after childbirth and continue—or appear—up to around a year after your baby is born.

> **IMPORTANT**: If you are having any thoughts of hurting yourself or hurting your baby, GET HELP IMMEDIATELY! Call 911, a suicide hotline, your doctor, a minister, rabbi, priest, or a child abuse prevention hotline. Take this very seriously! You can get help for how you feel, and any one of these resources will be able to help you.

Caring for a new baby is stressful, and like most new mothers, you may understandably be tired, anxious, and irritable. Experiencing some of these symptoms for a short period of time is common—it's known as the postpartum blues. But if you are regularly experiencing some of these symptoms for more than two weeks—and certainly if you have any thoughts at any point about harming yourself or the baby—you should immediately seek medical attention for treatment of PPD. The first year of your baby's life is far too important for you to spend it in a fog of sadness and depression, much less risk your life, or that of your child.

In addition to new and untreated thyroid conditions, and treated thyroid problems that require a dosage adjustment, there are other risk factors for developing PPD, including:

- Having type 1, type 2, or gestational diabetes
- A personal or family history of depression, anxiety, or postpartum depression
- A history of PMS or PMDD (premenstrual dysphoric disorder)
- Having had pregnancy or birth complications
- Experiencing difficulties with breastfeeding
- Having twins or other multiple births
- Having an infant who required treatment in the neonatal intensive care unit after delivery
- Having a pregnancy after infertility treatment
- Lack of support in caring for your baby
- Low confidence in your own ability to parent
- Having family members who express low confidence in your ability to parent
- Going through a major life stress or trauma—such as a job change, job loss, relocation, death of a loved one, financial stress, or marital stress—during pregnancy or after childbirth
- Not getting enough sleep

Treatment

First, if you are experiencing symptoms of PPD, it's important that you contact your doctor right away. Don't minimize the importance of getting help or delay treatment.

If you do not have a diagnosed thyroid condition, but are experiencing postpartum depression, the depression may actually be a sign of a thyroid condition not yet diagnosed. Our recommendation is that you start by having your physician test TSH, Free T4, Free T3, and TPOAb, and if your thyroid levels are not optimal, pursue treatment, as discussed earlier in the book.

If you are already on thyroid hormone replacement treatment, and are having signs of postpartum depression, that may indicate that your thyroid is not optimized. If you haven't already, this is a good time to get in to your doctor and have a check of your TSH, Free T4, and Free T3. If your thyroid levels are not optimized, pursue thyroid treatment as discussed earlier in the book.

If your thyroid levels are optimal, but you are still experiencing postpartum depression, you may want to have other hormones checked, specifically, progesterone levels. After delivery, levels of estrogen and progesterone plummet, and some women experience depression when levels of progesterone are very low. If that is the case for you, supplemental progesterone may help with your PPD symptoms.

If there are no other hormonal issues to address, talk to your doctor about counseling. Counseling is usually recommended for most cases of PPD, and can help with emotional support as well as goal setting and problem solving. If PPD is mild, counseling alone may be enough to help. Your doctor can recommend a licensed counselor trained in treating PPD. Feeling comfortable with the counselor is a must.

If you have moderate to severe PPD, your doctor or counselor will probably prescribe an antidepressant drug. If antidepressants are warranted, counseling should be used in conjunction to ensure the best outcome. Antidepressants are typically used for at least six months, sometimes longer. Most doctors recommend a year prior to tapering off the medicine, both to treat the PPD and then to prevent a relapse. If you are breastfeeding, talk to your doctor about the safety of continuing to breastfeed while taking the specific drug and dosage recommended.

Make sure that you are continuing with your omega-3 fatty acids and methylfolate supplementation. Some studies have shown that they may help with PPD.

Some other approaches that may help include the following:

- Parent coaching, which can help you feel more confident with baby care and your transition into parenthood
- Support groups—both in-person and online—where you can share experiences, and get support and understanding
- Learning and practicing infant massage, which can help you bond with your baby
- Regular exercise, which can help balance hormones and increase serotonin and dopamine, improving mood
- Stress reduction activities, such as meditation, gentle yoga, or breathing, to reduce your overall stress levels.
- Daily sunlight exposure, to help with mood and energy.

When you have PPD, it's also very helpful to ask for, and get, as much support and help as possible from your family and friends. In some cases, paid help with household tasks or childcare, or even a teenage mother's helper, can also be useful for women with PPD.

Rebecca's story is a classic case of PPD. She was being treated for hypothyroidism, and had such low milk supply with her first baby that she ended up having to use formula. The second time she became pregnant, Rebecca had twins:

As with my first baby, I had very low milk supply. I was depressed that I was failing as a mother—breastfeeding is so important, right? The twins were also not sleeping more than an hour at a time, and never at the same time. With my first baby, by 8 weeks, she was sleeping from 9 p.m. to 6 a.m. No matter what we tried, the twins would not settle into a routine. This time around, I had a little more help from my husband, my mom, and mother-in-law, but I just couldn't pull myself together. I was afraid that if I asked for too much help, I would look like a failure. One especially bad day, when the girls were about four months old, I put them into our minivan, and drove off, with my mom yelling at me not to leave—I was in no shape to be driving. I had just been sobbing over the fact that I was exhausted and that they never stopped crying. I obviously was a horrible mother, even though they were thriving at their well-baby checkups. Unfortunately, I was falling apart. I remember listening to them scream from their car seats, and as I looked at the oncoming bridge overpass I thought, *If I just turn my wheels a little to the right, this could all be over*. A voice in my head told me "Don't. Rachel—my older daughter—is not here and you CAN'T leave her without a mother!" Something in me snapped and I didn't turn the wheel. Instead, I cautiously got off of the freeway and drove home. I got the girls inside the house, and immediately called my GP and told her I needed help. I went in for a checkup and she told me she was pretty sure I was suffering from postpartum depression, and we agreed that I would try Zoloft (an antidepressant). I was also extremely sleep deprived, so she told me I had to get help at home too. We ended up hiring a postpartum doula who specialized in twins and multiples, and after only a few visits—that was all we could afford—she had the girls sleeping for a few hours at a time (swaddling—who knew?). Not only that, but she also taught me to set up all the bottles at night so all I had to do was grab them and go during those 2 a.m. feedings. Plus, she told me how truly exhausting it was to care for multiples. I had gone into the pregnancy thinking I'd done it once before with one—how hard could two be? Much. It took a long time for both of the twins to sleep through the night (they were two years old!), but eventually I was able to wean myself off of Zoloft, with my doctor's blessing. That was a time I'd never wish on anyone, or want to relive. Again, as with my issues with breastfeeding, not one doctor told me my Hashimoto's could have anything to do with my exhaustion or depression.

Breastfeeding Difficulties and Issues

There's no question that for the benefit of your baby, breast milk is considered superior to formula. Breastfed infants reportedly have fewer infections, lower rates of obesity later in life, and better overall health in general. Breastfeeding also helps reduce your own risk of breast cancer, and may help you return to your prepregnancy weight more quickly.

After the birth of your baby, one of the challenges that you may face when trying to breastfeed is low milk supply. Low milk supply is often the reason a woman gives up trying to breastfeed entirely.

If your newborn isn't gaining weight after the first week, and isn't having the requisite number of soiled and wet diapers each day, he or she might not be getting enough milk due to low milk supply. Some specific signs that you have low milk supply include:

- Your baby fusses, or continues to root for the breast, after nursing
- Your baby is using less than 5 to 6 soaking-wet disposable diapers (7 to 8 cloth diapers) per day
- Your baby is having fewer than 2 to 5 yellow, runny bowel movements each day in the first month. (After that point, your baby may normally cut down to one bowel movement a day, even a few times each week.)
- Your baby fails to gain about 0.5 ounce a day.

The hormone prolactin is responsible for the production of breast milk. It is stimulated by thyrotropin-releasing hormone (TRH), which in turn also stimulates TSH. When your levels of TRH are low, as they frequently are in hypothyroid women, prolactin is insufficient, and as a result, you may have difficulty producing enough breast milk to nourish your baby. Still, a thyroid condition doesn't prevent breastfeeding. Many women who are hypothyroid, for example, and optimized on thyroid hormone replacement, can successfully breastfeed. Being hyperthyroid also does not prevent breastfeeding in most cases.

If you do not have a diagnosed thyroid condition, but are experiencing low milk supply, it may be a sign that you have an undiagnosed thyroid condition. Our recommendation is that you start by seeing your physician and testing your TSH, Free T4, Free T3, and TPOAb, and if your thyroid levels are not optimized, pursue treatment, as discussed earlier in the book.

This was the case for Emma, who struggled to breastfeed, and didn't realize her thyroid could be the cause:

> Everything was good for the first 3 days. But when my milk was supposed to come in, it didn't. I would sit there feeding for half an hour swapping sides and still when I stopped, she would scream! At the end of the week, I had sat there for a few hours at a time, feeding my baby and only giving in to formula at night, when my husband brought it to me for a break. We all get a bit hormonal in those first few weeks but this was something else. My baby had a perfect latch, and I wasn't sore, but it didn't seem to be enough. But I was consumed with guilt. The midwife came to see me and I was hiding the formula bottles. I didn't understand. One day, I was feeding my baby and realized I had been sitting there for 5 hours! Just ridiculous. I tried medications, but was never able to breastfeed exclusively. Months later, I was diagnosed with thyroid problems. There is such a stigma attached to feeding babies. Health care professionals push "Breast is best," but if they are going to do that, they should at least know what to test for when it doesn't happen!

If you are already on thyroid hormone replacement treatment, and have a low milk supply, that may be a sign that your thyroid is not optimized. If you haven't already, this is a good time to get in to your doctor and have a check of your TSH, Free T4, and Free T3. If your thyroid levels are not optimized, pursue thyroid treatment as discussed earlier in the book. This may help you restore your milk supply to normal levels.

Thyroid Hormone Replacement and Breastfeeding

One of the common questions about breastfeeding with hypothyroidism is whether you should continue taking your thyroid hormone replacement drugs when you're breastfeeding. New mothers are warned about the dangers of taking various drugs while breastfeeding, and for that reason, some women may be concerned or confused about whether that applies to thyroid hormone replacement drugs.

When provided in proper dosage level, thyroid hormone drugs cross into breast milk in only minute quantities and have no adverse effect on the baby. In fact, treatment and maintenance of optimal thyroid function are essential for you to successfully breastfeed. If you take too much thyroid hormone, however, excess thyroid hormone can pass into your breast milk and negatively affect your baby. For this reason, take medication only as prescribed by your physician, and have periodic testing—usually at least every three months—while breastfeeding to ensure that you are not overmedicated.

Radioactive Scans While Breastfeeding

Radioactive thyroid scans using iodine—sometimes used to help diagnose Graves' disease and thyroid cancer—cannot be done while you are breastfeeding. The radioactive iodine can show up in your breast milk for weeks, concentrate in your baby's thyroid, and cause damage to the baby's gland. Graves' disease and hyperthyroidism will need to be diagnosed using blood tests, ultrasound, and clinical examinations.

If a scan absolutely needs to be done, experts recommend that radioactive technetium be used, instead of radioactive iodine. Technetium has a short half-life of six hours. So half the technetium leaves your body within six hours, and all of it is gone within thirty hours. If you are breastfeeding, you can "pump and dump"—pump milk and dispose of it—for the thirty hours after the technetium injection. After that point, you can safely resume breastfeeding.

Antithyroid Drugs and Breastfeeding

It's not common for a woman who is being treated with antithyroid drugs to deliberately plan a pregnancy, and doctors recommend that you be in remission—or have a more permanent treatment such as RAI or surgery—before attempting to conceive. However, the period after having a new baby is a time when some women's symptoms of Graves' disease and hyperthyroidism first appear. If you develop symptoms postpartum, and are diagnosed with hyperthyroidism/Graves' disease—or have a recurrence after previously being in remission—your doctor will likely recommend that you take antithyroid drugs.

In the past, women taking antithyroid drugs were told to completely avoid breastfeeding. In recent years, doctors have become less concerned, and have prescribed either the drug methimazole or propylthiouracil, called PTU. PTU used to be the preferred drug while breastfeeding, but recent studies comparing the various risks on both mother and baby of different antithyroid drugs while breastfeeding have caused experts to switch to methimazole as the preferred drug. In particular, PTU poses a potential risk for liver damage.

Generally, women with hyperthyroidism who are using methimazole should not be discouraged from breastfeeding, because the benefits to the baby considerably outweigh the very minimal risk posed to the baby by the small amount of methimazole that crosses into the breast milk. Daily doses of methimazole should not exceed 30 mg per day. If you are a nursing mother taking methimazole, the guidelines do recommend that your dosages of medication be divided and taken at times of day that occur after you've breast-fed. It is also recommended that your baby be periodically screened—ideally, every three months—for thyroid dysfunction.

Other Approaches

If you've ensured that your thyroid treatment is optimized, and are still having low milk supply issues, your next step is to get professional breastfeeding advice. A certified lactation consultant can check the baby's latch on to the nipple, offer ideas about various nursing positions, and suggest other ways to help you increase your milk supply. You can find a certified lactation consultant at your hospital, a birthing center, or through a recommendation from your OB or pediatrician. You may also wish to contact your local La Leche League, and/or attend a local La Leche meeting, as this organization may be able to provide advice and support in your efforts to successfully breastfeed.

A few additional tips to help milk supply:

- Stay well hydrated. You need to drink a fair amount of liquid—ideally water—to help maintain and increase your milk production.
- The more times you breastfeed, the more milk your body is stimulated to produce, and so frequency of nursing helps maintain and increase milk supply.
- You can practice switch nursing, also called "burp and switch nursing." With this method, you allow the baby to feed on one breast until he or she lessens in intensity and gets sleepy. Then switch her or him to the other breast. Try to make sure that the baby nurses twice at each breast during each feeding. This method can help increase milk production.
- You can also try double feeding—where you nurse your baby until he or she is satisfied; keep the baby upright and awake; burp, and 10 to 20 minutes later, nurse again. This technique can help increase your milk production.
- Try skin-to-skin contact with your baby during breastfeeding, which reportedly helps stimulate the let-down of milk.
- Pump. Even if you are breastfeeding, pumping milk can help increase milk supply. Some women pump for a few minutes after every feeding, to help stimulate increased milk production. You may also want to pump between nursing sessions to help increase supply. If your baby is unable to effectively nurse from the breast, you can also pump and give the milk to the baby using a bottle or dropper, to make sure your baby gets the benefits of breast milk.

Galactagogues

You can talk to your pediatrician or physician about the drug metoclopramide (Reglan). Metoclopramide is a galactagogue, a drug that helps increase milk production. If your doctor prescribes this drug, the typical dose is 10 to 15 mg, three times a day, and it's usually taken for no more than four weeks.

You can also talk to your physician, lactation consultant, nutritionist, or herbalist about herbal galactagogues. Some of the most common herbal galactagogues include:

- Fenugreek—available in capsule form, or as a tea, which is not quite as potent as the capsules. The typical dose is 2 to 3 capsules (580–610 mg each), taken three times daily. Some women achieve results quite rapidly—often in as little as a day or two, while others report a longer waiting period, or no effect on milk supply.
- Blessed thistle—which herbalists say stimulates blood flow to the breast. The tincture form is preferred, and as many as 20 drops, two to four times a day, is said to be the best dose for increasing milk production. (Note: Do not use blessed thistle if you are allergic to plants in the daisy family, and do not go over the recommended dose, as overdosing can cause nausea and vomiting.)
- Alfalfa—sometimes recommended as a galactagogue, either by itself or in combination with fenugreek and blessed thistle

When You Need to Use Formula

If you want to breastfeed and are unable to produce enough milk, you may have to supplement with formula, or use formula exclusively. Please don't feel guilty, or inadequate, or that you are not doing your best for your baby!

If you do use infant formula, make sure that you use one that has supplemental DHA. Also, many integrative experts recommend that soy formula only be used if your baby is allergic to every other form and brand of formula, due to concerns about the hormonal effects of an all-soy diet on infants. (It's interesting to note that in some countries, soy formula is restricted, available only by prescription, and is only prescribed when a baby cannot tolerate any of the other formulas available.)

Hair Loss

It's common in the weeks and months after pregnancy to have a larger-than-usual amount of hair loss. Many women experience an increase in hair volume and growth while pregnant, and the hormonal changes after delivery can then trigger loss of that extra hair. So, some heavier shedding of hair after childbirth is normal, and can be expected.

Significant hair loss, however—typically defined as more than 150 to 200 hairs per day—and/or loss of the hair on the outer edge of the eyebrows can be signs of a thyroid imbalance.

If you do not have a diagnosed thyroid condition, but are experiencing an unusual amount of hair loss after childbirth, or your eyebrows are thinning, it may be a sign of an undiagnosed thyroid condition. Our recommendation is that you start by seeing your physician and having TSH, Free T4, Free T3, TPOAb, and ferritin tests, to start, and if your thyroid and ferritin levels are not optimized, pursue treatment, as discussed earlier in the book.

Note: If you are experiencing hair loss, your ferritin levels should be at about the 80th percentile of the reference range at your lab. Lower levels can contribute to or trigger hair loss.

If you are already on thyroid hormone replacement treatment and are having heavy hair loss, that may be a sign that your thyroid is not optimized. If you haven't already, this is a good time to go to your doctor and check your TSH, Free T4, Free T3, and ferritin levels. If your thyroid and ferritin levels are not optimized, pursue thyroid treatment and iron supplementation, as discussed earlier in the book.

If your thyroid and ferritin levels are optimal, but you are still experiencing heavy hair loss, there are some other things you can do:

- Add a hair vitamin—a good hair vitamin may help calm down hair loss over time, and even start to encourage regrowth. One brand that we recommend is Cooper Complete Dermatologic Formula.
- Add an evening primrose oil supplement—at levels of around 1,500 mg a day, the oil can help slow down hormonal imbalances that contribute to rapid hair loss. Most experts consider evening primrose oil to be safe to use while breastfeeding, but there has not been a great deal of research on the use of this supplement while breastfeeding. It's best to discuss this with your physician before use.
- Use minoxidil (Rogaine)—this topical treatment, available over the counter, may help calm down your hair loss. While it's not thought to be a danger to nursing mothers, it does pass into breast milk, and you probably ought to avoid it if you are breastfeeding. **Note: The prescription hair-loss drug finasteride (Propecia) should never be used during**

pregnancy, or while breastfeeding, because of its ability to cause birth defects in a fetus, and health problems for your baby.

- Try lysine supplements—one study found that 90 percent of women with thinning hair were deficient in iron and the amino acid lysine. Lysine is the most difficult amino acid to get enough of via diet. Lysine helps transport iron, which is the most important element in the body and essential for many metabolic processes. When lysine and iron levels are low, the body switches some hair follicles off to increase levels elsewhere. Meat, fish, and eggs are the only food sources of lysine, but if you are experiencing hair loss, consider taking a lysine supplement. Lysine is considered safe during pregnancy.

A comprehensive listing of supplements and other approaches that can help with hair loss can be found in the book *Hair Loss Master Plan* by Mary Shomon and Brent Hardgrave.

If you continue to have significant hair loss, it's time to see a dermatologist who is experienced in hair loss. A good dermatologist can run additional tests that may identify the causes.

Weight Loss Challenges

It's common in the weeks and months after pregnancy to find it hard to lose the baby weight. Most women are not like celebrities, who are back to a size 2 when their babies are just a few weeks old—maybe with the help of full-time trainers, nannies, and unhealthful diet regimes! For the rest of us, there's a saying—it takes nine months to get there, and nine months to get it off.

Unfortunately, even that may not be true for women with an undiagnosed or undertreated thyroid condition. A complete inability to lose weight after childbirth, or postpartum weight gain despite a healthy diet and exercise, can be signs of a thyroid imbalance.

If you are dealing with stubborn weight challenges after pregnancy, it may be a sign that you have an undiagnosed thyroid condition. Our recommendation is that you start by seeing your physician, checking your TSH, Free T4, Free T3, TPOAb, and fasting glucose, to start, and if your levels are not optimized, pursue treatment, as discussed earlier in the book. If you are diagnosed with hypothyroidism, you may also want to get a copy of Mary Shomon's *Thyroid Diet Revolution* to provide more detailed guidance on how to successfully lose weight.

If you are already on thyroid hormone replacement treatment and are having weight issues, that may be a sign that your thyroid is not optimized. If you haven't already, this is a good time to get in to your doctor and have a check of your TSH, Free T4, and Free T3, to start. If your thyroid levels are not optimized, pursue thyroid treatment as discussed earlier in the book.

Other Hormones

Once your thyroid is optimized, if you still continue to gain weight, or are failing to lose weight with proper diet and exercise, integrative physician Kent Holtorf recommends that you have two key hormones—leptin and Reverse T3—checked, due to their important role in regulating weight and metabolism. According to Dr. Holtorf:

> Leptin is secreted by fat cells, and the levels of leptin increase with the accumulation of fat. The increased leptin secretion that occurs with increased weight normally feeds back to the hypothalamus as a signal that there are adequate energy (fat) stores. This stimulates the body to burn fat rather than continue to store excess fat, and stimulates thyroid-releasing hormone (TRH) to increase thyroid-stimulating hormone (TSH) and thyroid production. Studies are finding, however, that the majority of overweight individuals who are having difficulty losing weight have varying degrees of leptin resistance, where leptin has a diminished ability to affect the hypothalamus and regulate metabolism. This leptin resistance results in the hypothalamus sensing starvation, so multiple mechanisms are activated to increase fat stores, as the body tries to reverse the perceived state of starvation.

For elevated leptin levels, Dr. Holtorf in some cases recommends medications, such as metformin, which are used to increase insulin sensitivity in type 2 diabetes. When Reverse T3 is elevated, he typically recommends that T3 be included in the thyroid treatment, if it is not already being taken, or the dosage increased.

You should also consider having your physician check for signs of elevated blood sugar and insulin resistance by testing your fasting glucose and hemoglobin A1C. Insulin resistance can make weight loss difficult or impossible. A knowledgeable integrative physician, nutritionist, or endocrinologist can work with you to help reverse insulin resistance.

Other Key Recommendations

There are other things that you can do to help promote weight loss.

- Get enough sleep. That's easy enough to say when you're a new mother! But sufficient sleep is a crucial factor for weight loss. One study showed that women who slept 5 hours per night were 32 percent more likely to experience major weight gain (an increase of 33 pounds or more) and 15 percent more likely to become obese over the course of the 16-year study, compared to those who slept 7 hours a night.

- Increase your movement. One important way is to build muscle. Muscle cells are up to eight times more metabolically active than fat cells, and muscle burns more calories than fat. Adding weight-bearing or resistance exercise, such as weightlifting or exercise bands, to your regular workout is one of the only known ways to increase your metabolism, which can be lower than normal in women who are being treated for hypothyroidism. You should also increase your aerobic activity. Aerobic exercise that increases your heart rate can raise your metabolism while you're exercising. Some experts believe that aerobic exercise also boosts resting metabolism for several hours, as muscles burn calories to recover and repair themselves.

- Stay hydrated. Dehydration can contribute to an inefficient metabolism by affecting your body temperature and slowing detoxification. When you are dehydrated, your body temperature drops slightly, and causes your body to store fat as a way to help raise or maintain the temperature. Make sure you drink enough liquids, from 0.5 to 1 ounce of water for every pound of body weight, per day, to avoid this metabolic pitfall.

- Timed eating. Limit yourself to two to three meals a day and avoid snacks. Also, avoid eating after eight p.m. These changes can help lower leptin levels, and shift the body into fat-burning mode.

- Practice mindfulness when eating. Eating while under stress encourages fat storage. You can try taking three deep cleansing breaths before each meal and snack, as well as a deep breath between bites. Eat slowly and chew your food thoroughly. Also, don't multitask while eating—don't eat standing up, in your car, while reading, watching TV, nursing your baby, or while talking on the phone.

- Increase your fiber intake. Getting a good amount of fiber is one of the basic, effective tactics thyroid patients can employ to foster weight loss. Fiber has so many benefits for people with hypothyroidism who are trying to lose weight, and it can come from food, supplements, or both. One tip is to use psyllium capsules, taken with each meal, to ensure that you are getting a regular dose of fiber. Keep in mind, however, that you should take any fiber supplements only two to three hours after or before taking your thyroid medication. And if you start a high-fiber diet or supplement regimen, you should have your thyroid rechecked, since major changes in fiber intake can affect thyroid medication absorption rates.

Dietary Changes

Some additional dietary changes to consider include the following:

- Consider switching to a gluten-free diet. Many people find that gluten-free eating makes weight loss easier.
- Consider a low-glycemic/carbohydrate-controlled diet to balance blood sugar. One diet whose guidelines you can get, free on the web, is the healthy, anti-inflammatory, carbohydrate-controlled Rosedale Diet. It has been shown to lower blood sugar levels, lower cholesterol, and help with weight loss. You can also explore other doctor-developed balanced diets recommended to lower blood sugar and combat insulin resistance.
- Avoid any foods that you are allergic to, which may include common allergens, such as dairy, eggs, nuts, and other common food triggers.
- Eat sufficient protein (poultry, meat, fish, and eggs). If you are a vegetarian or vegan, you should consider consulting with a good nutritionist to determine the best way to get sufficient protein and still lose weight.
- Minimize or eliminate processed foods, refined sugars, refined carbohydrates, and high-fructose corn syrup.
- Minimize or eliminate sweets and desserts, including soft drinks.
- Minimize or eliminate honey, molasses, and all forms of sugar, including fruits. For some people, even fruit needs to be limited to several servings a week, and then, the lower-sugar fruits, such as berries, are recommended.
- Eat anti-inflammatory dietary fats (fatty fish, avocados, olives, olive oil).
- Take a daily probiotic supplement and eat probiotic-rich foods (kombucha, miso, kimchi, yogurt, kefir, sauerkraut).
- Avoid high-carb foods, such as grains, legumes (beans or peas), vegetables high in carbs, sugars, or starch (corn and most root vegetables, such as potatoes, carrots, beets).
- Eliminate diet drinks and the use of artificial sweeteners.
- Minimize or eliminate caffeine.
- Don't drink excessive alcohol.

For a comprehensive look at losing weight with hypothyroidism, we recommend you read Mary Shomon's book *Thyroid Diet Revolution*.

Your Healthy Pregnancy Plans from Preconception to Postpartum

How To Use Part 3:
Your Healthy Pregnancy Plans

We have designed Part 3 of this book as a set of stand-alone chapters that provide you with the essential action steps to take right now on your path to a healthy baby, given the particular thyroid condition or disease you have. If you wish to read an in-depth description of the science and rationale behind the action plans we've included in this section, you can refer back to Part 2.

If you are currently pregnant and reading this book, we do recommend that you nevertheless read Chapter 9 on preconception as well, because many of the tips are important during pregnancy too.

Our hope is that every person reading this book will read Chapter 9 and then read the chapter in Part 3 specific to her type of thyroid disease. Chapter 13 is devoted to postpartum health. Those struggling with infertility despite taking all the necessary steps to get thyroid healthy should also read Chapter 14.

9

Preconception

No matter what type of thyroid disease you have, there are certain common factors to consider and steps to take when you are considering pregnancy.

1. Choosing a Doctor

Find an integrative physician to manage your thyroid care. Integrative physicians are medical doctors (MDs), naturopathic doctors (NDs), or osteopathic physicians (DOs) who use both conventional and holistic/alternative approaches to help you achieve optimal health. The goal is to find a healthcare practitioner who treats you as a whole person and considers all the options for you. See Appendix A for resources to help you locate a good thyroid doctor.

Once you get pregnant, you will also need to find an obstetrician (OB) to monitor your pregnancy and deliver your baby.

2. Identify Your Fertile Window

Identify your fertile window, the days in your menstrual cycle when you are most likely to conceive. The number of days will vary. The fertile window is generally described as the five days before ovulation and the day of ovulation, though the fertile window is actually narrower in most cases; the majority of pregnancies occur during three days of the cycle: the two days before ovulation and the day of ovulation.

Watch for these three major fertility signs to identify your fertile window:

- At your most fertile your cervical fluid will become wet and slippery, like egg white.

- Your waking basal body temperature will typically range from about 97° to 97.5°F, with postovulatory temperatures rising to about 97.6°F and higher. The temperature shift is a good sign of ovulation.
- Your cervix's position will become soft, high, open, and wet around ovulation.

Watch also for secondary fertility signs as ovulation approaches. These may include "mittelschmerz" (a dull pain from follicular swelling or a sharp pain when the egg breaks through the ovary's wall), ovulatory spotting, increased libido, abdominal bloating, swollen vulva, and breast tenderness.

Such devices as OPKs (ovulation prediction kits) or fertility monitors may also help determine ovulation.

Have intercourse often during your fertile window. The missionary position is typically considered optimal when you are trying to conceive.

After intercourse, remain lying down for ten to twenty minutes, to give the sperm enough time to swim into the cervix rather than leaking out. Place a pillow under your hips to elevate your pelvis to maximize the effects of gravity.

Since sexual lubricants can affect sperm motility, if extra moisture is needed, use the Pre-Seed brand of lubricant, which will not limit or harm sperm like other sexual lubricants.

Avoid scented tampons, scented pads, vaginal sprays, and douches.

3. Chart Your Cycles

Use free or fee-based online services and apps to chart your cycle, or use the one we provide on our website at http://www.ThyroidPregnancyBook.com. Here are steps to chart your cycles manually. A blank chart is included in Appendix D.

Fertility expert Toni Weschler offers these instructions on how to chart your cycle:

1. Take your temperature first thing upon awakening, before you perform any other activities, such as drinking, talking on the phone, or getting up to use the bathroom.
2. You should take your temperature at about the same time every morning, give or take about an hour.
3. If using a digital thermometer, wait until it beeps, usually about a minute. Some women may prefer to leave it in another minute beyond to be absolutely sure it reflects your correct temperature.

4. Take your temperature orally. (If you find that you don't get a clear temperature pattern, you may want to switch to taking it vaginally. Just be aware that it's important to be consistent and always take it the same way throughout the cycle because vaginal temps tend to be higher than oral temps.)

5. Record your temperatures on a fertility chart specifically designed for recording temps and cervical fluid.

6. If your temperatures don't reflect an obvious thermal shift, you will want to draw a coverline—a horizontal line marking a temperature rise of at least two tenths of a degree above the highest temperature in the cluster of the preceding six temperatures. Highlight the last six temperatures before the rise and draw a coverline one tenth above the highest temperature of that cluster.

7. Your temperatures before ovulation will probably range from about 97° to 97.5°F. If they tend to remain in the 96s or 98s, it could be an indication of hypothyroidism or hyperthyroidism.

8. Normally, temperatures after ovulation will remain high for at least 10 days before you get your period. If they don't, you may have a short luteal phase that could be an indication that you are at risk for infertility or miscarriages.

4. Be Prepared for Your First Preconception Visit

Things to bring to your appointment:

- Copies of any blood work, saliva, or nutritional testing you have had done in the past two years
- A list of all prescription drugs and supplements you are currently taking, with the dosages
- A food diary, showing what you eat in a typical week
- Your fertility charts

Things to discuss with your doctor:

- Optimizing your thyroid levels for fertility
- Testing for and addressing any other hormonal issues, such as sex hormones, and adrenal health
- Testing for and balancing any nutritional deficiencies
- Dietary changes

- Addressing autoimmunity and inflammation
- The safety of antibiotics, antidepressants, antihistamines, anti-inflammatories, blood pressure medications, cold medications, antidiarrheal medications, pain medications, sleeping pills, antifungal treatments, migraine medications, and all supplements, in terms of their effects on conception and/or pregnancy
- Lifestyle changes

5. The Basics

Supplements and Nutrient Testing

Note: Always consult with your doctor before taking any supplements or herbs during pregnancy and lactation.

Start taking a prenatal vitamin as early as possible.

Take prenatal vitamins three to four hours apart from thyroid hormone replacement medication.

Select prenatal vitamins that contain methylfolate instead of traditionally used folic acid. Some brands that have made this switch are Thorne Prenatal Vitamins, NéevoDHA, and both Optimal Prenatal Vitamin and Optimal Prenatal Powder by Seeking Health. Check labels of any other brand you're considering for the names of forms of biologically active methylfolate, such as L-methylfolate, levomefolic acid, or L-5-MTHF (also called L-5-methyltetrahydrofolate). The book's website, http://www.ThyroidPregnancyBook.com, includes recommendations for brands of the supplements mentioned throughout the book.

Consider MTHFR genetic testing to determine whether you have the most common MTHFR genetic mutations C677T and A1298C. MTHFR, a genetic mutation affecting half of the population, makes the body's use of folic acid less effective. Contact your insurance to see whether this test is covered. Check the book's website for lab companies that offer MTHFR testing.

Not all prenatal vitamins contain iodine, so be sure to check that your prenatal contains at least 150 mcg of iodine and take it through pregnancy and breastfeeding.

Consult with an iodine-literate health-care provider to get iodine testing in preconception.

If you are a Hashimoto's patient, use caution with higher doses of iodine. Speak with your doctor to ensure you are taking sufficient selenium while supplementing with iodine.

Also check your prenatal vitamin for the dosage of selenium included. The optimal dosage is 200 mcg in the selenomethionine form, so you may need to supplement with additional selenium beyond what the vitamin provides. However, note that you should not take more than 400 mcg of selenium per day.

For sufficient omega-3 fatty acids, take 2,000 to 3,000 mg of a combined EPA-DHA supplement from a trusted brand, such as Nordic Naturals.

Take an active probiotic supplement—typically probiotics will need refrigeration—that contains the bacteria *Lactobacillus rhamnosus* GG, *Bifidobacterium bifidum*, *Lactococcus lactis*, and *Bifidobacterium breve*.

Ensure full iron testing is done, including measures of ferritin, serum iron, total iron-binding capacity (TIBC), and transferrin saturation. Have iron levels tested at preconception and then again in the second and third trimesters and in the early months of postpartum. The optimal level of ferritin—the stored form of iron—is between 75 and 100. Select a supplement with the iron glycinate form of iron. Iron supplements, including prenatal vitamins with iron, must be taken three to four hours apart from thyroid hormone replacement medication. Excessive iron supplementation is not safe, so speak to your doctor about the ideal dosage for you.

Your vitamin D level should be tested preconception. An ideal vitamin D score on a scale of 32 to 100 would be 50 or above.

Vitamin B_{12} should be tested preconception. The optimal level is near the top end of the "normal" range, 800 to 900. Ensure that your prenatal vitamin contains vitamin B_{12} and if you need to supplement this amount, be sure to obtain it in the form of methylcobalamin, not cyanocobalamin. Supplemental vitamin B_{12} is best absorbed sublingually.

Magnesium should also be tested preconception. Request testing of RBC (red blood cell) magnesium instead of the traditionally done serum magnesium. Optimum magnesium level is 5.5 to 6.5. Magnesium deficiency can be corrected through supplementation and/or transdermal absorption. Check supplement labels for bioavailable forms of magnesium, such as magnesium glycinate, magnesium taurate, magnesium citrate, magnesium malate, magnesium chloride, or magnesium carbonate. Transdermal magnesium is applied topically to the skin by using either magnesium oil, gel, lotion, or magnesium bath salts.

Supplement with 750 to 1,000 mg of phosphathidylcholine. One good brand is Optimal PC.

Supplement with 100 mg of coenzyme Q10 (CoQ10), preferably with the bioavailable form ubiquinol.

Dana's Experience

I fought an uphill battle to find a good thyroid doctor and I made it. I am blessed to have met Dr. Adrienne Clamp.

I was shocked to discover that I was severely deficient in many of the key nutrients essential for thyroid health, including vitamins B$_{12}$ and D, magnesium, iodine, selenium, and ferritin. It took finding a good doctor who did comprehensive nutrient testing for the first time in my life to find this out. It was not enough in my case to take a prenatal vitamin because I had severe deficiencies in certain nutrients and the prenatal alone was not sufficient to get me to the optimal levels for those nutrients. So, in addition to my prenatal vitamin I took additional supplements guided by nutrient lab testing that Dr. Clamp ran regularly while I was trying to conceive, then throughout pregnancy and postpartum. Nutrient testing continues to be an important part of my visits today and it should be part of your workup, too.

I'll never forget the day I was in Dr. Clamp's office in early pregnancy, sharing my deepest fear that I would miscarry again. She looked at me and said, "You will not lose your baby on my watch."

Other Key Basics

Moderate your intake of caffeine.

Stay hydrated by drinking water equivalent to half your body weight in ounces each day.

Control your weight. Read Mary Shomon's book *Thyroid Diet Revolution* if you are struggling with weight gain.

Begin or continue a moderate-intensity exercise routine. Avoid excessive amounts of exercise.

6. Optimize Your Thyroid

Ensure you are optimally treated before trying to conceive. Once optimized, give yourself several months of stability before trying to conceive.

Laura Kay lost her second child at 20 weeks, and was then diagnosed with Hashimoto's. She was told to wait until her TSH was below 2.0 to get pregnant:

This is not what a mom who was blindsided by losing her baby wants to hear. I wanted a baby in my belly ASAP! But I complied. I was put on the standard Synthroid and sent on my way. After three months of being on Synthroid, I was given the green light to try again. We used the natural family planning method, so I knew exactly when I was most fertile and when to time things. After four months, things weren't happening. So, I convinced the doctor to check me out. I had a laparoscopy and endoscopy done, which set me back a couple months as well. Of course, he found nothing. No reason for infertility. I was about to start insemination the next cycle. But I felt pregnant! The new OB had me come in so early, at 5 weeks, because of my history. Of course, they didn't see what they wanted to in the ultrasound. They tried to prepare me for the fact that I might have to abort, by taking pills. I cried and cried. They told me to come back in a week for a follow up ultrasound. Thank goodness, when I did, there was a heartbeat and she was in the right place. Needless to say, I changed OBs once again, to a more natural doctor, with less stress! I ended up staying on Synthroid, eating as gluten free as possible, and I had a healthy baby girl.

Request full thyroid testing and always get a copy of your lab results. Also check that your scores are not just normal, but *optimal*. While each person is unique and what is optimal is individual, these are generally the numbers to look for:

- Thyroid-stimulating hormone (TSH)—1.0 or lower
- Free thyroxine (Free T4)—top half of the reference range
- Free triiodothyronine (Free T3)—top half or top 25th percentile of reference range
- Reverse T3—low end of normal range
- Thyroid peroxidase antibodies (TPOAb) (to test for Hashimoto's)—within reference range
- Thyroglobulin antibodies (TgAb) (to test for Hashimoto's)—within reference range

- Thyroid-stimulating immunoglobulins (TSI) (to test for Graves' disease)—within reference range

If your doctor is unwilling to run these tests, get a second medical opinion. Appendix A provides a list of resources to help you locate a good thyroid doctor in your area.

Another option is to order your own thyroid lab tests through online laboratories. Some good laboratories are included in Appendix A, as well as on the book's website, http://www.ThyroidPregnancyBook.com, where we also provide links.

Hypothyroidism/Hashimoto's Disease

Hypothyroid women planning pregnancy should have their dose adjusted by their doctor to optimize TSH around 1.0, with Free T4 and Free T3 both in the top half of the reference range.

Patients previously treated for thyroid cancer on suppressive therapy should continue with their suppressive dose, as long as your TSH is not 0, and you have a detectable—even if very low—TSH level.

Do not wait for a missed period to confirm your pregnancy. To confirm your pregnancy as soon as possible, start using pregnancy tests as early as seven days after you have possibly conceived, and test daily, until you either get a positive result or start your menstrual cycle. Get thyroid testing immediately upon confirmation of pregnancy.

Make a plan with your doctor in advance to increase your thyroid medication dosage the very day you confirm your pregnancy. Some integrative doctors suggest that you add two levothyroxine pills a week, as soon as you confirm pregnancy. If you are on a T4/T3 or NDT drug, discuss the proposed increase in dosage with your doctor.

Hyperthyroidism/Graves' Disease

Wait until your thyroid function is stabilized before getting pregnant. The Pregnancy Guidelines strongly recommend that women with Graves' disease use contraception until a euthyroid state is achieved—meaning that thyroid hormone is at normal levels.

Consult with an alternative-minded health-care practitioner, such as a functional medicine practitioner, to see whether natural approaches to reduce autoimmunity and manage hyperthyroidism—which can include supplements, herbs, dietary changes, and treatments such as low-dose naltrexone—can put you into remission without RAI or antithyroid medications prior to conception. It can take as long as eighteen months to regulate and control Graves' disease hyperthyroidism using natural approaches.

If natural approaches have failed to put your Graves' disease and hyperthyroidism into remission, you have three options:

Antithyroid medications: The drug methimazole is normally used during preconception to achieve a remission of your symptoms, normalization of your blood work, and lowering of your antibodies. Around 30 percent of Graves' patients will achieve remission using methimazole, and it can take a number of months.

It is not recommended to attempt to get pregnant while actively taking antithyroid drugs.

The Pregnancy Guidelines recommend that if you are taking antithyroid medications and become pregnant, that you be switched to propylthiouracil (PTU) as early as possible in the first trimester to reduce risks of birth defects and then switch back to methimazole for the second and third trimesters. If you are taking methimazole, confirm your pregnancy as early as possible so that the switch to PTU can be done quickly in the first trimester.

Radioactive iodine treatment (RAI): RAI can be performed during the preconception period; however, be sure your doctor gives you a pregnancy test 48 hours prior to the RAI administration to ensure that you are not pregnant.

After RAI or surgery, the 2011 "Guidelines of the American Thyroid Association for the Diagnosis and Management of Thyroid Disease During Pregnancy and Postpartum," or Pregnancy Guidelines, recommend women wait for six months before conceiving, to allow them to get on a stable dose of thyroid hormone replacement medication. However, finding a stable dose may take longer than six months. Some experts recommend that you wait a year to protect your developing fetus from any residual radiation. As thyroid patient advocates we err on the side of caution and recommend waiting one year after RAI or surgery to conceive.

Thyroid surgery: Since antibody levels tend to rise after RAI and may remain elevated, the Pregnancy Guidelines recommend surgery for a woman who has high TSI antibody levels and who plans to get pregnant within two years.

Surgery may also be indicated if you are allergic or sensitive to antithyroid drugs, antithyroid drug treatment didn't work, or you prefer not to have RAI.

If you have surgery wait at least six months until you have had a history of several sets of blood tests showing optimal thyroid hormone replacement.

Even if you have been treated previously for Graves' disease with RAI or surgery, you may still have high thyroid antibody levels in your bloodstream. You should have TSI antibody testing prior to becoming pregnant.

Thyroid Cancer

Do not plan pregnancy while being actively treated for thyroid cancer.

If you have been previously treated for thyroid cancer with surgery and radioactive iodine, wait one year before attempting to get pregnant to reach optimal thyroid hormone replacement treatment.

If you have been previously treated for thyroid cancer on suppressive therapy you should continue with your suppressive dose, as long as your TSH is not 0 and you have a detectable—even if very low—TSH level.

7. Balance Other Hormones

Have your estrogen and progesterone levels tested. Some experts recommend a four-point salivary hormone test during the luteal phase, around Day 21 of your cycle, which measures estradiol, progesterone, DHEA, testosterone, and cortisol. Pregnenolone is another test done by integrative physicians.

Given the association between PCOS and thyroid disease, your doctor should evaluate you if you have symptoms of PCOS, including a history of irregular periods, weight gain, facial hair, adult acne, male-pattern baldness, ovarian cysts, and fertility problems.

Consult with an integrative physician about a 24-hour saliva cortisol test to measure your adrenal health. Adrenal dysfunction may be treated preconception with various approaches, including B complex, pregnenolone, DHEA, adrenal glandulars, hydrocortisone, vitamin C, licorice, chromium, adrenal cortex extract, adaptogenic herbs, magnesium, phosphatidylserine, phosphatidylcholine, 5 HTP or GABA, and lifestyle changes. Adaptogenic herbs include ashwagandha, rhodiola, Siberian ginseng (*Eleutherococcus*), holy basil, and American ginseng.

Since many of the treatments for adrenal fatigue are not to be used during pregnancy, one safe approach while you are actively trying to conceive is to take the adrenal support supplements and herbs during the preovulation phase of your cycle, then stop taking them at ovulation (using basal body temperature charting, ovulation predictor kits, or fertility monitors to determine ovulation) and resume only when your period starts. Adrenal support is then stopped throughout pregnancy and resumed when the baby is born to support you through the stressful experience of postpartum.

Have your hemoglobin A1C and fasting glucose tested.

8. Minimize Exposure to Toxins

Heavy Metals

Speak with your doctor about any necessary heavy metal testing, especially if you think you have been exposed to greater than normal levels of heavy metals. Possible causes of heavy metal toxicity include having an occupation or hobby that exposes you to heavy metals, eating a large quantity of fish from contaminated waters, having mercury dental amalgams, living near a landfill, or living in an older home with lead-based paint, pipes, or solder. According to the United States Environmental Protection Agency (EPA), if your home was built before 1978, old lead paint on your walls, doors, windows, and sills may be dangerous. The EPA also warns that lead pipes and lead solder were commonly used in household plumbing materials until 1986, and many water systems are still affected. Metals commonly tested include lead, mercury, arsenic, cadmium, and chromium. If elevated levels are found, your physician can recommend various forms of chelation therapy, to help detox and clear these levels from your body.

Avoid Food Toxins
- Choose organic, hormone-free, and pesticide-free foods whenever possible.
- Choose only grass-fed, organic meats and poultry.
- Avoid raw meat and poultry.
- Avoid deli meats.
- Avoid raw seafood, including shellfish and sushi.
- Avoid fish with high mercury levels (e.g., shark, swordfish, king mackerel, and tilefish).
- Avoid smoked seafood.
- Avoid locally caught freshwater fish that may have high levels of polychlorinated biphenyls (PCBs) (e.g., bluefish, striped bass, freshwater salmon, pike, trout, and walleye).
- Avoid raw eggs.

- Avoid unpasteurized milk and soft cheeses, such as Brie, Camembert, Roquefort, feta, Gorgonzola, and Mexican queso blanco, unless they are pasteurized.
- Avoid pâté.

Water/Fluoride
- Test your water for heavy metals, bacteria, and fluoride levels.
- Use only filtered water or use a reverse osmosis water system.
- Avoid fluoridated products, such as toothpastes and mouthwashes.

Air quality
- Use indoor HEPA air filters.

Chemicals
- Avoid endocrine-disrupting chemicals.
- Avoid polychlorinated biphenyls (PCBs) and phthalates.
- Avoid flame-retardant cloth and spray-on flame retardants.
- Avoid paints and adhesives that contain these ingredients.
- Avoid Teflon and nonstick coated pans.
- Avoid spray-on fabric protectors and stain-resistant carpets.
- Avoid new plastic shower curtains.
- Avoid canned foods.
- Check water bottles, food packaging, and other plastics, looking for the specific resin code on the bottom, usually located in a triangle of arrows. Avoid those numbered 1, 3, 6, or 7 (PC).
- Never use plastic in the microwave or with hot food.
- Discard plastics when they begin to have signs of wear and tear.
- Look for personal care products with the USDA Certified Organic Seal.
- Avoid products containing parabens, phthalates (DEHP, BBP, DBP, DMP, DEP), DMDM hydantoin, fragrance, triclosan, sodium lauryl/laureth sulfate, DEA (diethanolamine) and TEA (triethanolamine), formaldehyde, PEGs (polyethylene glycol), and anything with "glycol" or "methyl."
- Use only nontoxic, chemical-free natural cleaning products in your home.

Detoxification

Your practitioner may recommend a detoxification regimen if you have been exposed to toxins. Gentle therapies include castor oil packs, dry brushing, dry sauna therapy, coffee enemas (in moderation), rebounding (exercising on a mini-trampoline) and regular daily movement. Note that regular use of saunas, coffee enemas, and castor oil packs is not recommended during pregnancy.

9. Eat a Fertility-Friendly Diet

- Address food allergies and food sensitivities.
- Eliminate soy.
- Eat the rainbow: consume a green, yellow, orange, red, and purple vegetable or fruit every day.
- Ensure that your diet is heavy on iron-rich foods, such as spinach, Swiss chard, kale, and other dark leafy greens (cooked or steamed).
- Be careful not to eat large quantities of raw goitrogens (such as broccoli, kale, cabbage, cauliflower, collards, and spinach). Eat goitrogens in moderation, best steamed or cooked to reduce the goitrogenic effect.
- Balance blood sugar throughout the day by eating small, frequent meals. Eat foods low on the glycemic index. Eat protein with each meal. Include healthy fats. Avoid sugar and refined carbohydrates.
- If you are diabetic, get your blood sugar levels under control before you conceive.
- Limit caffeine.
- Avoid alcohol.

Jacqueline's experience shows the benefits of eating well:

I had the classic symptoms: gaining weight when eating like a sparrow, cold all the time, constipated, exhausted, and depressed. After being treated, all the symptoms just melted away, along with 30 excess pounds. Years later, I had moved away, my doctor had retired, and I had stopped taking thyroid medication. I got married and wanted to start a family, but I did not get pregnant, even after years of trying. I finally went to a fertility "expert" who did some blood tests and told me that my thyroid was a little "low" and I was not ovulating. He talked me into taking fertility drugs, not even addressing the low thyroid issues I had. I did not get the connection between infertility and low thyroid, and neither did he, apparently! After eight months of the infertility drugs, he pronounced me "barren" and told me to adopt. I do not know what guided me, but I went home and began reading everything I could get my hands on regarding conception, pregnancy, and nutrition. I changed my diet and began taking quality supplements. I did this for a year, and then went for a checkup with a new doctor. All my blood tests came back "normal." He encouraged me to continue taking vitamins and eating well, especially foods that contained iodine and folic acid. After a few months of fish, kelp, and leafy greens, I became pregnant! I had a healthy pregnancy and easy delivery and my son was healthy, too! Fast forward four years when I was blessed again with a healthy daughter.

10. Address Autoimmunity/Reduce Inflammation

- Consult with an alternative-minded doctor, such as a functional medicine physician, to address the immune system in autoimmune diseases, such as Hashimoto's and Graves' disease, before conception. Make sure you discuss safety of treatment methods during pregnancy and lactation.

- Heal a leaky gut by doing an elimination diet to determine your particular food sensitivities. Typical sensitivities include gluten/grains, dairy, soy, eggs, sugar, nightshades, and nuts. After a period of elimination, reintroduce the foods slowly one at a time, and assess your reactions. Eliminate any foods to which you react from the diet for a certain period of time to allow the immune system to heal. While the importance of healing a leaky gut is not a widely accepted concept in mainstream medicine, several of the integrative physicians we interviewed for this book emphasized its importance. For more information about leaky gut and elimination diets, read the online articles "9 Signs You Have a Leaky Gut" by Amy Myers, MD; "Is Your Digestive System Making You Sick and Fat?" by Mark Hyman, MD; and "How An Elimination Diet Can Change Your Health" by Jill Carnahan, MD.

- Speak with your doctor about supplements to heal the gut, such as L-glutamine, digestive enzymes, betaine hydrochloric acid (HCL), slippery elm, aloe vera, and marshmallow root.

- Eat lacto-fermented foods and beverages, such as kefir, yogurt, kimchi, kombucha, and beet kvass, and/or take a high-quality, multispecies probiotic.

- Include foods high in soluble fiber in your diet and/or take a prebiotic. If you start eating or supplementing with a lot more fiber, get your thyroid rechecked, because fiber intake may change your body's level of absorption of your thyroid hormone replacement medication.

- Consult with an integrative physician about additional supplements for autoimmune modulation, such as N-acetyl cysteine, alpha-lipoid acid, polyphenols (green tea, grapeseed, pine bark), resveratrol, glutathione, and curcumin.
- Test for intestinal pathogens such as parasites, Candida overgrowth, and small intestinal bacterial overgrowth (SIBO).
- Consider diets that may be helpful for autoimmune patients, including autoimmune paleo, GAPS, and the specific carbohydrate diet (SCD). The GAPS diet is based on the work of Natasha Campbell-McBride, MD, author of the book *Gut and Psychology Syndrome*. The GAPS diet was derived from the specific carbohydrate diet created by Dr. Sidney Valentine Haas. SCD gained great popularity after a mother, Elaine Gottschall, healed her own child of ulcerative colitis and became an advocate for SCD. Elaine Gottschall is author of the book *Breaking the Vicious Cycle: Intestinal Health Through Diet*. For more information on the autoimmune paleo diet, read *The Paleo Approach: Reverse Autoimmune Disease and Heal Your Body* by Sarah Ballantyne, PhD. (For more info on these specific diets, see Appendix A.)
- Look into low-dose naltrexone (LDN) to modulate the immune system. On its website, the nonprofit organization LDN Research Trust provides a list of LDN prescribing doctors and LDN pharmacists around the world. For more information about LDN, read Julia Schopick's book *Honest Medicine: Effective, Time-Tested, Inexpensive Treatments for Life-Threatening Diseases*.
- Supplement with 200 mcg per day of selenium in the form of selenomethionine. You should not take more than 400 mcg of selenium per day.
- Identify and treat chronic infections including Epstein-Barr virus (EBV), *Yersinia enterocolitica*, *Helicobacter pylori*, hepatitis C virus, *Borrelia burgdorferi* (Lyme disease), yeast overgrowth (*Candida*), cytomegalovirus, staph and strep, *Rickettsia*, Q fever, HTLV-1, herpes 1, 2, and 6, rubella/rubeola (measles), Coxsackie B virus, and parvovirus B-19.

11. Make Lifestyle Changes

- Stop smoking.
- Get adequate sleep: 8 hours a night. For insomnia, consider up to 3 mg of melatonin taken an hour before bedtime or eleven p.m., whichever is earlier. Melatonin may also help fertility.

- Get some sun exposure every day.
- Take a vacation in a sunny climate a month before you start trying to get pregnant.
- Include 15 to 30 minutes a day of stress-reducing activity. Consider:

  o Meditation
  o Guided imagery, relaxation CDs
  o Breath work, paced breathing, or pranayama breathing
  o Prayer
  o Tai chi
  o Qi gong
  o Slow, contemplative walking
  o Needlework
  o Coloring
  o Massage
  o Yoga

Hypothyroidism and Hashimoto's

Risks and Symptoms

Push for thyroid screening and evaluation if you have risk factors and common hypothyroidism/Hashimoto's symptoms but no current diagnosis. We include a list of risk factors and symptoms in this chapter, but you can also find a more comprehensive list at the book's website at http://www.Thyroid PregnancyBook.com. You can assess yourself, print it out, and take the list to your doctor's office to document your symptoms. The 2011 "Guidelines of the American Thyroid Association for the Diagnosis and Management of Thyroid Disease During Pregnancy and Postpartum," or Pregnancy Guidelines, encourage physicians to use a case-finding approach to identify women at risk for thyroid disease in pregnancy, but given that over half of people with thyroid disease worldwide remain undiagnosed, this is not a dependable approach. It is up to you to be informed and insist on proper testing and treatment during pregnancy.

If you haven't been diagnosed, the following risks/symptoms checklist can help you identify and communicate your symptoms to your doctor. If you've already been diagnosed, this checklist can help you determine whether you are being optimally treated.

Hypothyroidism/Hashimoto's Risks/Symptoms Checklist

My risk factors for hypothyroidism include:
- ☐ I have a family history of thyroid disease
- ☐ I have had my thyroid "monitored" in the past to watch for changes
- ☐ I had a previous diagnosis of goiters/nodules
- ☐ I currently have a goiter/enlargement in my thyroid and/or thyroid nodule
- ☐ I was treated for hypothyroidism or hyperthyroidism in the past
- ☐ I had postpartum thyroiditis in the past
- ☐ I had a temporary thyroiditis in the past
- ☐ I have a family history of autoimmune disease
- ☐ I have another autoimmune disease
- ☐ I am pregnant now, or I have had a baby in the past nine months
- ☐ I have a history of miscarriage
- ☐ I have had part/all of my thyroid removed due to cancer
- ☐ I have had part/all of my thyroid removed due to nodules
- ☐ I have had part/all of my thyroid removed due to Graves' Disease/hyperthyroidism
- ☐ I have had radioactive iodine due to Graves' disease/hyperthyroidism
- ☐ I have been prescribed anti thyroid drugs due to Graves' disease/hyperthyroidism

I have the following symptoms of hypothyroidism:
- ☐ I am gaining weight inappropriately
- ☐ I am unable to lose weight with diet/exercise
- ☐ I am constipated, sometimes severely
- ☐ I have hypothermia/low body temperature (I feel cold when others feel hot, I need extra sweaters, etc.)
- ☐ I feel fatigued, exhausted
- ☐ I feel run down, sluggish, lethargic
- ☐ My hair is coarse and dry, breaking, brittle, falling out
- ☐ My skin is coarse, dry, scaly, and thick
- ☐ I have a hoarse or gravelly voice
- ☐ I have puffiness and swelling around the eyes and face
- ☐ I have pains, aches in joints, hands, and feet
- ☐ I have developed carpal-tunnel syndrome, or it's getting worse
- ☐ I am having irregular menstrual cycles (longer, or heavier, or more frequent)
- ☐ I am having trouble conceiving a baby
- ☐ I feel depressed
- ☐ I feel restless

☐ My moods change easily
☐ I have feelings of worthlessness
☐ I have difficulty concentrating
☐ I have more feelings of sadness
☐ I seem to be losing interest in normal daily activities
☐ I am more forgetful lately

I also have the following additional symptoms, which have been reported more frequently in people with hypothyroidism:
☐ My hair is falling out
☐ I can't seem to remember things
☐ I have no sex drive
☐ I am getting more frequent infections that last longer
☐ I'm snoring more lately
☐ I have/may have sleep apnea
☐ I feel shortness of breath and tightness in the chest
☐ I feel the need to yawn to get oxygen
☐ My eyes feel gritty and dry
☐ My eyes feel sensitive to light
☐ My eyes get jumpy/tics in eyes, which makes me dizzy/vertigo and have headaches
☐ I have strange feelings in neck or throat
☐ I have tinnitus (ringing in ears)
☐ I get recurrent sinus infections
☐ I have vertigo
☐ I feel some lightheadedness
☐ I have severe menstrual cramps

Kaitlin's experience shows the importance of knowing about the various symptoms. After having an uneventful pregnancy with her first child, she had difficulty getting pregnant with her second and was undergoing fertility treatments:

After several failed attempts, I was diagnosed with low progesterone, and was able to get pregnant. At my eight-week appointment, they did blood work and checked my thyroid. Everything looked good to them. But I was exhausted, my skin was awful, and I had no appetite, and wasn't gaining weight. My son was born three weeks early. He had to be in the NICU for breathing problems. And after delivery, I had a bad hemorrhage. I never had any idea that my thyroid could cause all these issues with pregnancy until I saw the article on the Hypothyroid Mom website "300+ Hypothyroidism Symptoms . . . Yes REALLY." I had many of them, but in the reproductive category, I had eight different symptoms—hemorrhaging, breastfeeding issues, and more.

Thyroid Panel

Ensure that your thyroid evaluation includes a full medical history, physical examination, symptoms evaluation, and comprehensive thyroid lab panel. Your future child's father should have a workup, too, if he presents with common symptoms and risk factors.

Be aware that the Pregnancy Guidelines recommend a narrower TSH reference range and lower upper limit of the range for pregnant women than for the nonpregnant population. Given that many endocrinologists and obstetricians are not current on the guidelines, it is critical that thyroid patients obtain copies of their lab results to check that they have had the full battery of tests and that their scores are optimal. If a laboratory has not established its own trimester-specific reference ranges for TSH for pregnant women, the following reference ranges should be used.

- First trimester: 0.1 to 2.5 mIU/L
- Second trimester: 0.2 to 3.0 mIU/L
- Third trimester: 0.3 to 3.0 mIU/L

The lab you use should do the full battery of thyroid tests. In mainstream medical practice, testing for thyroid-stimulating hormone (TSH) is the gold standard for determining thyroid function. The Pregnancy Guidelines also make mention of testing for Free T4. However, there is more to thyroid testing than these two lab tests. While conventional doctors consider it controversial, many integrative physicians include tests for Free T3, Reverse T3, thyroid peroxidase antibodies (TPOAb), and thyroglobulin antibodies (TgAb) as part of comprehensive testing for hypothyroidism.

Check that your lab scores are not just normal but *optimal*. A lab score in the normal range doesn't necessarily mean that score is optimal for you. We are all unique and one size does not fit all. Here is a list of thyroid lab tests and optimal ranges used by many integrative physicians for pregnant hypothyroid women. This list is helpful for the diagnosis of hypothyroidism during pregnancy. It is also helpful for hypothyroid patients who are already diagnosed

> **Dana's Experience**
>
> I trusted that my well-trained, highly credentialed doctors would know how to manage my hypothyroidism during pregnancy. I didn't know enough about thyroid disease in pregnancy to advocate for myself and my baby. Throughout my first trimester, my TSH remained higher than the 2.5 mIU/L recommended in this book, soaring as high as 10.0 mIU/L. I felt so unwell and didn't know what to do. My doctor said that everything was fine and that TSH was only a concern in pregnancy if it went above 10.0 mIU/L.
>
> Wait . . . rewind . . . yes you read that correctly.
>
> My doctor was not concerned about TSH levels below 10.0 in pregnancy, because she was not aware of the danger to pregnancy with a TSH at that high range, and I wasn't aware of it either.
>
> She had clearly never read the Pregnancy Guidelines, and I miscarried.

and treated to determine whether their treatment is optimal. Chapter 2 provides detailed descriptions of the thyroid lab tests and what they indicate.

- TSH—typically 1.0 or lower
- Free T4—top half of the reference range
- Free T3—top half or top 25th percentile of reference range
- Reverse T3—low end of normal range
- TPOAb—within reference range
- TgAb—within reference range

Caroline's experience shows how often doctors are not aware of the recommended TSH ranges for pregnancy. She became pregnant after trying for six months.

In the first few months of pregnancy I felt tired and gained 25 lbs. I didn't think anything of it. At my first trimester appointment, I did tell the doctor I felt a lump in my throat. The doctor ran a thyroid panel and told me that my thyroid felt enlarged. I started spotting during the time I waited for my results. I got an ultrasound and the heartbeat of the baby was only 78 beats per minute, and the baby measured 2 weeks behind. They told me I must have had my dates wrong. My TSH results came back at 5.8, and my doctor started me on levothyroxine. I was spotting, and had another ultrasound, which showed an even slower heartbeat. I asked what was going on, but the doctor told me to calm down. The bleeding became heavier, and I ended up in the ER, where another ultrasound showed that my uterus was empty. I asked my OB if hypothyroidism had anything to do with the miscarriage. He said my TSH was only 5.8, so it was not likely. He said it was probably a chromosomal abnormality.

Contact your doctor if symptoms of overmedication arise, including feeling nervous or jittery, heart palpitations, weight loss, insomnia, rapid or irregular heartbeat, excessive sweating, diarrhea, tremors, muscle weakness, increased appetite, shortness of breath, and heat intolerance.

Lower than normal TSH readings may mean the patient is overmedicated, but not in all cases. If you are taking the proper dosage of thyroid hormone replacement, you may experience complete relief of symptoms but have suppressed TSH (readings below normal). TSH alone is not a reliable indicator of adequacy of treatment. Consult with an integrative physician to determine the optimal dosage for you.

If you have been previously treated for thyroid cancer using suppressive therapy, you should continue with your suppressive dose, as long as your TSH is not 0, and you have a detectable—even if very low—TSH level.

Should you find yourself symptomatically hyperthyroid on thyroid hormone replacement medication, speak with your doctor about testing your adrenals and iron. Ensure preconception that your adrenal function (ideally tested using a 24-hour saliva test) and iron (full iron panel testing will evaluate ferritin, serum iron, total iron binding capacity—TIBC—and transferrin saturation) are tested and treated if needed. See Chapter 4 for treatment options.

Medication Dose Changes During Pregnancy

Have a plan with your doctor in advance to increase your thyroid medication dosage the very day you confirm your pregnancy. Some integrative doctors suggest that you add two levothyroxine pills a week, as soon as you confirm pregnancy. If you are on a T4/T3 or NDT drug, discuss the amount by which to increase dosage with your doctor.

Request a lab requisition form for your thyroid lab tests in advance and save it until you confirm pregnancy.

Start testing for pregnancy as early as seven days postconception, since TSH can rise dramatically as early as two to three weeks postconception and require an increase in medication dosage.

> **Dana's Experience**
>
> After my miscarriage I was fortunate to stumble upon Mary Shomon's book *Living Well with Hypothyroidism*. Her book was so fabulous that I scheduled an individual thyroid consultation with her. I will forever remember Mary's tip during one of my phone consultation sessions with her. She told me to buy the biggest box of pregnancy tests I could find. She recommended that I try to confirm my pregnancy as early as possible and to contact my doctor as soon as possible for thyroid testing. You bet I followed her instructions, and I went out and bought boxes and boxes of pregnancy tests. As soon as I started trying to conceive, my goal was to confirm my pregnancy *as early as possible*. I don't believe my son Hudson would be here today if I had waited for thyroid testing at my first prenatal visit that was scheduled for 8 weeks gestation.

Call your doctor as soon as you confirm your pregnancy.

Get thyroid testing the same day you confirm your pregnancy or as soon as possible. Thyroid hormone replacement medication dosage may need to be increased more than once during early pregnancy to reach an optimal dosage for a healthy pregnancy. By 4 to 6 weeks gestation, pregnant hypothyroid women typically require an increase in their dosage of 30 to 50 percent above preconception dosage. The increase may be greater in women without residual functional thyroid tissue, such as patients who have undergone radioiodine ablation or total thyroidectomy.

Cathy, diagnosed with hypothyroidism as an infant and treated for years, became pregnant for the first time at thirty-five.

> I kept asking my OB-GYN when they would check my thyroid level and they kept putting it off. Eventually they encouraged me to ask my primary care physician. She boosted me 50 mcg just to be on the safe side. At thirty-two weeks and five days I woke with light spotting, which turned out to be a placental abruption. I ended up with an emergency C-section, and my son spent the next few weeks in the NICU. The doctors were baffled. I was checked for drugs, interviewed to rule out spousal abuse—they had no idea why this happened.

Ensure your thyroid is monitored regularly throughout pregnancy, approximately every four weeks during the first half of pregnancy and at least once between 26 and 32 weeks, at minimum.

Should you find yourself with new or worsening symptoms, don't hesitate to contact your doctor at any time during pregnancy.

Nicole and her husband started trying for a baby, but given that she was in her midthirties already, after six months, she went to see an infertility specialist.

I was already on medication for my hypothyroidism and was overweight. I went through IVF and was unsuccessful twice. We were devastated to say the least. We took a break for a while, and figured we would try on our own, but I didn't really hold out much hope considering my doctor told me I had "old eggs." But I got pregnant all on my own!!! Words can't describe how overjoyed we were. I was 40 years old at the time. I had been taking care of my thyroid and was taking my meds like I was supposed to. As soon as I found out I was pregnant (I was five weeks) I went to see my endocrinologist. She confirmed my pregnancy and immediately upped my meds. She said it was better to be a little hyper rather than hypo during pregnancy. I went back to see her every month during the first months of my pregnancy, then it was every two months. I had to double my normal dosage but my numbers were perfect. I went on to have a wonderful pregnancy. I carried to full term and my son was born very healthy.

Watch your body for symptoms listed in the checklist and contact your doctor right away if you experience new or worsening symptoms. Always listen to your body and push for medical attention. This is a time in your life to be overprotective of yourself and your baby, even if it means calling the doctor's office over and over again. Don't hesitate to seek a second medical opinion if your doctor refuses to listen to your symptoms or reevaluate your treatment.

After erratic menstrual cycles, a miscarriage, and being diagnosed afterward with hypothyroidism, Jennifer took a pregnancy test after every single missed period.

I finally got a positive, but there was this undercurrent of fear. I was terrified I was going to miscarry again. I immediately contacted my doctor's office, who sent me to an OB. I was extremely lucky, because my OB had experience with hypothyroid moms and religiously checked my levels. And he checked them better than my primary care doctor! He did TSH,

<table>
<tr><td>

Dana's Experience

</td><td>

Morning sickness? Nausea? Toxicity? There isn't a word that accurately describes the sick feeling I felt during the pregnancy that I lost. I actually said to family members,

</td></tr>
</table>

"Something is wrong with the baby. I feel there is toxicity inside me." My body was whispering (actually it was more like shouting) that something was very wrong during the pregnancy. The fatigue was deepening, the constipation was worsening, my skin was drying and cracking, and I felt an overall unwell "toxic" feeling. I knew that something wasn't right. I had called the doctor's office several times explaining that I wasn't feeling well and each time my symptoms were dismissed. I worried that I was being a nuisance. After all, doctor knows best, I thought.

I miscarried several days later.

I felt that same sick toxic feeling develop in early pregnancy around 6 weeks pregnancy with my second son. This time my gut instincts told me it was a red flag that my hypothyroidism was not optimally treated and I rushed to call my new thyroid doctor. She increased my thyroid hormone replacement medication for the second time that first trimester (I had already increased my dosage the same day of my positive pregnancy test at three weeks) and that awful toxic feeling thankfully went away.

I had an "Aha!" moment during the interview I conducted with certified nutritionist Kim Schuette for this book. She explained, "When the liver is unable to efficiently clear excess hormones, morning sickness often ensues. This can often be due to a sluggish liver and thyroid. Low thyroid hormones often result in impaired clearance of toxins in the liver."

Hmmm . . . I knew my body better than I realized.

Always listen to your instincts carefully. You are, after all, the expert on your body.

Free T4, and Free T3 levels. Twice he had to increase my levothyroxine dosage. It was a tough pregnancy; I had hyperemesis gravidarum and couldn't even keep water down. I often would throw up my pill right after I took it. After six hospitalizations (where they often forgot to give me my medicine) and multiple middle-of-the-night panicked calls, my OB had a PICC line inserted into my arm and I had a Zofran pump and IV fluids through home health. This continued until I gave birth. My rainbow baby is now a beautiful fourteen-month-old girl who has a lot of sass and is the joy of her parents' lives.

Thyroid Hormone Replacement Medication

Be aware of the various thyroid hormone replacement medication options described in Chapter 5, including levothyroxine (synthetic thyroxine/T4), liothyronine (synthetic triiodothyronine/T3), and natural desiccated thyroid (natural combination of T4/T3 hormone).

While the Pregnancy Guidelines indicate that the synthetic form of the T4/thyroxine hormone, known generically as levothyroxine, is the only treatment to be used in pregnancy, we recommend that you find an integrative, holistic, or alternative physician who will explore all the treatment options to find what is right for you. The majority of experts we interviewed explained that optimizing thyroid function on a T4/T3 combination therapy as well as NDT is safe in pregnancy. They tend to use whichever combination works best for each patient.

Melissa had a very different experience with her first pregnancy on levothyroxine, and later pregnancies on NDT.

> During my first pregnancy, I was taking levothyroxine. I was exhausted, gained a great deal of weight, and went into premature labor at 36 weeks. My baby needed to stay in the NICU for several days, but he was thankfully otherwise healthy. Postpartum I lost my eyebrows, couldn't lose weight and was excruciatingly tired. I was diagnosed with Hashimoto's, and switched to Nature-Throid. I had two wonderfully easy pregnancies and subsequent births of my two sons in 2012 and 2015. I was on Nature-Throid before and throughout both pregnancies. I was completely in tune with what my body required in terms of thyroid medication and when my levels were off. Both boys were born full term and postpartum recovery was minimal. The differences among my three pregnancies were substantial in terms of energy and bounce back after my Hashimoto's diagnosis. I'm now six months postpartum after my third and feel like I have all the energy in the world.

Find your optimal thyroid medication type and dosage ideally before pregnancy. It can take several months of careful experimentation with a good doctor to reach optimal level. Experimentation is not ideal during pregnancy when your developing baby is depending on you for thyroid hormone.

Contact your doctor if you experience allergic reactions to new thyroid medications. Every brand includes different fillers, binding agents, and dyes, and your body is unique in how you react to these different ingredients.

Choose brand names for levothyroxine over generic levothyroxine whenever possible, to ensure consistent dosing. If due to cost considerations or insurance coverage you must use a generic levothyroxine, there are a few things to keep in mind:

- If you are stabilized on a generic levothyroxine, find out who the manufacturer is. While your doctor can't prescribe a particular generic manufacturer's levothyroxine, if you have a relationship with your pharmacist, your pharmacist may be able to ensure that you get levothyroxine from the same generic manufacturer with each refill. (Note: This is harder—or impossible—with large chains and mail-order pharmacies, however.)
- Get a large supply, such as three months' worth. Make sure it doesn't expire during your usage time, however.
- If you can't ensure refills from the same manufacturer, pay close attention to your symptoms, and if you notice them worsening after a refill, ask your doctor to check your levels.

Thyroid Medication: Practical Tips

Take Your Thyroid Medication Properly

- Always double-check your prescription to make sure that you have the prescribed drug, at the correct dosage, and that you've been given the full amount of the prescription. Also verify that generics have not been substituted for brand names when your physician has specified "dispense as written" (DAW) or "no substitution."
- Take thyroid medication on an empty stomach first thing in the morning or as advised by your doctor.
- Wait at least one hour before eating and before drinking coffee (including decaf).
- Take vitamins or supplements, including prenatal vitamins that include iron and calcium, as least 3 to 4 hours apart from your thyroid medication.
- Take antacids at least 3 to 4 hours apart from your thyroid medication.
- Drink calcium-fortified beverages (e.g., orange juice or nondairy milks) at least 3 to 4 hours apart from thyroid medication.
- Be consistent about a high-fiber diet. If you start or stop eating high fiber, get your thyroid rechecked.

- If you feel nauseated during pregnancy such that you have to eat as soon as you get up, wait at least one hour after you eat before taking thyroid medication.
- Speak with your doctor about when to take your thyroid medication. While first thing in the morning is normally advised for levothyroxine, many integrative doctors recommend breaking up your daily dosage of T4/T3 combination or NDT over the course of the day, and may prescribe taking half of the dosage twice a day.
- Also speak with your doctor about the option of taking your thyroid medication before bedtime. However, some people on T3 or NDT may have difficulty sleeping if they take it at night.
- If you make a change to how you take your thyroid medication, request thyroid testing after several weeks.

Remember to Take Your Medication Every Day

- Use a weekly pillbox with separate compartments for each day or time of day, or use a service lik PillPack.
- Consider electronic pillboxes that will alert you to take your next dose of medication with an audible sound and a visual LED lighting system.
- Take your medication at the same time each day along with another daily event, such as getting out of bed or washing your face.
- Leave your medication in an easy-to-spot place, such as beside your alarm clock.
- Create e-mail or text alerts to remind yourself to take your medicine.
- Consider signing up for a text, call, or e-mail reminder service.
- Use electronic medicine schedules online.
- Use a reminder app for your medications.
- Include a reminder to take your medication on your calendar.
- Leave notes to remind yourself.
- Wear a wristwatch with an alarm.
- Ask a loved one to help you to remember to take your medication every day.

Store Your Thyroid Medication Properly

- Check the storage information on the insert of your medication and/or with your pharmacist.
- Store your thyroid medication in a cool area away from humidity and moisture. Your bathroom is not the best place.

- Always carry your medication in the original containers with pharmacy labels with you on an airplane, instead of storing them in your checked luggage.
- If you are traveling by car, keep medications with you, not stored in the trunk. Do not leave your medication in a hot car for extended periods.
- Speak with your pharmacy about whether it turns off air-conditioning when the store is closed evenings and/or weekends during warm seasons of the year.
- If you order your medications from a mail-order pharmacy, request overnight delivery.
- If you notice unusual symptoms during summer months, speak with your doctor about retesting your levels.
- Request a new refill if you suspect your medication has been damaged by heat.

Hashimoto's Disease

Ensure thyroid peroxidase antibodies (TPOAb) and thyroglobulin antibodies (TgAb) are tested.

If you have elevated antibodies but are not receiving thyroid hormone replacement medication, ensure your thyroid is monitored every four to six weeks during pregnancy until mid-pregnancy, then at least once between weeks 26 and 32 of pregnancy, so as to start thyroid hormone replacement treatment if necessary.

Consult with an alternative-minded physician, such as a functional medicine physician, for guidance on caring for your immune system in light of Hashimoto's. Discuss the safety of treatment methods in pregnancy and lactation. See the Autoimmunity section of Chapter 4 for autoimmune treatment methods safe during preconception.

Eat lacto-fermented foods and beverages, such as kefir, yogurt, kimchi, kombucha, and beet kvass, and/or take a high-quality, multispecies probiotic.

Include foods high in soluble fiber in your diet and/or take a prebiotic. If you start eating high fiber, get your thyroid rechecked because it may change the absorption of your thyroid hormone replacement medication.

Balance blood sugar throughout the day by eating small, frequent meals. Eat protein with each meal along with healthy fats. Avoid sugar and refined carbohydrates.

Look into low-dose naltrexone (LDN) to modulate the immune system. On its website, the nonprofit organization LDN Research Trust provides a list of LDN prescribing doctors and LDN pharmacists around the world.

Supplement with 200 mcg per day of selenium in the form of selenomethionine. You should not take more than 400 mcg of selenium per day.

Consider diets that may be helpful for Hashimoto's, including autoimmune paleo, GAPS, and the specific carbohydrate diet (SCD).

Melanie was thirty-four when she was diagnosed with Hashimoto's.

> I had antibodies levels in the thousands, and my endocrinologist said I shouldn't try to conceive because it would either end up as a miscarriage or a baby with neurological issues. I was devastated and depressed for weeks. I took his prescription of Synthroid but I also researched going gluten-free before my next visit. He laughed at all my research and the idea of going gluten free. I tried it anyway. While my antibodies didn't reduce in the numbers I had hoped, they did go down. I got pregnant with twins right away. Both babies are extremely bright and could sing their ABCs by their first birthday. I changed doctors, but I'd love to take the babies to his office to show him that he needs to do some more research of his own before he tells women not to try to conceive.

Additional Considerations

Note that over-the-counter, nonprescription glandular thyroid supplements made from pig, sheep, or cow thyroid glands are not prescription thyroid medication yet they can have a considerable effect on your thyroid health. Do not take without consulting your doctor.

Do not self-medicate.

If your doctor refuses to listen to your symptoms, or order the appropriate tests, consider other thyroid medications, or you have several options:

- Bring a checklist of hypothyroidism risks and symptoms, to back up your request.
- If your doctor reviews your checklist and refuses to order thyroid tests, ask the doctor to sign and date a copy of your checklist, indicating his or her refusal to test, and to put that in your medical record. Keep a signed copy for yourself. Send a copy to the HMO or insurance company's consumer liaison, along with your request that testing be approved.

- Consider having your tests done through a patient-directed, direct-to-consumer laboratory testing service. This book's website http://www .ThyroidPregnancyBook.com has recommendations for this service.
- If your doctor thinks that a TSH of 4 is fine, even during pregnancy, or refuses to test you for thyroid antibodies, bring in a copy of the Pregnancy Guidelines, showing the trimester-specific reference range. (You'll find the URL to the complete guidelines at http://www.ThyroidPregnancy Book.com.)
- Find an open-minded thyroid doctor who is open to running comprehensive thyroid lab tests, explores the treatment options to find what's right for you, and listens to you and your symptoms. See Appendix A for resources to help locate a good thyroid doctor in your location.

Always discuss supplements with your doctor and/or pharmacist during pregnancy and lactation. Look for supplements free of gluten, dairy, and soy.

11

Hyperthyroidism and Graves' Disease

Risk and Symptoms

Push for thyroid screening and evaluation if you have risk factors and common hyperthyroidism/Graves' disease symptoms but no current diagnosis. We provide a risks/symptoms checklist in this chapter, but check the book's website at http://www.ThyroidPregnancyBook.com for a more comprehensive checklist. You can assess yourself, print it out, and take the checklist to your doctor's office to document your symptoms. The 2011 "Guidelines of the American Thyroid Association for the Diagnosis and Management of Thyroid Disease During Pregnancy and Postpartum," or Pregnancy Guidelines, encourage physicians to use a case-finding approach to identify women at risk for thyroid disease in pregnancy, but given that over half of people with thyroid disease worldwide remain undiagnosed, this is not a dependable approach. It is up to *you* to be informed and insist on proper testing and treatment during pregnancy.

If you have not yet been diagnosed, this risks/symptoms checklist can help you identify symptoms. If you are already diagnosed and treated for hyperthyroidism/Graves' disease, use the checklist to help assess whether or not your thyroid treatment is optimal.

Hyperthyroidism/Graves' Risks/Symptoms Checklist

My risk factors for hyperthyroidism include:
- ☐ I have a family history of thyroid disease.
- ☐ I have had my thyroid "monitored" in the past to watch for changes.
- ☐ I had a previous diagnosis of goiters/nodules.
- ☐ I currently have a goiter/enlargement in my thyroid and/or thyroid nodules.
- ☐ I was treated for hyperthyroidism in the past.
- ☐ I had postpartum thyroiditis or hyperthyroidism during a previous pregnancy.
- ☐ I had a temporary thyroiditis in the past.
- ☐ I have a family history of autoimmune disease.
- ☐ I have another autoimmune disease.
- ☐ I am pregnant now, or I have had a baby in the past nine months.
- ☐ I have a history of miscarriage.
- ☐ I have had radioactive iodine in the past due to Graves' disease/hyperthyroidism.
- ☐ I have taken antithyroid drugs in the past due to Graves' disease or a diagnosis of hyperthyroidism.

I have the following symptoms of hyperthyroidism:
- ☐ My heart feels like it's skipping a beat, racing, and I feel like I'm having heart palpitations.
- ☐ My pulse is unusually fast.
- ☐ My pulse, even when resting or in bed, is high.
- ☐ My blood pressure is high.
- ☐ My hands are shaking and/or I'm having hand tremors.
- ☐ I feel hot when others feel cold; I am feeling inappropriately hot or overheated.
- ☐ I am perspiring more or excessively.
- ☐ I am losing weight inappropriately.
- ☐ I am losing or maintaining weight but eating more.
- ☐ I feel like I have a lot of nervous energy that I need to burn off.
- ☐ I am having diarrhea or loose or more frequent bowel movements.
- ☐ My eyes are dry/blurry vision/a noticeable "stare" or bulging eyeballs.
- ☐ My skin looks or feels thinner.
- ☐ My muscles feel weak, particularly the upper arms and thighs.
- ☐ I am having difficulty getting to sleep, staying asleep, or going back to sleep after awakening in the middle of the night.
- ☐ I feel fatigued, exhausted.

☐ I have difficulty concentrating.
☐ My hair is coarse and dry, breaking, brittle, falling out.
☐ My skin is coarse, dry, scaly, thin.
☐ I have a hoarse or gravelly voice.
☐ I have pains, aches in joints, hands and feet.
☐ I am having irregular menstrual cycles (shorter, less frequent, lighter, or not at all).
☐ I am having trouble conceiving a baby.
☐ I have had one or more miscarriages.
☐ I feel depressed.
☐ I feel restless, nervous, irritable, or anxious.
☐ I experience panic attacks.

Special Considerations

Never plan to get pregnant while you are hyperthyroid or thyrotoxic due to any cause. Ensure your thyroid levels are optimized *before* trying to conceive.

Ensure that the cause of your hyperthyroidism is determined. See the section "Hyperthyroid Conditions" (page 201). Get a specific diagnosis and treatment plan prior to conception. Common causes of hyperthyroidism to investigate include:

- Graves' disease
- Toxic adenoma and toxic multinodular goiter
- Transient hyperthyroidism of hyperemesis gravidarum (THHG)
- First-trimester HCG elevation
- Hyperthyroid phase of Hashimoto's
- Painless thyroiditis
- Gestational transient thyrotoxicosis (GTT)
- Factitious hyperthyroidism due to thyroid hormone replacement over-medication for hypothyroidism

If you become pregnant while hyperthyroid or you develop hyperthyroidism during pregnancy, get a specific diagnosis and treatment plan as soon as possible. If you are diagnosed with Graves' disease or have uncontrolled or severe hyperthyroidism during pregnancy, consult with a perinatologist—an obstetrician who specializes in high-risk pregnancy. These doctors are also sometimes called "maternal-fetal medicine" or "high-risk pregnancy" specialists.

Diagnosis

Insist on a clinical evaluation to check for enlargement of your thyroid; eye symptoms, such as bulging of the eyeball; weight loss; rapid pulse; or higher blood pressure.

Understand the blood tests used for diagnosis of hyperthyroidism:

- TSH value less than 0.01 mIU/L
- Elevated Free T4 (Note: Free T4, *not* Total T4, should be measured.)
- Elevated Free T3
- Elevated thyroid-stimulating immunoglobulin (TSI), sometimes called TSH receptor antibody (TRAb)

Note: In nonpregnant patients, radioactive iodine uptake (RAIU) is used to evaluate the cause of hyperthyroidism. RAIU is never done during pregnancy.

Your baby's father should also have a thyroid evaluation if he presents with common symptoms and risk factors, or if he has a prior history of hyperthyroidism/Graves' disease.

Treatments

If you are pregnant with mild or subclinical hyperthyroidism and few symptoms, your doctor may recommend that your treatment be deferred until after pregnancy. Treatment is almost always required for moderate to severe hyperthyroidism.

Radioactive Iodine

Never receive RAI during pregnancy or while breastfeeding. Wait at least four weeks after nursing has ceased.

Wait six months to one year after RAI, and only after thyroid levels are stabilized, before attempting to conceive.

Antithyroid Drugs

Antithyroid drugs are almost always the first course of treatment in pregnancy. Propylthiouracil (PTU), methimazole (MMI), and carbimazole are effective in pregnant women.

PTU is typically recommended during the first trimester due to the rare risk of congenital birth defects with the other drugs.

Discontinue PTU after the first trimester around 13 weeks and switch to MMI to decrease the risk of liver disease associated with PTU. Recheck your thyroid levels two weeks after the switch.

Take MMI during the first trimester or take PTU during the second and third only in cases of allergies, sensitivities, or side effects from the other anti-thyroid drugs.

If you are diagnosed during the first trimester, start on the lowest possible dose of PTU, then retest thyroid levels every two weeks until levels normalize.

The Pregnancy Guidelines recommend antithyroid treatment during pregnancy to achieve a Free T4 at the top or slightly above the reference ranges and TSH in the low-normal range. Optimal thyroid treatment, however, is unique to the individual.

Avoid higher doses, such as more than 200 mg a day of PTU or 30 mg of MMI.

Ensure monitoring of thyroid levels every two to four weeks after levels are normalized.

Contact your doctor immediately if you experience any of the following symptoms:

- Fatigue
- Weakness
- Abdominal pain
- Loss of appetite
- Skin rash or itching
- Easy bruising
- Yellowing of the skin or whites of the eyes, called jaundice
- Persistent sore throat
- Fever

Beta-Blockers

Beta-blockers are frequently prescribed in nonpregnant patients.

If you have very elevated blood pressure or heart rate, or palpitations, a short course of beta-blockers may be prescribed for no longer than two weeks during pregnancy.

Do not take beta-blockers during the end of pregnancy.

Surgery

If you are not pregnant, surgical removal of the thyroid, known as thyroidectomy, is performed if antithyroid drugs can't be tolerated or RAI is ineffective.

Surgery is typically not done in pregnancy unless necessary. Some reasons for surgery during pregnancy:

- You have allergic reactions or side effects from antithyroid drugs.
- You require extremely high doses of antithyroid drugs (more than 30 mg of MMI or 300 mg of PTU).
- Your condition is not responding to antithyroid drugs.
- Your fetus is showing evidence of thyroid dysfunction due to antithyroid drugs (such as slow fetal heart rate or slowed bone development).

If surgery is required during pregnancy, it is recommended that the surgery be done during the second trimester.

After two miscarriages that were attributed to hyperthyroidism, Samantha's third pregnancy was off to a terrible start, and surgery was the best solution:

Because I was hyperthyroid during this pregnancy, I had high blood pressure, weekly adjustments of my medication, an emergency total thyroidectomy at 24 weeks pregnant, a placental abruption, and kidney failure. I had to have an emergency C-section at 35 weeks. But thanks to my medical team of seven specialists and one kick-ass maternal fetal medical physician, my gorgeous daughter is now five. She had no ill effects, and is healthy. And I am now hypothyroid with minimal struggles.

Speak with your doctor about a short course of potassium iodine solution and testing of antibody levels prior to surgery.

Two possible complications of thyroid surgery:

- Damage to the laryngeal nerves, resulting in temporary or permanent hoarseness or loss of voice. In rare cases tracheotomy is needed if both nerves are damaged.
- Damage to the parathyroid glands resulting in low calcium levels in the blood.

Ensure frequent monitoring of your thyroid levels postsurgery to determine optimal thyroid hormone replacement medication.

If you were previously treated or have a current diagnosis of Graves' disease, insist on monitoring of your antibodies.

Read Chapter 7 for tips on finding a good thyroid surgeon, what to expect from thyroid surgery, and the recuperation process.

Iodine Therapy

Consult with an integrative physician about the use of iodine therapy for hyperthyroidism in preconception and during pregnancy as an alternative to antithyroid drugs, RAI, and surgery.

Low-Dose Naltrexone (LDN)

Consult with an integrative physician about the use of low-dose naltrexone for Graves' disease in preconception and during pregnancy.

Hyperthyroid Conditions

Ensure that the cause of your hyperthyroidism is identified.

Graves' Disease

Check that your doctor has taken your family history and medical history, discussed your symptoms, and done a clinical examination looking for classic signs, such as goiter, high pulse rate, and eye-related symptoms.

Know the lab testing used for diagnosis:

- TSH value less than 0.01 mIU/L
- Elevated Free T4 (Note Free T4, *not* Total T4, should be measured)
- Elevated Free T3
- Elevated antibody thyroid-stimulating immunoglobulin (TSI)

In nonpregnant patients, radioactive iodine uptake (RAIU) is used for diagnosis. However, RAIU is never done during pregnancy.

Read treatment section above.

A complete thyroid panel, including TSI, should be checked around the midpoint of pregnancy, from between 20 and 24 weeks gestation.

If your TSI levels have dropped, your doctor may start tapering down your dosage. Most doctors will not discontinue antithyroid drug treatment until after the 32nd week of pregnancy.

If you have elevated levels of TSI your fetus should be checked for thyroid dysfunction, explained in the section titled "Fetal and Neonatal Hyperthyroidism" (page 207).

Toxic Adenoma/Toxic Multinodular Goiter

In nonpregnant patients, RAIU is used for diagnosis, but RAIU is not performed during pregnancy.

During pregnancy, diagnosis will typically be made using several criteria:

- Blood work that shows hyperthyroidism, but does not show thyroid antibodies
- Symptoms
- Visible nodules or visible enlargement of your thyroid
- Palpation of your neck, and ability to feel a nodule or nodules
- Ultrasound imaging that shows a nodule or nodules

During pregnancy, antithyroid drugs are the primary treatment. If the hyperthyroidism can't be controlled and poses a danger to you or your baby, or the nodule(s) are threatening your ability to breathe or swallow, surgery may be recommended.

After a miscarriage, followed by a successful pregnancy, Courtney wanted her son to have a little brother or sister.

We started trying when our son was about 18 months old and I got pregnant right away. I noticed that this pregnancy was way different than the other two. I was nauseous all the time and threw up about once a day. I started having crazy heart palpitations and dizzy spells. My heart was at 150 at rest lying down. This really freaked me out! My doctor put me on heart medications. I lost the baby at 12 weeks. That was a year ago. Since I lost our baby, I've been on the warpath with doctors. I finally found a doctor that listens to me. In the past, I had seen an ENT surgeon, since my endocrinologist wouldn't listen to me. They discovered nodules on my thyroid but said they were benign. They wouldn't put me on thyroid meds because my levels were always in the "normal" range. The ENT doctor offered to remove my thyroid. I agreed. He removed my thyroid and discovered at least a dozen noncancerous nodules. I just wish a doctor would have listened to me before I lost my two babies when I kept telling them I didn't feel well. It wasn't all in my head like they thought.

Following childbirth, and after you conclude breastfeeding, if your nodule(s) continue to cause hyperthyroidism or significant symptoms, your doctor may recommend RAI treatment or surgery.

Transient Hyperthyroidism of Hyperemesis Gravidarum (THHG)

If you develop hyperemesis gravidarum—persistent vomiting—during your pregnancy, have your thyroid function evaluated, including TSI levels. In some cases, this condition is associated with a short-term hyperthyroidism known, logically enough, as transient hyperthyroidism of hyperemesis gravidarum, or THHG.

THHG presents with free T4 usually only slightly elevated and the T3 level typically normal.

Some factors distinguish THHG from other types of hyperthyroidism in pregnant women:

- The presence of severe vomiting, not characteristic of typical hyperthyroidism
- Significant weight loss, which is not characteristic during pregnancy
- The lack of typical Graves' disease symptoms, including goiter (enlarged thyroid) and eye-related symptoms
- The lack of other "classic" hyperthyroidism symptoms such as tachycardia (a rapid heart rate greater than 100 beats/minute), diarrhea, muscle weakness, or tremor

Some cases of THHG require no thyroid-specific treatment, and the thyroid abnormalities will spontaneously resolve by the end of the second trimester.

If your symptoms are severe, you may receive a short course of antithyroid drugs, usually PTU, during the first trimester. If you are also diagnosed with Graves' disease, you should be treated with antithyroid drugs as clinically necessary. You may require hospitalization to receive intravenous fluids and nutrition. In some severe cases, medications, including metoclopramide (Reglan), antihistamines, and antireflux medications, may also be prescribed.

If your symptoms are mild, treatment usually involves dietary changes, rest, and antacids. Consider alternative treatments including acupressure, herbal remedies such as peppermint and ginger, and hypnosis.

HCG Elevation

If you have HCG-elevated hyperthyroidism, which normally presents around 13 weeks, you should have your thyroid levels monitored monthly through your pregnancy until levels return to normal.

No treatment is normally needed since this condition usually returns to normal during the second and third trimester.

Hashimoto's Disease/Hyperthyroid Phase

If you are diagnosed with Hashimoto's and develop hyperthyroidism symptoms during your pregnancy, have your TSH, Free T4, Free T3, TPOAb, TgAb, and TSI checked.

Your thyroid hormone replacement medication may need to be lowered. Have your thyroid levels rechecked every two weeks because your thyroid may quickly shift back into hypothyroidism and your dose will again need to be increased.

If you are not being treated with thyroid hormone replacement medication, depending on how elevated your thyroid levels are and on the severity of your symptoms, your doctor may recommend a short course of antithyroid drugs. Have your levels rechecked every two weeks, as it's possible that within weeks, your thyroid may shift back into hypothyroidism, and you will need a reduction in the dosage of antithyroid drugs, or even to stop taking them entirely.

Painless Thyroiditis

Painless thyroiditis usually presents with low TSH, elevated Free T4, and the absence of thyroid antibodies. Have your thyroid levels monitored throughout pregnancy. Treatment is most likely not needed.

Gestational Transient Thyroiditis (GTT)

Diagnosis of GTT is made when you have no history of previous hyperthyroidism, no goiter, no thyroid antibodies, but low TSH and elevated Free T4 and Free T3 levels.

Typically, no treatment is needed for GTT. In the rare case of severe GTT—having a Free T4 level that is above the reference range and a TSH less than 0.1—you may need a course of treatment with antithyroid drugs.

Factitious Hyperthyroidism

Your doctor will lower your dose of thyroid hormone replacement medication, since this condition is caused by overmedication for hypothyroidism. You should be retested within several weeks, and continue adjusting your dosage and rechecking until the hyperthyroidism resolves, and blood test levels return to normal.

Thyroid Storm

If you suspect that you are going into thyroid storm, you must go immediately to an emergency room, as this is a life-threatening condition that can develop and worsen quickly. You must be treated within hours to avoid fatal complications such as stroke or heart attack.

Untreated Graves' disease and/or hyperthyroidism are particular risk factors, as are being female, and pregnant. Even when Graves' disease has been diagnosed and is being treated, certain other factors raise the risk of thyroid storm:

- Infection: lung infection, throat infection, or pneumonia
- Blood sugar changes: diabetic ketoacidosis, insulin-induced hypoglycemia
- Recent surgery to the thyroid
- Abrupt withdrawal of antithyroid medications
- Radioactive iodine (RAI) treatment of the thyroid
- Excessive palpation (handling/manipulation) of the thyroid
- Severe emotional stress
- An overdose of thyroid hormone
- Toxemia of pregnancy and labor

The symptoms of thyroid storm include:

- Fever of 100 to as high as 106
- A high heart rate that can be as high as 200 beats per minute
- Palpitations, chest pain, shortness of breath
- High blood pressure

- Confusion, delirium, and even psychosis
- Extreme weakness and fatigue
- Extreme restlessness, nervousness, mood swings
- Exaggerated reflexes
- Difficulty breathing
- Nausea, vomiting, diarrhea
- Recent dramatic weight loss may have taken place
- Profuse sweating, dehydration
- Stupor or coma

Thyroid storm is treated on an emergency basis with a combination of antithyroid drugs, blockade iodine drug, beta-blockers, and treatment for any underlying nonthyroidal illness or infection that may be contributing to the thyroid storm.

Natural Approaches to Treating Hyperthyroidism

Hyperthyroidism during pregnancy requires careful treatment. Natural treatments may take time and some treatments including herbs may not be safe in pregnancy. Before you conceive, however, is an ideal time to explore natural treatment options with an experienced practitioner.

Consult with a holistic practitioner to discuss natural approaches that are safe during pregnancy given your own individual situation. The approaches your practitioner recommends may include:

- Eating more goitrogenic foods
- Taking such supplements as selenium, magnesium, omega-3 fatty acids, vitamin D, B vitamins, iodine, lithium, and l-carnitine
- Taking herbs such as lemon balm (*Melissa officinalis*), bugleweed, eleuthero, passionflower, and motherwort
- Reducing stress

If you have been diagnosed with Graves' disease, consult with an integrative physician who looks at the immune system. He or she may investigate root causes of autoimmunity, including food sensitivities (in particular, gluten), leaky gut, blood sugar imbalance, chronic inflammation, environmental toxins, chronic infections, allergies, gut flora imbalance, adrenal dysfunction, and nutrient deficiencies, including too-low levels of vitamin D and selenium.

For more information on addressing an underlying autoimmune condition, read the "Autoimmunity" section in Chapter 9.

Fetal and Neonatal Hyperthyroidism

Your baby is at risk of developing thyroid dysfunction if:

- You had Graves' disease in the past and had RAI or surgery to treat it (no matter how long it has been since you had RAI or thyroidectomy).
- You developed Graves' disease during the pregnancy and are being treated with antithyroid drugs.
- You developed Graves' disease during the pregnancy and had surgery to treat it.

If you have a past or current history of Graves' disease, make sure that you consult with a pediatric endocrinologist, a maternal-fetal medicine specialist, a perinatologist, or a high-risk OB with expertise in fetal and neonatal thyroid issues, to ensure that your baby is properly monitored and treated before and after birth.

If you have a past or current history of Graves' disease, notify your OB, endocrinologist, the attending physicians, pediatricians, and nurses at the hospital.

Monitoring During Pregnancy

If you have a past or current history of Graves' disease, ensure that your TSI is measured at 20 to 24 weeks gestation.

If you have Graves' disease/hyperthyroidism during pregnancy, or have a history of Graves' disease, ensure that your baby is screened for fetal thyroid dysfunction during the fetal anatomy ultrasound done between weeks 18 to 22, and rescreened every 4 to 6 weeks thereafter, or as clinically indicated. The screening will assess fetal heart rate (fetal thyrotoxicosis is suggested when the baby's heart rate is more than 160 beats per minute), and the ultrasound will be examined for any signs of thyroid enlargement, goiter, growth retardation, hydrops, or accelerated bone maturation.

If your unborn baby is determined to be hyperthyroid, you may be prescribed the antithyroid drug methimazole, whether or not you yourself are hyperthyroid, to help normalize your baby's thyroid function before birth.

Neonatal Hyperthyroidism

If you had elevated antibodies during your third trimester or your newborn is suspected to be hyperthyroid, ensure that your pediatric endocrinologist or specialist tests the newborn's TSH and Free T4 levels right after birth.

Watch your newborn for symptoms of hyperthyroidism. Signs and symptoms of hyperthyroidism in a newborn include:

- An unusually small head circumference
- An unusually prominent forehead
- A dangerous accumulation of fluid under the skin (known as fetal hydrops)
- Enlarged liver and/or spleen
- Low birth weight
- Premature birth
- Warm, moist skin
- High blood pressure
- Fast heartbeat
- Irregular heart rhythms
- Irritability, hyperactivity, restlessness, poor sleep
- An enlarged thyroid (goiter)
- Difficulty breathing due to goiter pressing on the windpipe
- Excessive or normal appetite, with poor weight gain
- Bulging eyes, stare
- Vomiting
- Diarrhea

Get testing done immediately if you see any of these symptoms in your baby.

Treatment for neonatal hyperthyroidism should be started as soon as it's diagnosed. Typically, an antithyroid drug is used, along with a beta-blocker, such as propranolol, to help control muscular and heart overactivity. In some cases, iodine in the form of Lugol's solution or potassium iodide may be given to help inhibit the release of thyroid hormones. If your baby is extremely hyperthyroid, your doctor may prescribe glucocorticoid drugs.

Your baby should have weekly thyroid function tests to monitor progress. Once the condition starts to improve, the dosages of medications can be gradually decreased, and ultimately discontinued. This usually takes place between 3 and 12 weeks, as your antibodies disappear from your baby's circulation.

There are some rare cases, however, where neonatal hyperthyroidism has continued for as long as six months or more in an infant.

Fetal and Neonatal Hypothyroidism

If you are being treated with antithyroid drugs during pregnancy, there are two key risk factors that can increase the risk of your baby's developing fetal or neonatal hypothyroidism:

- Poor control of your hyperthyroidism throughout your pregnancy
- High doses of antithyroid drugs

If your specialist confirms fetal hypothyroidism as a complication of your treatment, they will likely reduce your dosage of antithyroid medications.

As part of the postbirth "heel-stick test," babies born in the United States are automatically tested for hypothyroidism at birth. However, you should ensure that not only this test, but also a more detailed panel of thyroid tests, are done on your newborn, if you have any risk factors, or your newborn shows any of the following symptoms of neonatal hypothyroidism:

- A dull expression
- Puffiness in the face
- A thickened tongue
- A tongue that sticks out of the baby's mouth
- Episodes of choking
- Constipation
- Jaundice
- Poor feeding
- Excessive sleepiness or lethargy
- Lack of muscle tone
- Unusually short height
- Decreased muscle tone
- Failure to grow
- A hoarse cry
- Large soft spots on the skull

If neonatal hypothyroidism is diagnosed, your baby should start thyroid hormone replacement treatment immediately. Regular follow-up is necessary, because if the hypothyroidism is transient, the baby will eventually be able to stop taking the thyroid medication. But if the thyroid gland has been permanently damaged, then thyroid hormone replacement treatment will need to continue indefinitely.

Your Monitoring Timeline

Given the number of tests and retests needed to monitor women with hyperthyroidism/Graves' disease during pregnancy and their babies, we've created a suggested timeline to discuss with your doctor. Always call your doctor right away, even before scheduled checkup appointments, if symptoms worsen or new symptoms develop. In the case of suspected thyroid storm, go immediately to the emergency room.

Preconception

Test TSH, Free T4, Free T3, and TSI for women who have a past or current history of hyperthyroidism/Graves' disease. Women who have risk factors and common hyperthyroidism/Graves' disease symptoms but no current diagnosis should also seek testing preconception.

RAIU, if needed, is safe preconception, but not safe during pregnancy.

RAI and surgery are options in preconception. RAI is not safe during pregnancy. Surgery is recommended only for second trimester.

Wait 6 to 12 months, and only after thyroid levels are stabilized after RAI, to try to conceive.

Preconception is an ideal time to consult with an integrative physician about natural treatments.

Positive Pregnancy Test

Test TSH, Free T4, Free T3, and TSI.

Switch to PTU as soon as possible for the first trimester if you are on another antithyroid medication.

If you are newly diagnosed in the first trimester, start PTU and have testing every 2 weeks until normalized.

Week 5

Recheck thyroid levels TSH, Free T4, and Free T3. Continue rechecking every 2 to 4 weeks after levels have normalized.

Week 7

Recheck thyroid levels TSH, Free T4, and Free T3.

Week 10

Recheck thyroid levels TSH, Free T4, and Free T3.

Week 13

Recheck thyroid levels TSH, Free T4, and Free T3.
Switch from PTU to MMI.

Week 14

Surgery, if needed, is recommended in the second trimester (beginning at week 14 after your last menstrual period through week 27 of pregnancy).

Ensure frequent monitoring of your thyroid levels, including TSI, post-surgery to reach optimal thyroid hormone replacement.

Week 15

Recheck thyroid levels TSH, Free T4, and Free T3 (two weeks after switch from PTU to MMI).

Week 18

Recheck thyroid levels TSH, Free T4, and Free T3.

If you have Graves' disease/hyperthyroidism during pregnancy or have a history of Graves' disease, ensure fetal thyroid dysfunction is screened during the fetal anatomy ultrasound done between weeks 18 to 22, and rescreened every 4 to 6 weeks or as clinically needed.

Week 22

Recheck thyroid levels TSH, Free T4, and Free T3, as well as TSI between 20 to 24 weeks if you have a past or current history of Graves' disease.
Screening for fetal thyroid dysfunction.

Week 26

Recheck thyroid levels TSH, Free T4, and Free T3.
Screening for fetal thyroid dysfunction as clinically needed.

Week 30

Recheck thyroid levels TSH, Free T4, and Free T3.
Screening for fetal thyroid dysfunction as clinically needed.

If you have elevated antibodies during the third trimester or your newborn is suspected to be hyperthyroid, contact a pediatric endocrinologist, a maternal-fetal medicine specialist, a perinatologist, or a high-risk OB with expertise in fetal and neonatal thyroid issues in the hospital where you plan to deliver in advance to ensure your newborn is tested right after birth.

Week 34

Recheck thyroid levels TSH, Free T4, and Free T3.
Screening for fetal thyroid dysfunction as clinically needed.

Week 38

Recheck thyroid levels TSH, Free T4, and Free T3.
Screening for fetal thyroid dysfunction as clinically needed.

Baby's Birth

Ensure your baby receives the "heel-stick test" postbirth to test for neonatal hypothyroidism at the hospital.

If you had elevated antibodies during your third trimester, or your newborn is suspected to be hyperthyroid, have a pediatric endocrinologist, a maternal-fetal medicine specialist, a perinatologist, or a high-risk OB with expertise in fetal and neonatal thyroid issues test your newborn's thyroid function right after birth.

Watch your newborn for signs of thyroid dysfunction for several weeks after birth.

12

Thyroiditis, Goiter, Nodules, and Thyroid Cancer

Thyroiditis

In nonpregnant patients a radioiodine uptake is often used to identify the type of thyroiditis; however, this test should not be done in pregnancy. Diagnosis during pregnancy is made by symptoms, clinical examination, blood tests, imaging tests, or in some cases, fine-needle aspiration biopsy, which is considered safe in pregnancy.

Painless Thyroiditis/Silent Thyroiditis/Lymphocytic Thyroiditis

You will most likely not need treatment because this tends to be a short-term, transient condition.

Speak to your doctor if you are on any of the following medications that can trigger painless thyroiditis—interferon-alfa, interleukin-2, amiodarone, and lithium.

De Quervain's Thyroiditis/Granulomatous Thyroiditis/Painful Thyroiditis/Subacute Thyroiditis

This type of thyroiditis typically starts out with a period of hyperthyroidism that may last from four to six weeks. Thyroid hormone levels then start to drop, becoming normal for about four weeks, and then continue to decline toward a hypothyroid phase, which again lasts around four to six weeks.

In nonpregnant patients, pain or swelling is treated with nonsteroidal anti-inflammatory drugs, such as aspirin or ibuprofen. Since these drugs are not recommended during pregnancy, consider non-medication-based treatments, such as hot or cold compresses.

Beta-blockers may be prescribed if you are experiencing significant hyperthyroid symptoms during pregnancy for no longer than two weeks. Do not take beta-blockers during the end of pregnancy.

Thyroid hormone replacement medication may be needed in a hypothyroid phase during pregnancy, to ensure that your TSH is within the range appropriate for your trimester. See Chapter 5 for pregnancy treatment considerations for hypothyroidism.

Ensure that your diagnosis is included in your medical records, and request that a comprehensive thyroid panel be part of your annual checkup.

Acute Suppurative Thyroiditis

This type of thyroiditis is usually caused by a bacterial infection that can lead to an abscess in the thyroid gland.

Treatment steps may include:

- Ultrasound of the thyroid, to determine whether there are any abscesses to be treated. Ultrasound is safe during pregnancy.
- Fine-needle aspiration (FNA) of the mass in your thyroid; the fluid or material will be cultured to identify infection. FNA is considered safe in pregnancy.
- Blood tests to evaluate thyroid function (TSH, Free T4, and Free T3), and to look for signs of infection
- Prescription of an antibiotic medicine that will treat the particular type of infection. (There are antibiotics that are considered safe to take during pregnancy.)
- Drainage of the mass or lump
- Surgical drainage or removal of the gland in rare cases

Postpartum Thyroiditis

There are a few different, typical courses of postpartum thyroiditis:

- Mild hypothyroidism that typically starts around two to six months after delivery, and then normalizes
- Mild hyperthyroidism that typically starts around one to four months after delivery, and then normalizes

- Mild hyperthyroidism, beginning one to four months after delivery, lasting around two to eight weeks, shifting into mild hypothyroidism, which can last for weeks or months, and then normalizes

To differentiate between the hyperthyroid phase of postpartum thyroiditis and Graves' disease, ensure testing of the antibody thyroid-stimulating immunoglobulin (TSI), which is typically positive in Graves' disease, and evaluation of clinical signs of Graves' disease, including goiter and ophthalmopathy/thyroid eye disease.

If radioactive iodine uptake (RAIU) is needed and you are breastfeeding, insist that iodine-123 or technetium be used instead of iodine-131. Pump and discard milk for several days, before resuming breastfeeding.

Antithyroid drugs are not typically recommended for the hyperthyroid phase. Speak to your doctor about a beta-blocker, such as propranolol at the lowest possible dose, to relieve symptoms. Propranolol is considered safe while breastfeeding.

If you are in the hypothyroid phase and have severe symptoms or if you are planning to try to get pregnant again, have a complete thyroid panel, including TSH, Free T4, Free T3, TPOAb, and TgAb rechecked every four to six weeks. If your thyroid levels are not optimal and you are symptomatic, treatment should be considered.

Given that women with Graves' disease in remission and women who became hyperthyroid after a previous pregnancy are at higher risk to develop postpartum thyroiditis, request thyroid screening at three and six months postpartum.

If you have a prior history of PPT ensure you receive annual thyroid testing to evaluate for permanent hypothyroidism.

Start supplementation with 200 mcg per day of selenium in the form of selenomethionine during preconception, and continue through the first year after pregnancy. Some studies have shown that supplemental selenium may help prevent postpartum thyroiditis in women who are positive for thyroid peroxidase antibodies (TPOAb). Check your prenatal vitamin to determine the dose of selenium included, and if needed add on an individual selenium supplement to total 200 mcg per day. You should not take more than 400 mcg of selenium per day.

Goiter/Enlarged Thyroid

Your physician will assess the cause of the goiter to determine the course of treatment. Possible causes to investigate include:

- Iodine deficiency
- Hashimoto's disease
- Graves' disease
- Multinodular goiter
- Large nodule
- Thyroiditis
- Thyroid cancer

Diagnostic tests include:

- Blood tests—TSH, Free T4, Free T3, TPOAb, TgAb, and TSI
- Urinary iodine test
- Ultrasound
- Fine-needle aspiration (FNA) biopsy
- Radioactive scans are used in nonpregnant patients, but are not done during pregnancy

If surgery is necessary due to pain, impaired breathing or swallowing, surgery will be scheduled for the second trimester or after pregnancy. Thyroidectomy will render you hypothyroid requiring lifelong thyroid hormone replacement medication.

Nodules/Lumps/Cysts

Consult an endocrinologist with expertise in thyroid disease and thyroid nodules.

A thyroid ultrasound will be performed.

Nodules larger than 1 cm should be biopsied during pregnancy, and nodules from 5 mm to 1 cm in size should be biopsied if you have any thyroid cancer family risk or suspicious findings on the ultrasound.

If the nodules are not causing physical symptoms, have no suspicious characteristics of cancer, and/or have been shown to be benign after biopsy, most doctors recommend monitoring them periodically with ultrasound. If they remain the same size, periodic monitoring continues.

Speak to your doctor about percutaneous ethanol injection (PEI) for benign cystic (fluid-filled) nodules during pregnancy.

If surgery is required for a benign nodule, it is recommended that the surgery be performed in the second trimester or after delivery.

If a benign thyroid nodule is producing thyroid hormones (known as a "toxic" nodule), RAI is not given during pregnancy or breastfeeding. See Chapter 11 for hyperthyroidism treatments safe during pregnancy and lactation.

Speak to your doctor about radiofrequency thermal ablation.

All nodules found during pregnancy should be fully evaluated, including blood work, ultrasound, and if there are any suspicious characteristics or family history of thyroid cancer, a fine-needle aspiration (FNA) biopsy.

Consider Afirma Thyroid FNA Analysis for inconclusive or indeterminate thyroid nodules.

Thyroid cancer expert Jennifer Sipos shared:

> During pregnancy the biggest question is: If the FNA biopsy comes back malignant, what are we going to do with that information? For most patients who have a thyroid cancer diagnosis during pregnancy, we wait until after they deliver. We will usually say to the patient, "We're not going to do any kind of surgery for this cancer until after you deliver, so do we want to know if it's cancer or not during the pregnancy, and do you want to live with the potential stress of that during the pregnancy? Or do you want to wait until after delivery for us to do the FNA?" If I were in that position, I would probably just watch the nodule during pregnancy and wait until after delivery to do the FNA.

If your FNA biopsy determines that you have thyroid cancer, ensure that your practitioner is not just an endocrinologist but an endocrine thyroid specialist who has particular expertise in thyroid cancer.

Thyroid Cancer

Testing

Testing for thyroid cancer during pregnancy typically involves:

- Blood work, including TSH, Free T4, Free T3, and thyroglobulin (Tg) levels
- Testing calcitonin levels if you have a family history of medullary thyroid carcinoma or multiple endocrine neoplasia (MEN) 2
- Thyroid ultrasound
- FNA biopsy
- Radioactive uptake test, usually done in a nonpregnant patient but not done in pregnancy

Thyroid Cancer Risks and Symptoms Checklist

☐ I have a family history of thyroid cancer.
☐ I have had radiation treatments to my neck area.
☐ I have had exposure to radiation or nuclear accidents, especially in childhood.
☐ I have a lump or nodule in the neck, especially in the front of the neck, in the area of the Adam's apple.
☐ I have an enlargement of the neck.
☐ I have enlarged lymph nodes in the neck.
☐ I have hoarseness, difficulty speaking, voice changes.
☐ I have difficulty swallowing, or a choking feeling.
☐ I have difficulty breathing.
☐ I have pain in my neck or throat or discomfort with neckties, turtlenecks, scarves, necklaces.
☐ I have a persistent or chronic cough not due to allergies or illness.
☐ I have asymmetry in the thyroid.

Types of Thyroid Cancer

Papillary and Follicular Cancer

For well-differentiated thyroid cancer found during pregnancy, the 2011 "Guidelines of the American Thyroid Association for the Diagnosis and Management of Thyroid Disease During Pregnancy and Postpartum," or Pregnancy Guidelines, suggest that surgery may generally be deferred until after delivery. However, neck ultrasounds should be performed each trimester to assess for rapid nodular growth or lymph node metastases, which will require surgery. Your doctor will, however, likely recommend increasing your thyroid hormone dosage to achieve a suppressed TSH below normal, 0.1 to 1.5 mIU/L, to help prevent the cancer from spreading.

For metastatic or late-stage papillary and follicular thyroid cancer during pregnancy, you will need to consult with a thyroid cancer specialist to discuss the safety and potential concerns regarding the radiation treatments, drugs, and chemotherapy that are used for nonpregnant patients.

While surgery is generally deferred until after pregnancy, if surgery is necessary, the second trimester is typically recommended.

> **Choosing a Surgeon**
>
> When it comes to picking your surgeon, make sure you select someone with extensive experience in thyroid surgery.
> - Ask how many thyroid surgeries he or she performs each year. (100+ should be minimum.)
> - Consider traveling to a university hospital or medical center that specializes in thyroid surgeries.
> - Surgical specialists can be either head/neck surgeons or surgical oncologists. Find one that specializes in endocrine surgery.

Thyroid Hormone Replacement Medication

All patients receiving a total thyroidectomy and the majority of patients receiving subtotal thyroidectomy (partial removal of the thyroid gland) will require lifelong thyroid hormone replacement treatment, often at suppressive levels to keep the TSH below the level that is the normal range for someone without thyroid cancer to prevent recurrence. See Chapter 5 or 10 for pregnancy treatment considerations for hypothyroidism.

Medullary Thyroid Cancer

For medullary thyroid cancer, surgery is recommended during pregnancy if there is a large primary tumor, or extensive spread to the lymph nodes. The surgery would typically be performed during the second trimester, but based on the stage and aggressiveness of the cancer, the need for immediate surgery may outweigh the risks, and the surgery could be performed any time during the pregnancy.

The treatment for medullary cancer is typically to remove the thyroid, and lymph nodes, if affected. RAI is not used, as this type of cancer does not take up iodine. Follow-up with thyroid hormone replacement is necessary.

These are the specialists involved in MTC treatment:

- Head/neck surgeons or surgical oncologists who specialize in endocrine surgery
- Endocrinologists
- Radiologists
- Medical oncologists for advanced cases

Medical oncologist Dr. Scot C. Remick advises:

> If it's a complex thyroid case, it's important to avail yourself of multidisciplinary care at a major medical center to coordinate what is the optimal approach. See if there are any trials and coordinate the different modalities of therapy. That does not necessarily need to be immediately at a university center or a National Cancer Institute NCI-Designated Cancer Center. There are many prominent, large community hospitals that have multidisciplinary tumor boards.

For advanced medullary thyroid cancer during pregnancy, consult with a thyroid cancer specialist.

Anaplastic Thyroid Cancer

Treatment for anaplastic thyroid cancer typically includes a full thyroidectomy. Because this is an aggressive and invasive cancer that may affect the trachea (windpipe), patients may also need a tracheostomy. A thyroid cancer expert will need to make further recommendations regarding radiation, drug, or chemotherapy treatments for this type of thyroid cancer during pregnancy.

Surgery Follow-up

Thyroidectomy renders patients hypothyroid, meaning they will require lifelong thyroid hormone replacement medication.

All thyroid cancer patients undergo regular monitoring of thyroid levels via blood test, to make sure that the thyroid hormone replacement dose is optimal and that TSH levels are suppressed if necessary. Follow-up may also include:

- Physical examinations
- Neck ultrasound
- RAI scan—Not done during pregnancy or while breastfeeding
- Thyroglobulin (Tg) blood tests
- Antithyroglobulin antibodies (TgAb) test
- MRI of the head/neck/chest area—Not typically done during pregnancy or while breastfeeding.

If you want more information on life after a thyroidectomy or have further questions, contact the Thyroid Cancer Survivors' Association (ThyCa). See Appendix A for its contact information.

Treating Hypothyroidism in Pregnant Thyroid Cancer Survivors

According to the Pregnancy Guidelines, in women who have persistent thyroid cancer, TSH can be maintained below 0.1 mIU/L during pregnancy. In women who are free of thyroid cancer but who had a high-risk tumor in the past, suppression should be maintained at TSH levels between 0.1 mIU/L and 0.5 mIU/L. In low-risk patients with no signs of thyroid cancer, TSH can be kept at the lower end of the normal range (0.3–1.5 mIU/L).

Typically, pregnant women who are on thyroid hormone replacement after thyroid cancer require a smaller dose increase compared to women who are hypothyroid due to other disorders. The guidelines recommend that in these women, TSH be monitored every four weeks during pregnancy until 16 to 20 weeks of gestation and once between 26 and 32 weeks of gestation.

Wait six months to one year after RAI to ensure optimal thyroid hormone replacement treatment and to confirm remission of thyroid cancer before trying to conceive.

If a woman has had a previously treated differentiated thyroid cancer, and undetectable thyroglobulin (Tg) levels, no special monitoring is needed during pregnancy. However, the guidelines recommend an ultrasound be performed during each trimester in a woman previously treated for differentiated thyroid cancer who has high Tg levels or any evidence of persistent disease.

13

Postpartum

Postpartum is a time when women are vulnerable to developing a new thyroid condition or the worsening of an existing one. Push for a comprehensive thyroid workup, including Free T4, Free T3, Reverse T3, TPOAb, and TgAb, if you are not currently diagnosed but have symptoms of thyroid disease. Schedule regular thyroid monitoring, usually at least every three months, throughout the first postpartum year.

Keep taking your prenatal vitamin all the way through postpartum for as long as you are nursing your child and possibly longer.

Request comprehensive nutrient assessment, including vitamin D, ferritin, vitamin B_{12}, magnesium, iodine, and selenium, during postpartum. Continue to supplement for nutrient deficiencies as advised by your doctor.

And take care of yourself. Postpartum is a challenging time for every mom, but for thyroid patients there is the added complexity of shifting hormones and in many cases worsening of symptoms. Rest whenever possible. Ask for help from friends and family. For the first three months, minimum, get help with household chores, laundry, cooking, cleaning, and so forth. Hire a doula or a mother's helper if you can. Don't feel guilty about accepting or paying for help.

Hypothyroidism/Hashimoto's

If you have, or have had hypothyroidism, have thyroid testing, including TSH, Free T4, Free T3, Reverse T3, TPOAb, and TgAb, done no more than two weeks after delivery, and any necessary medication dosage adjustments made.

Get your thyroid rechecked no more than eight weeks later and thereafter every eight weeks, until you are stabilized at optimum thyroid levels.

Dana's Experience

The postpartum year after my first son, Benjamin, was born was the most challenging year of my life. My hypothyroidism symptoms raged high but I remained undiagnosed until the end of that year. I didn't know that I was battling a health condition that was robbing me of my energy and I felt like a bad mother. I struggled every single day that year just to stay awake. I don't know how I survived that difficult time.

When I was pregnant with my second son, I knew better. I prepared myself for postpartum. I hired helpers in advance to assist me in the early months with chores and babysitting so I could catch up on missed sleep. I called a lactation consultant and scheduled visits with her in advance. I rented a hospital-grade electric breast pump to arrive on the day I came home from the hospital. I had my doctor give me a lab requisition form in advance of my delivery so that I could go in a few days postpartum to have my thyroid lab tests drawn. I had meals ready in the freezer and a file full of great take-out options ready. Family flew in from out of town to stay with me for the first few weeks. My acupuncturist was actually waiting for me in the lobby of my building the day I came home from the hospital with my baby, to give me treatments to restore my health and build up my milk supply.

If there is one piece of advice that I have for postpartum women with thyroid disease it is to *be good to yourself.*

For Hashimoto's patients, ensure your TSH is kept in the lower end of the reference range around 1.0, to help avoid the risk of antibody flare-up in the months after childbirth.

If you had elevated thyroid peroxidase antibodies (TPOAb) before or during pregnancy and did not receive treatment due to normal thyroid levels, you are at risk of becoming hypothyroid after pregnancy. Ensure your thyroid is regularly monitored and watch yourself for symptoms postpartum, using the checklist provided in Chapter 10.

Hyperthyroidism/Graves' Disease

If you have hyperthyroidism postpartum, methimazole is the first choice of treatment. If you are breastfeeding, doses up to 20 to 30 milligrams of methimazole a day—taken as divided doses after breastfeeding—are considered safe for you and your baby.

Propylthiouracil (PTU), because it is associated with an increased risk of liver toxicity, is the second choice for antithyroid medication after pregnancy, at doses up to 300mg a day.

RAI or surgery may be performed if you are allergic or sensitive to antithyroid medication or your hyperthyroidism does not respond to medications. RAI is not safe while breastfeeding.

Consult with an alternative-minded health-care practitioner to see if natural approaches to reducing autoimmunity and managing hyperthyroidism—which can include supplements, herbs, dietary changes, and such treatments as low-dose naltrexone—can put you into remission without RAI, surgery, or antithyroid medication. Discuss the safety of these treatments while breastfeeding. It can take as long as eighteen months to regulate and control Graves' disease hyperthyroidism using natural approaches. See Chapter 6 for an in-depth look at hyperthyroidism testing and treatment.

Emma had a difficult pregnancy, with many symptoms, and postpartum, she learned just in time that she was suffering from hyperthyroidism:

> I had a terrible time breastfeeding my baby girl. It just didn't happen. I got to 6 weeks postpartum. I tried to book in with my GP for the six week postnatal checkup and was told they couldn't fit me in for another 4 weeks and to phone back. I was starting to feel more and more unwell. Things just weren't right. I was exhausted. Things got worse and when I phoned back for an appointment I was told I'd have to wait again! My baby was 10 weeks old by this time. I was terrified I had postpartum depression, and I needed blood work to help me figure out what I was dealing with! The doctor did blood work, and put me on beta-blockers, which landed me in the emergency room a few days later. I was not right. I turned into a verbally violent, almost psychotic, bag of rage! I screamed at my poor husband and there was nothing anyone could do. I got a phone call a few days later from the doctor telling me I needed to start medication immediately and there was no time to wait! Turns out, I was close to a thyroid storm! My levels were that high. I am very upset that thyroid testing is not an essential test during and after pregnancy! I could have died, and so could my baby. This could wreck lives even without the prospect of losing a child. It hurts me to think of everyone else going through it, not knowing to demand.

Postpartum Thyroiditis

Know the three typical potential courses of postpartum thyroiditis:

- Mild hypothyroidism, which typically starts around two to six months after delivery, and then normalizes
- Mild hyperthyroidism, which typically starts around one to four months after delivery, and then normalizes
- Mild hyperthyroidism, beginning one to four months after delivery, lasting around two to eight weeks, then shifting into mild hypothyroidism, which can last for weeks or months and then normalizes

To differentiate between the hyperthyroid phase of postpartum thyroiditis and Graves' disease, ensure testing of the antibody thyroid-stimulating immunoglobulin (TSI), which is typically positive in Graves' disease, and evaluation of clinical signs of Graves' disease including goiter and ophthalmopathy/thyroid eye disease.

If radioactive iodine uptake (RAIU) is needed and you are breastfeeding, insist that iodine-123 or technetium be used instead of iodine-131. Pump and discard milk for several days, then you can resume breastfeeding.

Antithyroid drugs are not typically recommended for the hyperthyroid phase. Speak to your doctor about a beta-blocker such as propranolol at the lowest possible dose to relieve symptoms. Propranolol is considered safe while breastfeeding.

If you are in the hypothyroid phase of postpartum thyroiditis and have severe symptoms or if you are planning to try to get pregnant again, have a complete thyroid panel including TSH, Free T4, and Free T3 rechecked every four to six weeks. Ensure testing of both TPOAb and TgAb to differentiate between postpartum thyroiditis and Hashimoto's disease. Hashimoto's can come with swings up and down in TSH with both hypothyroid and hyperthyroid symptoms. If your thyroid levels are not optimal and you are symptomatic, treatment should be considered.

Women with Graves' disease in remission and women who became hyperthyroid after a previous pregnancy are at higher risk to develop postpartum thyroiditis. If you are at higher risk for one of these reasons, request thyroid screening at three and six months postpartum.

If you have a prior history of postpartum depression (PPD), ensure that you receive annual thyroid testing to evaluate for permanent hypothyroidism.

Start supplementation with 200 mcg per day of selenium in the form of selenomethionine preconception and continue through the first year after pregnancy. Some studies have shown that selenium supplemental may help prevent postpartum thyroiditis in women who are positive for TPOAb. Check your prenatal vitamin to determine the dose of selenium included and if needed add an individual selenium supplement to total 200 mcg per day. You should not take more than 400 mcg of selenium per day.

Postpartum Depression

Contact your doctor right away if you are experiencing symptoms of postpartum depression (PPD).

Push for comprehensive thyroid testing that includes Free T4, Free T3, Reverse T3, TPOAb, and TgAb, and pursue thyroid treatment as discussed earlier in the book. If your doctor won't run testing, immediately find a doctor who will. See Appendix A for a list of resources to help you locate a good thyroid doctor.

Be careful, however, that if you haven't been diagnosed with a thyroid problem, your doctor doesn't automatically assume you have PPD without also doing a complete thyroid evaluation.

When Hayley's first son was born, it triggered what she now knows ten years later was her thyroid problem:

I think the symptoms had been sneaking up quietly for a few years! I thought I was dying, I honestly did. I was so sick by the time my son was

---

Dana's Experience

I sat exhausted, barely able to keep my eyes open during my postnatal checkup. I was describing my excessive fatigue, rapid weight gain, hair loss, dry cracked feet, constipation, unusually heavy menstrual periods, and insomnia when my doctor passed me a prescription for an antidepressant and told me that I had postpartum depression. I looked at her in disbelief. I graduated from Columbia University with my master's degree in psychological counseling. I knew she was wrong.

A few months later I landed in the emergency room with excruciatingly painful kidney stones. The emergency room doctor thankfully ran comprehensive lab testing. I was diagnosed with hypothyroidism in the ER that day.

three months old. My GP was convinced I had postpartum depression, but luckily I have worked all my adult life with people who have suffered various mental health issues and I KNEW that's not what it was. I fought against them until my health visitor suggested a blood test, and it turned out that I was hypothyroid. I had four more beautiful babies while suffering from hypothyroidism. All breastfed and all perfect. I know I am super lucky and blessed but there is hope!

If your thyroid levels are optimal, but you are still experiencing postpartum depression, there are a number of recommended tests and treatments to discuss with your doctor, including:

- A full hormone assessment done, including progesterone, estrogen, and cortisol levels.
- Testing for anemia, including complete blood count (CBC) and full iron panel (ferritin, serum iron, total iron binding capacity [TIBC], and transferrin saturation).
- Testing for vitamin D. The best test is 25-OH vitamin D.
- Taking a high-quality probiotic. Culturelle and Bio-Kult are two good brands.
- Identifying food sensitivities by doing an elimination diet. Typical sensitivities include gluten/grains, dairy, soy, eggs, sugar, nightshades, and nuts. After a period of elimination, reintroduce the foods slowly one at a time, and assess your reactions.
- Using a supplement of omega-3 fatty acids; 2,000 to 3,000 mg of a combined EPA-DHA supplement from a trusted brand, such as Nordic Naturals, is recommended
- Taking B-vitamin supplements.
- Taking bioidentical progesterone.

> If you are having any thoughts of hurting yourself or hurting your baby, GET HELP IMMEDIATELY! Call 911, a suicide hotline, your doctor, or a child abuse prevention hotline.

Breastfeeding Difficulties and Issues

If you do not now have a diagnosed thyroid condition, but are experiencing low milk supply, see your physician for thyroid testing, including TSH, Free

T4, Free T3, TPOAb, and TgAb, to start. If your thyroid levels are not optimized, pursue treatment, as discussed earlier in the book.

If you are already on thyroid hormone replacement treatment, and your milk supply seems low, see your doctor for thyroid testing, including TSH, Free T4, Free T3, TPOAb, and TgAb, to start. If your thyroid levels are not optimized, pursue thyroid treatment as discussed earlier in the book.

Take your thyroid medication as prescribed by your physician and have periodic testing while breastfeeding, usually at least every three months, to ensure that you are not overmedicated. When provided in proper dosage level, thyroid hormone replacement crosses into breast milk in only minute quantities and has no adverse effect on the baby. Treatment and maintenance of optimal thyroid function are essential for you to successfully breastfeed.

If you are hyperthyroid, methimazole is the antithyroid drug recommended for breastfeeding women. Doses of methimazole should not exceed 30 mg per day taken as divided doses after breastfeeding.

If you are taking any antithyroid medications while breastfeeding, ensure regular monitoring of your infant's thyroid function, ideally every three months.

Do not have radioactive thyroid scans done while you are breastfeeding. If a scan absolutely needs to be done, insist that radioactive technetium be used instead of radioactive iodine. If you are breastfeeding, you can "pump and dump"—pump milk and dispose of it—for the 30 hours after the technetium injection. After that point, you can safely resume breastfeeding.

No RAI while breastfeeding. Stop breastfeeding at least four to eight weeks prior to RAI treatment.

Consult with a certified lactation consultant if you're still having low milk supply issues despite optimal thyroid treatment. Find a consultant at your hospital, birthing center, or through your local La Leche League, and/or attend a local La Leche meeting (see Appendix A).

Consider these additional tips to help milk supply:

- Stay well hydrated.
- Breastfeed frequently.
- Practice switch nursing, also called "burp and switch" nursing. Allow the baby to feed on one breast until the intensity of sucking diminishes and he or she begins to get sleepy. Then switch the baby to the other breast. Try to make sure that the baby nurses twice at each breast during each feeding.
- Try double feeding, where you nurse your baby until he or she is satisfied; keep the baby upright and awake; burp; and 10 to 20 minutes later, nurse again.

- Try skin-to-skin contact with your baby during breastfeeding.
- Pump. Some women pump for a few minutes after every feeding. You may also want to pump between nursing sessions. If your baby is unable to effectively nurse from the breast, you can also pump and give the milk to the baby using a bottle or dropper.
- Ensure that you are well nourished. Eat warm, cooked foods, such as stews, porridges, and bone broths, as well as iron-rich foods, such as meat and dark greens.
- Consult with an acupuncturist who specializes in women's health.

Talk to your physician, lactation consultant, nutritionist, or herbalist about trying one of the herbal galactagogues that help increase milk supply:

- Fenugreek—available in capsule form, or as a tea, which is not quite as potent as the capsules. The typical dose is 2 to 3 capsules (580–610 mg each), taken three times daily.
- Blessed thistle—the tincture form of this herb is preferred, and as many as 20 drops, two to four times a day, and it is said to be the best dose for increasing milk production. (Note: Do not use blessed thistle if you are allergic to plants in the daisy family, and do not go over the recommended dose, as overdosing can cause nausea and vomiting.)
- Alfalfa—sometimes recommended either by itself or in combination with fenugreek and blessed thistle.
- Additional herbs used in nursing teas include stinging nettle, marshmallow root, red raspberry leaf, anise, caraway, verbena, and coriander. Brands to consider include Traditional Medicinals Organic Mother's Milk or Weleda Nursing Tea.

Talk to your pediatrician or physician about the drug metoclopramide (Reglan). The typical dose is 10 to 15 mg, three times a day, and it's usually taken for no more than four weeks.

Supplement breast milk with formula or use formula exclusively if you are unable to increase milk supply. Use an infant formula with supplemental DHA. Do not use soy formula unless your baby is allergic to every other form and brand of formula, due to concerns about the hormonal effects of an all-soy diet on infants.

Alison believes she was hypothyroid before she got pregnant, but she had not been diagnosed. Breastfeeding problems, however, were a clue:

Mary's Story

When I was pregnant with my daughter, I did everything I could to ensure that my thyroid levels were stabilized. My baby was born healthy—though she was breech, which required a planned C-section. (Breech birth is a risk even in treated hypothyroid mothers.) In the first few days after delivery, I didn't become engorged. I had some milk, and nursed my baby, but she was fussy, and not sleeping well. I consulted my doula, who was a lactation expert, and she said that my daughter wasn't latching on well, and that it was possible I had low milk supply. I went to see the nurse practitioner at my OB's office—she was a certified lactation consultant. She suggested that I pump multiple times a day to help stimulate production, and take fenugreek. I pumped, using a hospital-grade pump, but still wasn't getting much milk. After a few days, very few wet diapers, and a very unhappy baby, we saw at the baby's checkup that she'd lost weight—not gained. At that point, the doctor recommended supplementing with formula. I was so mad and frustrated with myself and my body, but started the formula. We used a dropper, so that she wouldn't get too comfortable with a bottle and get "nipple confusion." Eventually, after exhausting myself with lengthy nursing sessions and multiple pumping sessions a day—which never got more than a small amount of milk—I realized that I was spending more time worrying about breastfeeding than enjoying my baby. While I pumped for six months, and gave her a small bottle of breast milk every day, I knew it was time to stop when an hour's pumping got one ounce of milk. I think the most important point is to understand that no matter what you do to optimize your thyroid, and help milk supply, and how many experts you consult, some of us simply don't have enough milk. Rather than beat yourself up, or feel guilty, find a safe and healthy formula, and spend your time loving and enjoying your baby!

I had blood work done at a health fair through work a year or so prior to becoming pregnant and my TSH levels came back high, but I had no idea what that meant. I was in my 20s and not concerned enough about my health to take that issue to a doctor. I honestly never thought of it again. Having said this, my first pregnancy was plagued with issues that in my opinion should have led to at least requesting this simple thyroid blood test. I could write you a book just on the pregnancy, but the biggest sign to me that a doctor could or should have at least looked at my thyroid were the issues I had with breastfeeding.

I immediately tried to breastfeed my son, and could not tell that I had any milk at all. Over the first two weeks at home my son lost weight while

I tried to breastfeed. I purchased a breast pump and could not pump enough milk to feed him sufficiently. I was basically pumping around the clock and still couldn't fill up a small bottle in double the recommended time. Several weeks in, I developed mastitis so severe that I was bedridden with a fever and was pumping bloody milk. At this point I gave up breast-feeding and went to formula. Finally my sweet baby began to gain weight. I felt horrible that I had been starving him. I felt like a failure as a woman and a mother that I couldn't do this one thing that having breasts is inher-ently supposed to mean. When my son was six months old, I was at a doctor's appointment with my gastroenterologist and he, not my OB-GYN, noticed my neck and sent me for my first official thyroid testing. I was on Synthroid for my second pregnancy, and felt well through the preg-nancy, but again, I had low milk supply. At least this time I knew and be-gan formula as a supplement to the breast milk from the start.

If you try, but still can't breastfeed, understand that this is a health-related issue for you, not a lack of trying. Your baby can be healthy with the right formula, and lots of love!

Hair Loss

If you experience significant hair loss, defined as more than 150 to 200 hairs per day, and/or the loss of the outer edge of the eyebrows, see your physician to test your TSH, Free T4, Free T3, TPOAb, TgAb, TSI (if you suspect hyper-thyroidism), and ferritin. For women experiencing hair loss, ferritin levels should be at the top end of the reference range.

If your thyroid and ferritin are optimal and you still experience heavy hair loss:

- Add a hair vitamin, such as Cooper Complete Dermatologic Formula.
- Add an evening primrose oil supplement, around 1,500 mg a day. It's best to discuss with your physician the safety of evening primrose oil while breastfeeding before use.
- Try lysine supplements. Lysine is considered safe during pregnancy.
- Check nutrient deficiencies, including vitamins D and B_{12}, iodine, zinc, and magnesium.
- Check for sex hormone imbalances, including testosterone and DHT (dihydroxytestosterone).
- Take an omega-3 fatty acid supplement.

- Test for adrenal fatigue, using a 24-hour saliva cortisol test.
- Use minoxidil (Rogaine). While it's not thought to be a danger to nursing mothers, minoxidil does pass into breast milk, and you probably ought to avoid it if you are breastfeeding.
- **Note: the prescription hair loss drug finasteride (Propecia) should never be used during pregnancy, or while breastfeeding, because of its ability to cause birth defects in a fetus and health problems for your baby.**

If your hair loss began with a change in thyroid medication brand or dosage, notify your doctor.

If you continue to have significant hair loss, see a dermatologist who specializes in hair loss.

For detailed protocols read the book *Hair Loss Master Plan* by Mary Shomon and Brent Hardgrave.

Weight-Loss Challenges

If you do not have a diagnosed thyroid condition, but are dealing with weight challenges after pregnancy, see your physician to test your TSH, Free T4, Free T3, TPOAb, and TgAb, to start. If your levels are not optimized, pursue treatment as discussed earlier in the book.

If you are already diagnosed, on thyroid hormone replacement treatment, and are having weight challenges, see your physician to test your TSH, Free T4, Free T3, TPOAb, and TgAb, to start. If your levels are not optimized, pursue treatment as discussed earlier in the book.

Get a copy of Mary Shomon's book *Thyroid Diet Revolution*.

If you continue to struggle with weight challenges despite optimal thyroid treatment, request testing for Reverse T3 and leptin.

Consult with an integrative physician regarding treatments for elevated leptin including metformin. For elevated Reverse T3, speak to your doctor about including T3 in your treatment or increase the dosage if it is already being taken.

Check for signs of elevated blood sugar and insulin resistance by testing fasting glucose and hemoglobin A1C.

Get seven to eight hours of sleep a night.

Increase aerobic activity, but be careful not to exhaust yourself. Exercise that is too intense for you can trigger adrenal fatigue which in turn can affect thyroid function.

Try high-intensity interval training (HIIT), which involves short intervals of high intensity exercise for 30 to 60 seconds, followed by one to two minutes of a low- to moderate-intensity interval.

Build muscle by adding weight-bearing or resistance exercise, such as weightlifting, exercise bands, or T-Tapp.

Drink from 0.5 to 1 ounce of water for every pound of body weight per day.

Limit yourself to two to three meals a day, and avoid snacks. Avoid eating after eight p.m.

Practice mindfulness when eating. Eat slowly and chew your food thoroughly. Take three deep cleansing breaths before each meal and snack, as well as a deep breath between bites.

Increase your fiber intake. Use psyllium capsules with each meal. Take fiber supplements two to three hours apart from your thyroid medication. If you start a high-fiber diet or supplement regimen, have your thyroid rechecked.

Try a gluten-free diet.

Avoid sugar, processed foods, allergens, refined sugars, refined carbohydrates, and high-fructose corn syrup.

Eat anti-inflammatory dietary fats (fatty fish, avocados, olives, olive oil).

Take a daily probiotic supplement and eat probiotic-rich foods (kombucha, miso, kimchi, kefir, sauerkraut).

Eat sufficient protein (poultry, meat, fish, and eggs).

Minimize or eliminate sweets and desserts, including soft drinks.

Minimize or eliminate honey, molasses, artificial sweeteners, and all forms of sugar, including fruits.

Minimize or eliminate caffeine.

Minimize or eliminate alcohol.

Fertility Challenges

nfertility can be a heartbreaking journey when you want more than anything to conceive a child. All the action items that we've mentioned for your particular thyroid disease diagnosis in Part 3 of this book are critical steps to conceiving. However, in some cases, you may have to go beyond those recommendations to have your babies.

Pursue Thorough Thyroid and Antibody Testing

As mentioned throughout Part 3, a comprehensive thyroid workup is essential for women with thyroid disease wishing to conceive. Testing should include the following:

- TSH
- Free T4
- Free T3
- Reverse T3
- Thyroid peroxidase antibodies (TPOAb) for Hashimoto's
- Thyroglobulin antibodies (TgAb) for Hashimoto's
- Thyroid-stimulating immunoglobulin (TSI) for Graves' disease

It is important to note, however, that traditional blood tests for thyroid antibodies do not identify one out of every five women who are actually antibody-positive. If your thyroid is optimal but you are still struggling, it may be that you have Hashimoto's or Graves' disease and don't know it. If you do have thyroid autoimmunity, then modulation of the immune system is an important component of your treatment plan as explained in Chapter 9.

If you test negative for antibodies, but have signs and symptoms suggestive of autoimmune thyroid disease, you may want to ask for more sensitive thyroid antibody tests—known as the enzyme-linked immunosorbent assay (ELISA), or gel agglutination tests. These can pick up the subset of autoimmune thyroid patients who do not test positive for antibodies.

Explore Other Autoimmune Hormonal Connections

Autoimmune thyroid disease is linked to a number of related autoimmune conditions that you should also investigate:

- Premature ovarian insufficiency (POI), also known as premature ovarian failure
- Endometriosis
- Polycystic ovary syndrome

Naturopath Dr. Fiona McCulloch explained:

Premature ovarian insufficiency has been strongly associated with immune dysregulation, or autoimmunity. Up to 50 percent of patients with POI have been found to have at least one autoimmune factor. Implantation failures with IVF and recurrent miscarriages have often been associated with immune dysregulation as well, and also with clotting disorders that can have an immune component. Patients with autoimmune disease such as Hashimoto's, lupus, rheumatoid arthritis, celiac disease, and type 1 diabetes have been found to have lower fertility rates. Endometriosis has strong autoimmune and inflammatory components. A study on 3,680 women with endometriosis found increased rates of thyroid disease, and of autoimmune diseases such as rheumatoid arthritis and lupus. Other research has found abnormal polyclonal B cell activation in women with endometriosis, a classic characteristic of autoimmune disease. PCOS also has very strong immune components. All women with PCOS have a type of inflammation that is chronic and systemic, related to fatty tissue inflammation and insulin resistance. This type of inflammation can dysregulate the entire immune system, and affect the way that the eggs develop in the ovary. PCOS is also associated with increased miscarriage risk.

Stacy and her husband tried for years to conceive, though test after test said "normal":

I had extreme exhaustion, weight gain, tingling in hands and feet, itching and eczema. Not to mention just how cold I was and my thinning hair and eyebrows. But one day I stubbed my toe badly and thought it was broken. I went to the clinic to see a doctor I have never seen before. He asked about my overall health and I shared tearfully. He asked if anyone in my family had thyroid issues. Yes! My mom, both aunts and both grandmas. He ordered lab testing that he felt warranted me to see a thyroid specialist, who diagnosed Hashimoto's. I was immediately put on medication and metformin to help with fertility. He contacted my OB-GYN and set a plan into action. They sent me to a fertility doctor and started Clomid. I spent three months getting my thyroid checked and semi-regulated or at the fertility doctor or getting some sort of testing done. After three months of Clomid, shots, pills, and patches, I was just done. We had been trying for five years and I felt I just couldn't do it emotionally anymore. But in that third month I found out I was pregnant! Three months later I started having severe cramping, and was put on bed rest for the rest of my pregnancy. My thyroid had gone out of balance, and they changed my dose. But I now have an amazing and healthy little boy. It took five years of trying to have a child while being undiagnosed with Hashimoto's. If I didn't stub my toe I don't know if anyone would have caught this.

Get an Infertility Evaluation

While thyroid treatment may be a simple breakthrough solution for infertility, be sure you also have a basic infertility evaluation.

A basic infertility evaluation should include:

- Medical history
- Physical examination
- Blood work
  - o Follicle-stimulating hormone (FSH)
  - o Luteinizing hormone (LH)
  - o Estradiol
  - o Progesterone
  - o Prolactin
  - o DHEA-S
  - o Testosterone
  - o Antimullerian hormone
  - o Complete thyroid panel

- Ultrasound
- Antral follicle count
- Fallopian tube assessment
- Semen analysis for the man

On Day 3 of your cycle, testing of FSH, LH, and estradiol.

On Day 21 of your cycle, testing of progesterone.

It may seem ridiculous, or even shocking, but many doctors, including infertility specialists, ***do not routinely test for thyroid disease in infertile patients!*** Never assume! Insist on a complete thyroid panel as part of your blood work.

You'll also want to ensure that your partner is given a full medical workup, including comprehensive thyroid testing and male hormones. And, yes, men can get thyroid problems, and in some cases, it can affect their fertility, too!

When Should You Pursue an Infertility Evaluation?

You will notice that the chart on page 239 is broken out by age. Age is a major factor in fertility. The probability of having a baby decreases by 3 to 5 percent each year after the age of thirty, and at a faster rate after forty. As women get older, the miscarriage rate also rises.

Infertility specialist Dr. Hugh Melnick shared some thoughts:

I believe that any woman with thyroid disease who is even remotely interested in the possibility of having a baby at some future time should have her fertility status evaluated by the age of 30. Such an evaluation is quite easy and can be done in a single visit to a doctor's office, scheduled during the time of a menstrual period. The evaluation consists of a vaginal sonogram of the ovaries and the uterus, and a blood draw. Using the sonogram, an estimation of the quantity of eggs that are remaining in the ovaries can be made. This is called the antral (resting) egg follicle count. In general, the more eggs seen, the higher the probability of pregnancy.

The most important blood test is the antimullerian hormone (AMH). The higher the AMH level, the more eggs are found in the ovaries. When there is a low antral follicle count and a low AMH level, the prognosis for conception is not good. Other hormones tested include FSH (follicle stimulating hormone), LH (luteinizing hormone), and estradiol (estrogen). Moderate elevations in the levels of FSH and LH, with a normal

Menstrual cycle chart			Irregular Menstrual Cycles (and You Want to Get Pregnant)
	Regular Menstrual Cycles		
	Under 35	*Over 35*	*Any Age*
Women Without Thyroid Disease	Try for a year before a basic infertility workup.	Try for six months before a basic infertility workup.	Have a basic infertility workup right away.
Women with Thyroid Disease	Try for six months before a basic infertility workup.	Have a basic infertility workup right away.	Have a basic infertility workup right away.

estrogen level, are not favorable signs and often predict the possibility of egg quality issues in the near future.

Although many women may be anxious about having their fertility potential tested, the information obtained from this testing is really invaluable for making some very important life decisions. For example, I have had patients in their early 30s, who were unexpectedly found to have low egg reserve, immediately decide to pursue pregnancy while their remaining eggs were still of good quality.

According to OB/GYN Thomas Moraczewski:

In women in their late 30s and early 40s desiring to conceive, "egg quality" becomes paramount. A man manufactures sperm every day in a 90-day life span, but the woman is born with all the ova (eggs) she will carry. There are some supplements that may help boost ovarian quality. Check out Fairhaven Health, a supplier of fertility-related products (fairhaven health.com).

Some supplements to consider include:

- *OvaBoost*: Supplement that promotes egg quality. Recommended for all trying-to-conceive women, and particularly women trying to conceive later in life and women with PCOS. Blend of 2,000 mg myo-inositol, methylfolate, melatonin, and antioxidants. 4 capsules daily.

- *FertiliTea*: Blend of plant-based products helpful in fertility and hormonal balance (red raspberry leaf, chasteberry, lady's mantle, nettle leaf, green tea, peppermint leaf). Drink 2 to 3 cups daily.
- *FertilAid*: Vitamins and herbal supplements that support menstrual cycle regularity and hormonal balance. 3 capsules daily.
- *FertileDetox*: Blend of supplements that help the body's detoxification systems eliminate harmful chemicals. For women and men. 3 capsules daily.

Single supplements that are useful to increase cellular energy of egg and blood flow include:

- CoQ10: 200 mg
- L-arginine: 500 mg
- Myo-inositol: Promotes hormonal balance, insulin sensitivity, and ovulation support. Dosage: 2,000 mg daily. Brand: *Pregnitude*. Caution: Do not combine with SSRI antidepressants or anticonvulsants.
- Vitamin D: Measure blood levels but most women need 6,000 IU daily.

Pursue Extensive Infertility Testing

If a basic infertility evaluation does not identify treatable issues, and/or if you have had multiple miscarriages, you should consider more extensive infertility testing. This may include:

- Hysteroscopy
- Laparoscopy
- Endometrial biopsy
- Cervical mucus testing
- Chromosome analysis/karyotype
- Infections testing, including:
  - Ureaplasma
  - Mycoplasma
  - Gonorrhea
  - Chlamydia culture
  - Syphilis
  - Toxoplasmosis
  - Cytomegalovirus (CMV)

o Hepatitis B or C
o HIV

Pursue Immunological Testing

If you have Hashimoto's or Graves' disease, are receiving optimal thyroid treatment, and have plotted your cycles and fertile window and attempted conception for a year (if you're under 30), or 6 months (if you're over 30) but have not conceived, you should request immunological testing.

When a person has an untreated autoimmune condition, such as Hashimoto's or Graves', disease, she is more vulnerable to develop other autoimmune conditions. Once the immune system has made the mistake of attacking one part of the body, it is more likely to attack others, including reproductive tissue and even the implanted embryo.

Immunologic testing is also recommended for women with the following indications or risk factors:

- Two miscarriages after the age of 35
- Two IVF failures after age 35
- Three miscarriages before age 35
- Three IVF failures before age 35
- Poor egg production (less than 6 eggs) from a cycle stimulated using fertility drugs
- One blighted ovum where a placenta develops, but there is no fetus visible on ultrasound at no later than around 6 weeks in the pregnancy
- Previous autoimmune/immune test results, i.e., tested positive for antinuclear antibodies or rheumatoid factor
- Previous pregnancies where the baby had intrauterine growth retardation
- One living child and more than one miscarriage while attempting to have a second child
- Diagnosis of another autoimmune disease, such as:
  o Type 1 diabetes
  o Multiple sclerosis
  o Celiac disease
  o Addison's disease
  o Cushing's disease
  o Alopecia areata
  o Sjögren's syndrome
  o Rheumatoid arthritis

o Pernicious anemia

o Systemic lupus erythematosus

o Sarcoidosis

o Scleroderma

o Vitiligo

o Psoriasis

Immunological Fertility Tests

If you test positive in the immunological fertility testing be sure to consult with an integrative physician to address modulation of the immune system as described in the "Autoimmunity" section of Chapter 9.

Antinuclear Antibodies (ANA)

Antinuclear antibodies attack the cell nucleus of foreign invaders in your body. The immune system may mistakenly target the egg as an invader and attack its nucleus. This condition is common in systemic lupus erythematosus, Sjögren's syndrome, and scleroderma. Treatment may include the corticosteroid prednisone, baby aspirin, or the blood thinner heparin.

Antiovarian Antibodies (AOA)

The immune system may mistakenly produce antibodies to attack the ovaries. This condition commonly occurs in thyroid disease, Addison's disease, and endometriosis. Treatment may include corticosteroids such as dexamethasone or prednisone.

Antisperm Antibodies (ASA)

Antibodies may be created by the body that target sperm. Both men and women should be tested for ASA. Treatment may include corticosteroids, intrauterine insemination (IUI), or in vitro fertilization (IVF) with intracytoplasmic sperm injection whereby each egg is injected with a single sperm.

Antiphospholipid Antibodies (APA)

All cells of the body, including blood cells and their membranes, contain phospholipids. APAs attach to the phospholipids making them sticky and clumped together, which can lead to the formation of clots and poor blood flow. Reduction in blood flow to the placenta or the endometrium can reduce oxygen and nutrients to the embryo. Treatment may include daily low-dose baby aspirin or blood thinners, such as warfarin or heparin.

Natural Killer Cells

Natural killer cells are a helpful part of the immune system, defending the body from foreign invaders, such as tumor cells and virus-infected cells. However, if there is malfunction of natural killer cells, they may mistakenly attack the embryo in pregnancy. The idea that elevated natural killer cells can cause miscarriage in some women is controversial in the medical world, but we feel worth investigating. Treatment may include a steroid such as prednisone, intravenous immunoglobulin, or intralipid infusions. Consult with an integrative physician about natural approaches to reduce inflammation, such as addressing food sensitivities, testing for vitamin D deficiency, avoiding high sugar and refined carbohydrates, and adding antioxidant-rich foods and such supplements as omega-3 fatty acids and curcumin.

When Surgery Is Needed to Treat Infertility

Some conditions, such as cysts, scar tissue, adhesions, and fibroids, warrant surgery to correct your anatomical or structural impediments to pregnancy. Some surgeries to treat infertility include:

- Tubal anastomosis (reversal of tubal ligation or sterilization)
- Fallopian tube reconstruction
- Surgery for endometriosis
- Surgical removal of uterine fibroids
- Surgery for adhesions/scar tissue
- Reconstructive surgery of birth defects involving the uterus and vagina
- Surgical treatment of ovarian cysts
- Repair or removal of hydrosalpinx/damaged fallopian tube
- Surgical removal of endometrial polyps
- Tubal cannulation, to unblock fallopian tubes

Try Assisted Reproduction Drugs

Not everyone will be able to get pregnant naturally. If you've followed the steps in this book and still have not conceived, a number of assisted reproductive technologies (ARTs) are available to you, including fertility drugs. Fertility drugs are particularly helpful for women who are not ovulating or ovulating irregularly. They are also helpful for women with PCOS.

Fertility drugs are also typically used as part of an ART program that includes such techniques as intrauterine insemination (IUI) or in vitro fertilization (IVF). Fertility drugs may be used also for male infertility. Discuss side effects and risks with an infertility specialist.

Clomiphene

The drug clomiphene citrate, common brand names Clomid and Serophene, can be used to stimulate ovulation. Clomiphene is given for five days, starting Days 3 to 5 of the cycle.

Gonadotropins

Gonadotropins also stimulate ovulation. They are administered by injection. They are not generally used unless a patient has not responded to clomiphene.

Brand names Follistim and Gonal-f are synthetic recombinant FSH identical in structure to human FSH. Brand names Menopur and Repronex are a mixture of FSH and LH made by obtaining and purifying the urine of postmenopausal women, and extracting the FSH and LH. The daily injections are typically given for seven to twelve days, starting on Day 2 or 3 of your cycle to stimulate the ovaries to produce multiple eggs. The ovarian follicles where eggs mature are monitored by blood tests and ultrasounds. Once the follicles are big enough, the injections stop, and you get a shot of human chorionic gonadotropin (HCG), brand names Pregnyl, and Novarel and Ovidrel, to trigger the release of the eggs from the follicles. Have sex 12 to 36 hours after the HCG shot, because ovulation usually occurs around 36 hours after receiving the HCG injection.

Women taking fertility drugs are at risk for ovarian hyperstimulation syndrome (OHSS), which can be severe enough to require hospitalization. Speak to your doctor about the warning signs to watch, including nausea and vomiting, abdominal pain, enlarged abdomen, shortness of breath, diarrhea, darker urine, excessive thirst, and rapid weight gain.

After several heartbreaking miscarriages, Ashlee was diagnosed with hypothyroidism.

It actually gave a little relief to my grief to know what had taken life from me . . . that I had done nothing wrong. But knowing that my body had betrayed me like this, was infuriating to me. My doctor put me on levothyroxine and began to treat me for what seemed like months to level out my hormones. After several months of grieving and healing, we decided to talk to my doctor to make sure my body was capable of carrying another child. After she gave us the go ahead, we began to try. It was the longest 2 1/2 years of my life. I didn't realize fertility was so complex. It needed calendars, prayers, ovulation tests, etc. After the first year of trying, my doctor began to do some more tests. I wasn't ovulating. So I was put on a medicine to make me have a normal period. After my period, she would then prescribe me something to make me ovulate. And then she would test to make sure it had worked. I spent a whole year having my arms poked and prodded, while testing my thyroid consistently and checking to make sure ovulation occurred, hormones raging from all of the medicine I was taking. After almost three years and on the verge of giving up, I saw so clearly the words "PREGNANT" on that stick. I have never cried, laughed, danced, hugged, and thanked God that much. The whole pregnancy was spent on pins and needles. I had nightmares of losing this child. After I found out I was having a baby boy, my heart finally calmed down. I began to prepare and enjoy the thought that one day soon, I would hold this tiny miracle in my arms. That day came. It was beautiful. Just me and this tiny human who I had longed for, for so long.

Try Assisted Reproduction Techniques

Intrauterine Insemination (IUI)

IUI is a fertility treatment that involves placing sperm into a woman's uterus without intercourse. Since only 1 of 2,000 sperm ejaculated into the vagina actually can make it to the fallopian tube, direct insemination can help improve the odds. IUI is also used in combination with fertility drugs.

In Vitro Fertilization (IVF)

IVF is the most common fertility treatment. It involves joining a woman's egg and a man's sperm outside the body in a laboratory dish. Injectable fertility drugs are given to stimulate the ovaries to produce multiple eggs, known as "superovulation." In some cases Lupron is prescribed to reduce the chance of premature release of the eggs. Ultrasounds and blood tests are used to determine when the follicles are big enough and an HCG injection is given. Thirty-six hours after the HCG shot, the eggs are retrieved by inserting a needle through the vaginal wall into the ovary under ultrasound guidance. The best-quality eggs and the man's sperm are placed together in a laboratory dish for the sperm to fertilize the egg. Intracytoplasmic sperm injection may be used to inject the sperm directly into the egg.

Donor Eggs

If you are unable to use your own eggs for conception, a donor egg is fertilized with sperm from your partner and implanted in your uterus.

Egg or Embryo Freezing

If you plan to have babies in the future and you wish to extend your fertility, another option is egg or embryo freezing, termed oocyte cryopreservation.

> **An important note:** Various studies have shown that in women with thyroid antibodies, or borderline hypothyroidism, treatment with thyroid hormone replacement medications make these assisted reproduction approaches more effective. Make sure that your thyroid treatment is optimized throughout the process. And keep in mind that drugs used to stimulate the ovaries may destabilize your thyroid medications, so get rechecked regularly while undergoing any assisted reproduction support.

Explore Natural Fertility Approaches

There are a number of natural approaches that may also aid in overcoming infertility.

Herbal Medicine

There is a long tradition of herbal medicine for fertility enhancement. If you are interested in herbal fertility help, consult with an herbal medicine practitioner with expertise in fertility treatment for specific guidelines and formulations unique to your own situation. Always consult with a skilled practitioner about the safety of herbs taken during pregnancy and breastfeeding. A few key points to keep in mind:

- Chaste tree berry (Vitex) is a hormone balancer that lowers prolactin and raises progesterone. It helps lengthen the luteal phase (starts after ovulation until before your period starts). It is used to treat amenorrhea (lack of menstruation), irregular cycles, low libido, low cervical mucus, PCOS, and uterine cysts. Traditionally used to prevent miscarriage associated with low progesterone. It is considered safe to take during your entire cycle, but stop if you become pregnant.

- Helonias-viburnum is considered a uterine tonic that is good for women with a history of miscarriage.
- Red clover blossom, high in calcium and magnesium, has some blood-thinning properties and is also thought to help make cervical mucous more favorable to longer survival of sperm.
- Stinging nettle is thought to thicken the endometrium and improve environment for implantation of a fertilized egg.
- Red raspberry leaf is a commonly used tonic for reproductive health that strengthens the uterine lining and lengthens the luteal phase. Used to treat endometriosis and uterine fibroids. It can be taken during your entire cycle but stop if you become pregnant.
- Motherwort is used to treat amenorrhea, painful menstruation, uterine fibroids, ovarian cysts, poor egg health, and endometriosis. Motherwort is best not used during your menstrual period. Do not use this herb during pregnancy because it stimulates mild uterine contractions.
- Dong quai root is a popular Chinese herb to help utilize estrogen properly, increase circulation to the uterus, regulate the menstrual cycle, improve egg health, and treat endometriosis, ovarian cysts, and uterine fibroids. It is a blood-thinning herb, so it should not be taken during your period. Stop using once you have ovulated and discontinue during your period and throughout pregnancy.
- Black cohosh helps relieve menstrual cramps and helps regulate ovulation. Used for amenorrrhea (absent period), uterine prolapse, uterine fibroids, ovarian cysts, and endometriosis. Take during the first of your cycle, from menstruation until ovulation.
- Wild yam increases production of progesterone, which is helpful for women with short luteal phases. Traditionally used to treat miscarriage, it should only be taken after ovulation or it may prevent ovulation if taken before. Do not use during pregnancy.
- Ginseng helps male fertility by raising testosterone, treating impotence, increasing sperm count, sperm mobility, and libido.
- Saw palmetto used by men with fertility issues can help correct male impotence, testicular atrophy, and low libido.

- Evening primrose oil helps increase cervical mucus and balance estrogen. It should not be taken after ovulation when trying to get pregnant as it promotes contractions of the uterus.
- False unicorn root strengthens the uterine wall, promotes follicle growth, and regulates menstruation. It is used in the treatment of uterine prolapse, low cervical mucous, uterine hemorrhage, endometriosis, PCOS, male impotence, miscarriage, and amenorrhea (absent menstruation). It should only be taken during the first half of your cycle from menstruation to ovulation. It should not be taken during pregnancy.

Traditional Chinese Medicine

There is a long tradition of using Traditional Chinese Medicine (TCM) for treatment of infertility. TCM typically includes a combination of both acupuncture and herbal treatments to help resolve imbalances and restore health. TCM is very customized for the individual, and so you would need to see a trained, reputable practitioner of this ancient art and science for customized treatment that helps to regulate the menstrual cycle and hormones, balance the endocrine system, strengthen the overall constitution, and prepare the body to support a pregnancy.

TCM can also be used to help support overall health, which can make assisted reproductive technologies more effective.

TCM is not a quick-fix approach, however. It can take several months of treatment to achieve some balance in a younger woman, and women closer to age forty, those who smoke, and those who have had more extensive fertility treatment—such as fertility drugs, hormonal supplements, assisted reproductive technologies, or who have hormonal conditions—all require from six months to a year before seeing some results.

According to New York City acupuncturist Suzanne Connole,

Most fertility clinics now accept that acupuncture may boost the success rates of IVF and other ART. Some even offer it in the office as part of the embryo transfer treatment. This is based on the results of a German study from *Fertility and Sterility* that showed that acupuncture before and after embryo transfer had a success rate of 42 percent versus 26 percent in the control group. These numbers are truly significant and have made many doctors think more about the use of acupuncture for their patients.

My own clinical experience after 12 years of practice and that of my colleagues is that acupuncture and Chinese medicine has much more to

Dana's Experience

I was months away from turning 40. I was optimally treated for my thyroid but still, month after month of trying to conceive, I was still not pregnant. There are a few key things that I believe made all the difference for me. First, I was charting my cycles and using ovulation predictor kits. I noticed that my cycles were not ideal. I had irregular cycles with a short luteal phase, and below-normal morning basal body temperature (which are common issues with hypothyroidism). With regular acupuncture appointments and Chinese herbs prescribed by my acupuncturist, Suzanne Connole, I watched my fertility charts literally normalize before my very eyes within a few months. Then, I read the book *Making Babies* by Dr. Sami David and Jill Blakeway and started the following fertility supplements under my doctor's guidance. I got pregnant within one month:

- 30 mg daily of coenzyme Q10 (CoQ10), which improves pelvic blood flow.
- Baby aspirin which improves blood flow.
- Royal jelly is what the queen bee feeds on to produce hundreds of eggs a day and is often referred to as the bees' own fertility drug! I took one teaspoon of Y.S. Organic Bee Farms' Fresh Royal Jelly every day. It is also used to increase sperm count in men.
- Chlorophyll is a high alkaline food. Cervical mucus must be alkaline, not acidic, for sperm survival. I added liquid chlorophyll to my morning smoothie.
- Red raspberry leaf tea to strengthen the uterine wall and lengthen the luteal phase of my cycle. I drank this tea during preconception, then stopped during pregnancy, then resumed postpartum.
- I also put a warm water bottle on my lower abdomen before ovulation, to improve blood flow to the uterus.

add to this, and we urge patients and doctors to begin treatment with Chinese medicine well before the IVF cycle starts. We have seen that the more treatment we can do before IVF, the stronger and more balanced the woman's body is, and the better her body responds to the drugs. In addition, Western medicine has little to offer in early pregnancy besides progesterone supplementation. While it is hard to quantify with research, we have seen many women with high risk of miscarriage or who have suffered multiple miscarriages, carry to full term.

Lifestyle Changes

There are some basic lifestyle changes you'll want to incorporate for enhanced fertility:

- Stop smoking—smoking impairs fertility, increases the risk of miscarriage, and if you do get pregnant, it's harmful to an unborn baby, not to mention your own health. Avoid secondhand smoke exposure as well.
- Avoid recreational drugs, such as marijuana, cocaine, and ecstasy.
- Be mindful of medications. Discuss with your doctor your use of antibiotics, antidepressants, antihistamines, anti-inflammatories, blood pressure medications, cough medicines and decongestants, diuretics, painkillers, sleeping pills, steroids, antifungal medications, and others.
- Avoid alcohol.
- Limit caffeine.
- Get adequate sleep.
- Minimize or avoid exposure to chemicals, such as those found in household cleaners and personal care products.

Weight and Exercise

Weight and exercise are both important issues for fertility. In terms of weight, you want to normalize your weight as much as possible for maximum fertility. Being overweight or underweight, especially by more than 15 percent, can hurt fertility.

Excessive exercise—such as training for a marathon or triathalon, being a professional athlete or gymnast, or participating in endurance sports—may cause amenorrhea, the lack of a period, or change hormone levels so as to make pregnancy very difficult to achieve. While you want to exercise for general health, flexibility, aerobic health, and muscle strength, avoid overexercising to enhance your fertility.

Mind-Body Approaches

Many experts point to the role of stress in fertility. Living in a state of stress or anxiety not only has a serious hormonal impact, as we've discussed throughout this book, but simply does not allow your body to function optimally, including your fertility and reproductive capabilities.

Some alternative practitioners recommend mind-body therapies for stress reduction and relaxation to help enhance fertility. Overall, mind-body techniques and the relaxation response have as their objective calming the mind; achieving a peaceful state; coping with stress; relaxing the body and mind; generating a "relaxation response"; expressing and clearing emotions; changing negative thoughts; and controlling physical functions, such as breathing.

There are many mind-body therapies to choose from, and you'll need to explore those that appeal most to you, but some of the suggested approaches include the following:

- Psychotherapy, counseling
- Biofeedback
- Guided imagery
- Hypnosis
- Yoga
- Tai chi
- Mindfulness-based stress reduction
- Prayer/spiritual healing
- Creative therapies—music therapy, art therapy, dance therapy
- Breathing exercises
- Support groups
- Reiki/energy work
- Qi gong
- Guided meditation CDs/MP3s. One we particularly recommend is "Hormonal Balance" from One Light One Spirit.

Into the Future

Saving Our Babies

15

Martin Luther King Jr. asked: "What happens when a man stands up and says enough is enough?"

What happens is, SHE takes action.

Both of us are motivated by stories like Brenda's:

> I had thyroid nodules, and an enlarged thyroid that was untreated for years. When I was pregnant, my doctor said my thyroid was functioning. Five months into the pregnancy, I had a scan that showed full spina bifida, and my baby boy only had a partial brain, and could not survive. I had to end the pregnancy. Afterwards, I was still not being treated for my "borderline" thyroid problem. Doctors just kept passing the buck. I had all sorts of problems, and in the end, I had to have a hysterectomy. I was still not being treated for my thyroid. Finally, after years of being told my thyroid was borderline, I finally started treatment last year. And I finally had a biopsy, which showed Hashimoto's thyroiditis. I lost my baby and yet not one doctor linked the Hashimoto's to what happened to my baby? It will always haunt me. What if I had been treated? Maybe my little boy would be here today.

Brenda and her baby deserved more. They deserved action.

In writing this book, we have taken action. Our hope is that you will turn around and take action as well—to help yourself, and your children, as well as women and children everywhere.

Because enough is enough. Things need to change.

Couples are going through expensive and invasive fertility testing and treatments, and still ending up childless.

Millions of those lucky enough to get pregnant suffer the sadness and loss of miscarriage.

Later in pregnancy, families are going through the agony of having still-born babies. Mothers are developing preeclampsia and placental abruptions, risking their lives and the lives of their babies, who are usually delivered prematurely. Women are having breech births—and having to recuperate from C-sections—just when they want to bond with their babies.

After delivery, postpartum hemorrhages endanger some new mother's lives. Postpartum depression can make a happy time a truly difficult one for some new mothers. And some mothers, no matter what they do, can't breastfeed and give their babies the healthiest start possible with breast milk.

Then there are the babies . . . our babies. Babies are being born prematurely, with numerous health problems—a terror for parents—and often require months of expensive hospitalization. There are babies with low birth weights who have to spend extra time in the hospital. There are babies who have birth defects. And at worst, there are babies born with mental retardation—that could have been prevented. As they get older, we see children who have cognitive problems, developmental issues, and learning disabilities. Children are being diagnosed with autism and ADHD at epidemic levels.

And much of it can be linked to undiagnosed thyroid problems. The thyroid is not the culprit in every case, but it is in many, and the lack of attention, the lack of understanding, and the obvious disregard for something so important has to stop.

Scientific research reveals that untreated or improperly treated thyroid disease during pregnancy increases the risk of all of these situations. This is why the most fundamental change that must happen is the adoption of universal thyroid screening in pregnancy.

Universal Thyroid Screening Is Essential in Pregnancy

Universal thyroid screening before or in early pregnancy is not currently the standard of care in the United States or most areas around the world. Surprisingly, thyroid screening during pregnancy remains *rare,* and is in some cases actually discouraged. Why? Our theory is that it is primarily an economic decision. Around 5 million women each year are pregnant and hoping to continue the pregnancy and have a healthy baby. If universal screening were adopted, those women would all need thyroid screening—the costs of which HMOs and insurance companies are reluctant to cover.

This puts the burden on women to seek out and push for screening and evaluation on their own. This book aims to find women who have fallen through the cracks of mainstream medicine and put them on a path to better health and healthy babies, but only you can get the testing you need, for your particular situation, before our recommendations will be useful to you. If you take only one thing away from this book, take this: **You need to ask for— even demand—thyroid testing.**

As many as 60 million people in the United States have thyroid conditions. The majority are women, and the majority of women are undiagnosed. They are unaware that they have a health condition that puts their fertility, their babies—and even their own lives—in danger. It is a tragedy.

The sad truth is that diagnosed thyroid patients receiving treatment also fare poorly in terms of fertility, successful pregnancy, and postpartum health. Many endocrinologists and obstetricians have *not* read the American Thyroid Association's and the Endocrine Society's guidelines, and have little understanding of the complexities or standards of care for pregnant thyroid patients and their babies. The burden is on the patient to push for comprehensive testing and optimal treatment. It is up to the patient to be well informed and advocate for herself and her babies.

How many babies have to needlessly suffer before there is an outcry for universal thyroid screening in pregnancy? Countless babies are lost and others harmed for life while there are reliable, inexpensive, readily available thyroid lab tests that could make this suffering avoidable.

An ongoing controversy among scientific societies regarding whether all pregnant women should be screened for thyroid dysfunction is going on right this very minute as you read this book. A growing number of studies show an association between maternal thyroid disease and adverse pregnancy outcomes, including impaired neurocognitive development in offspring. The argument made is that there is only limited evidence at this time and more studies are needed. *Yes*, absolutely, more studies are needed but we need them *right now*. Are the countless women around the world with thyroid disease and their babies expected to wait for more studies to be conducted?

A survey of endocrinologists found that 74 percent think there should be universal thyroid screening in pregnancy. But it is "not recommended" by the very professional groups that establish their guidelines.

The Endocrine Society is the world's oldest, largest, and most active organization of endocrinologists, representing more than eighteen thousand physicians and scientists across the globe. Since members could not reach agreement with regard to screening recommendations for all newly pregnant women, they recommend targeted screening of high-risk women only. In their pregnancy guidelines they openly shared that this case finding approach will miss

30 percent or more of women with overt or subclinical hypothyroidism. *This is not acceptable.*

We urge that every woman ask for and receive thyroid screening as soon as pregnancy is confirmed.

The ideal basic protocol would be a three-point thyroid screening process:

- Preconception
- As soon as pregnancy is confirmed
- A six-week postpartum checkup

We are not talking just about TSH tests, though that would be a start. But we believe that tests of TSH, Free T4, Free T3, and TPOAb, at minimum, are necessary to identify the most common thyroid issues that affect fertility, pregnancy, and postpartum health.

Prenatal Vitamins Need to Include Iodine and Methylfolate

It's been established that you need more iodine during pregnancy and breastfeeding. It's simple: 150 mcg iodine daily. So, why do some prenatal vitamins contain no iodine or contain less than the required amount? Many of the prenatal vitamins that do not contain iodine are the prescription vitamins! It's outrageous!

In early 2015, the Council for Responsible Nutrition (CRN) advised that all vitamins intended for pregnant women include 150 mcg of iodine. This is an important step, but how long will it take, and will the vitamin manufacturers listen?

Meanwhile, we also know about how crucial it is to take folic acid before and during pregnancy, to prevent neurological problems in the baby. At the same time, half the population has a genetic defect—MTHFR—that makes it difficult to absorb folic acid. It's unrealistic to call for mass screening for the MTHFR gene mutation. But there is a simple solution: All prenatal vitamins should include the methylfolate form of folic acid, so that it is properly absorbed by all women.

In the meantime, always check labels of prenatal vitamins or visit the book's website http://www.ThyroidPregnancyBook.com for a list of prenatal vitamins with adequate iodine and that include methylfolate.

Insist on Comprehensive Thyroid Evaluation

Conventional medicine's gold standard for the diagnostic testing of thyroid disease is the TSH test, but if you've read any section of this book, you know by now that it's not enough. Integrative physicians include Free T4, Free T3, Reverse T3, TPOAb, and TgAb in their thyroid screening panels, yet these tests are rarely performed by mainstream doctors.

If you don't know you have a thyroid problem, it can't be treated. If you don't know if you have antibodies, you can't explore immune-modulating treatments that may help calm inflammation and autoimmunity. If you haven't had an ultrasound, you don't know whether you have suspicious nodules—and early detection of thyroid cancer is important, given the increasing rate of thyroid cancer.

Always get a copy of your lab results and check both that you've had the right tests and that your levels are optimal not just normal.

Keri started her third pregnancy with low-normal T4 and a TSH of 4.99.

> My doctor didn't bother to give me the results, so I thought that the thyroid tests must have been normal. When I was four months postpartum, my primary care doctor ordered thyroid tests because I was gaining so much weight. My TSH was 275 and my T4 and T3 were very very low!! No wonder I felt horrible!

Tracy lost a baby at 25 weeks gestation: "The doctors thought it was due to drug abuse, although I didn't do any drugs. After running test after test trying to find a reason, I was diagnosed with hypothyroidism. My TSH was over 300 at that time. That's how I was diagnosed."

Laura Kay was almost 20 weeks into her second pregnancy when she went to a maternal fetal specialist to find out the sex of her baby:

> We were blindsided by the news that her heart was not beating. To this day, they say they don't know why this happened. Looking back at this pregnancy, I was beyond exhausted. I would wake up (after sleeping 8 hours), put cartoons on for my 1 1/2-year-old, and fall back asleep on the couch for two hours. I couldn't do the dishes or the most mundane task. I mentioned this to the OB, and she just said it was normal in pregnancy. After losing the baby, I tried my hardest to lose the baby weight (so I wouldn't have the constant reminder when I looked into the mirror). I was eating the Paleo diet, running in the morning, doing CrossFit workouts in the evening at least four times a week. After a month of that, at my follow-up OB appointment, I hadn't lost a pound. I knew something was wrong. I asked to get my thyroid checked and was told, "You are fine. Your TSH is within the normal parameters." (Of course it was 3.9, and 4.0 was the cutoff.) I started to see a

naturopathic doctor. She recommended getting a full thyroid panel done. That's when I was diagnosed with Hashimoto's, with antibody levels over 1,000. At that point, I was convinced Hashimoto's was my baby's killer. I went on a rampage researching the disease and reading blogs about hundreds of women who went through a similar experience. Hashimoto's also had me enraged to the point of switching OBs and making every mom-to-be that I know get a full thyroid panel run while pregnant.

We Need Doctors Who Explore Treatment Options

The goal is to be as thyroid-healthy as possible before trying to conceive. That means working with a doctor who is open to all the treatment options, including natural approaches, to find what is right for you.

Thyroid health is like a big puzzle with many related pieces. Droves of patients are out on the internet seeking answers to their persistent symptoms. Thankfully, many find their way to us, where they learn that there is more to thyroid health than thyroid testing and treatments used in mainstream medicine.

Here are some of the treatment challenges that infuriate us the most:

The gold standard for treatment of hypothyroidism is T4-only levothyroxine drugs, which work for some but fail for others, yet many doctors refuse to consider the alternatives, including synthetic T4/T3 combined or natural desiccated thyroid.

Hyperthyroid and Graves' patients are rushed into radioactive iodine treatment (RAI) to ablate their thyroid glands, leaving them hypothyroid for life, when there are alternative approaches—including antithyroid medications and natural treatments—that many have found effective.

Patients with indeterminate nodules are rushed into surgery—without being told of the Afirma test that can almost definitively diagnose or rule out thyroid cancer. Many thousands of needless thyroid surgeries—and lifetimes of hypothyroidism—could be avoided.

Thyroid cancer patients preparing for RAI suffer weeks of significant hypothyroid symptoms due to withdrawal of their thyroid medication to elevate their TSH to ensure RAI is most effective. If they are even told that there is another option—Thyrogen, which can be injected to quickly elevate their TSH without the need for weeks of torment—it is often too expensive or in "short supply." Interestingly, large academic centers seem to have plenty of Thyrogen for their patients.

There are key nutrients essential for thyroid hormone production, including vitamins D and B_{12}, iron, iodine, zinc, selenium, and magnesium. Comprehensive nutritional assessment is essential for thyroid patients yet rarely done in mainstream medical offices.

Thyroid, adrenals, and sex hormones are intricately connected. When one is off balance, the others may be thrown off balance as well. Many thyroid patients have low progesterone that can lead to miscarriage, but progesterone is not always tested. Given our modern, stressful lifestyles, adrenal dysfunction is common, yet rarely addressed. Integrative physicians use 24-hour saliva cortisol testing for adrenal function in preconception, yet adrenals are rarely tested in mainstream medicine. Adrenal fatigue is not even a recognized diagnosis in conventional medicine.

Hashimoto's and Graves' disease are more than thyroid diseases; they are autoimmune diseases. The immune dysfunction is often disregarded in mainstream medicine yet it's an important part of autoimmune treatment. Underlying root causes of autoimmunity investigated by integrative physicians include food sensitivities, chronic infections, leaky gut, blood sugar imbalance, toxicity, and nutrient deficiencies, including vitamin D and selenium.

Many practitioners, including infertility specialists, do not routinely test for thyroid disease in infertile patients. Rather than perform comprehensive thyroid testing and consider natural fertility approaches, infertility patients are rushed into assisted reproductive technologies (ARTs), such as IVF. ARTs put women and their babies at risk not to mention the exorbitant cost. In the United States, for example, IVF can cost on average $12,000, before fertility medications, which typically cost another $3,000 to $5,000, per cycle!

Be well informed about the full array of treatment options available to you. Don't hesitate to consult with two, three, four, even ten doctors until you find the one that helps you.

A Study of T4/T3 and NDT in Pregnancy Is Overdue

Speaking of treatment options, we need a double-blind, peer-reviewed study that compares women on T4/T3, NDT, or levothyroxine in terms of the pregnancy outcomes and impact on the children.

Unfortunately no one is going to design and carry out this study; as an ethical matter, we don't do this kind of testing on pregnant women. But a retrospective study can be done. Recruit doctors who use all three treatments. Have a protocol for monitoring and testing throughout pregnancy, with follow-up of their children. Evaluate the rates of miscarriage, preterm labor, preeclampsia, other pregnancy complications, breastfeeding problems, postpartum depression, and other postpartum issues. Evaluate the status of the subjects' children, in terms of growth milestones, and later, diagnosis of ADHD and autism. We may find that NDT or T4/T3 treatment has better outcomes for mother and/or baby—which would revolutionize the current standard of care.

Doctors Need to Listen and Learn

We urge physicians to look beyond thyroid lab results and listen to women and their symptoms. What is considered "normal" may not be "optimal" for that person. Many patients are not being treated because of "borderline" thyroid results despite obvious symptoms. We are more than our lab values.

Sandi had two healthy pregnancies, and when her children were two and four years old, became pregnant again.

> Everything went wrong. My heart started acting up, and they thought at 27 years old I was having a heart attack. They then started blood work and found my thyroid had stopped working and my TSH was in the hundreds! I have never felt so bad in my life. I had preeclampsia, and my son was delivered at 37 weeks. Several years later, I got pregnant, but lost it at five weeks. At that time, my TSH was 10, and I was told that my thyroid had nothing to do with my miscarriage. A year later, I was pregnant again, and lost the baby at six weeks. I learned that my TSH was a 5. Again I was told that my thyroid had nothing to do with it. Since that time, I've been reading. Everything I read says your thyroid should be under 2.5 in the beginning to have a healthy pregnancy! Why don't doctors know this stuff? Why didn't they do blood work to check my level the second I stepped foot in their door?

In February 2013 the American Association of Clinical Endocrinologists issued a press release stating that as part of its year-round thyroid awareness campaign, the association would educate the public about thyroid disorders during pregnancy.

This is a good start, but it is not enough. A press release simply can't have the desired impact, and the lack of awareness about thyroid disease in pregnancy remains pervasive.

We need better dissemination of thyroid pregnancy guidelines to patients and physicians including family physicians, OB/GYNs, endocrinologists, and infertility specialists by national and worldwide thyroid organizations, including the American Thyroid Association and the Endocrine Society.

We need doctors to keep current on thyroid disease, including reading the 2011 "Guidelines of the American Thyroid Association for the Diagnosis and Management of Thyroid Disease During Pregnancy and Postpartum," and the 2012 "Management of Thyroid Dysfunction during Pregnancy and Postpartum: An Endocrine Society Clinical Practice Guideline" or Pregnancy Guidelines. Maybe a few physicians will even read this book!

Be Empowered and Find Your Voice

Very few thyroid patients know the Pregnancy Guidelines themselves, so as to be sufficiently well-informed in their discussions with doctors. And remember, you can't assume that your physician will be knowledgeable about thyroid disease in pregnancy, either. Do the research so that you know *more* about thyroid disease than your doctor.

We know what girls have been taught:

Girls are taught that *good girls* are nice.
Girls are taught that *good girls* follow the rules, and keep the peace.
Girls are taught that *good girls* are polite and respectful of authority.
Girls are taught that *good girls* don't complain, brag, or call attention to themselves.
Girls are taught that *good girls* put everyone else before themselves.
Girls are taught that *good girls* don't challenge the status quo, and don't assert themselves.

Are you a "good girl"? Are you struggling to find your voice?

It's time to forget about being a good girl, and instead, be good to yourself, be a good mother, and be a good advocate! Speaking up for yourself and your baby is essential when it comes to thyroid disease in pregnancy.

Our hope is to create an army of well-informed thyroid patients in the world who will speak up for themselves and their babies—and help create change.

We love what infertility specialist Dr. Hugh Melnick had to say:

Since starting medical school in 1968, I have seen the transition from the "old country doctor" approach to the treatment of symptomatic hypothyroidism with NDT, to the ATA medical establishment's approach of advocating T4 monotherapy, determined solely by TSH levels. Fortunately, the pendulum is now swinging back to "old school" symptomatic treatment with NDT. I, for one, am totally in favor of going "old school" when it comes to helping people suffering with hypothyroidism! An immense amount of credit and recognition must go to the women who have made the pendulum swing back in the proper direction, through disclosure in their books and blogs, sharing their experiences and the invaluable lessons learned while suffering with hypothyroidism in the hands of uninformed and uncaring physicians. They have made public the problems encountered by a vast number of patients who are still denied treatment because their blood tests were normal, or had the reality of their symptoms and suffering negated because their doctors believed in TSH levels and T4-only therapy, rather than heeding their patients' symptoms as a cry for help. These women are today's real experts in the diagnosis and treatment of hypothyroidism and we as physicians have a lot to learn from them.

What Can You Do?

Contact thyroid organizations including the American Thyroid Association, the Endocrine Society, and the American Association of Clinical Endocrinologists, and push for universal thyroid screening in pregnancy. On our website for the book, http://www.ThyroidPregnancyBook.com, you'll find sample letters to guide you in writing to these groups.

Write to your HMO and health insurer to share your story about undiagnosed thyroid issues and your miscarriage, preterm labor, or impact on your baby. Again, we have a sample letter you can use as a starting point on our website.

Write to your members of Congress demanding protection for the babies of women with thyroid disease.

Reach out to people and groups in the media who would be interested in supporting change to help protect children and let them know about this book.

Visit the book's website to keep track of our advocacy efforts and to learn more about thyroid disease in pregnancy.

Speak up at your doctor's office. If you're not getting the help you need, don't hesitate to seek a second medical opinion. Never settle.

Share this book with people and groups in your social circles, because there is a good chance someone you know is struggling with thyroid disease.

Tell your family members, daughters, friends, co-workers—everyone you know who might become pregnant or who is pregnant—to demand comprehensive thyroid screening in early pregnancy.

Educate uninformed doctors—for example, those who think a TSH of 5 is fine for conception or during pregnancy. Bring them a copy of the Pregnancy Guidelines (see page 1 of Appendix A for links to printable versions of the guidelines). And bring them a copy of this book!

Keep Your Hope

Here we are at the very end of a book that we've felt compelled to write for years. We've spent hours thinking about this last chapter, wondering what last thing we wished to say . . . what one word might sum up what is in our hearts. . . and we've found it:

HOPE.

Dana's Experience

The day my second son was born, I felt that I had witnessed a miracle.

The child that doctors told me would never be mine had come.

I had my two beautiful boys, Benjamin and Hudson, and I, Dana Trentini, had come from the depths of sorrow to this place of joy.

I know there is hope because hope happened to me.

Appendix A
Resources and Support Groups

This section features a number of resources to help you obtain further information and support. Additional resources are also available at the website for this book, located at http://www.ThyroidPregnancyBook.com. At the site, you'll find current listings for organizations and their contact information, current website addresses, links to online sources where you can get more information about any books that are mentioned, products and services we've mentioned, experts featured in the book, and other helpful resources.

The Book
http://www.ThyroidPregnancyBook.com

Order Your Own Thyroid Tests and Panels
http://www.ThyroidPregnancyBook.com/tests

2011 Guidelines of the American Thyroid Association for the Diagnosis and Management of Thyroid Disease During Pregnancy and Postpartum
http://www.ncbi.nlm.nih.gov/pmc/articles/PMC3472679/

2012 Management of Thyroid Dysfunction During Pregnancy and Postpartum: An Endocrine Society Clinical Practice Guideline
http://press.endocrine.org/doi/abs/10.1210/jc.2011-2803 (see Full Text)

2007 Management of Thyroid Dysfunction During Pregnancy and Postpartum: An Endocrine Society Clinical Practice Guideline
http://press.endocrine.org/doi/pdf/10.1210/jc.2007-0141

The Authors

Dana Trentini

HypothyroidMom
http://www.hypothyroidmom.com
Facebook: https://www.facebook.com/HypothyroidMom
Twitter: https://twitter.com/HypothyroidMom

Mary Shomon

Thyroid.About.com
http://thyroid.about.com

Thyroid-Info.com
http://www.thyroid-info.com

Thyroid support from Mary Shomon:
Facebook: https://www.facebook.com/thyroidsupport
Twitter: https://twitter.com/ThyroidMary

Mary Shomon's other books:
Beautiful Inside and Out, coauthored with Gena Lee Nolin
Thyroid Diet Revolution, 2 editions
The Menopause Thyroid Solution
Living Well with Hypothyroidism, 2 editions
Living Well with Graves' Disease and Hyperthyroidism
Living Well with Autoimmune Disease
Living Well with Chronic Fatigue Syndrome and Fibromyalgia
The Thyroid Hormone Breakthrough
The Hair Loss Master Plan, coauthored with Brent Hardgrave

General Hormonal Health

Hormone Foundation
http://www.hormone.org
> Educational resources based on the clinical and scientific expertise of the Endocrine Society, the world's largest organization of endocrinologists, representing more than eighteen thousand physicians and scientists.

You & Your Hormones
http://www.yourhormones.info
> Information on hormones and hormone diseases for patients, parents, students, and teachers. Produced and managed by the Society for Endocrinology.

Endocrinology, Thyroid, Autoimmune Disease

American Autoimmune Related Diseases Association
http://www.aarda.org

AARDA is a nonprofit health agency dedicated to the eradication of autoimmune diseases and the alleviation of suffering and the socioeconomic impact of autoimmunity through fostering and facilitating collaboration in the areas of education, public awareness, research, and patient services in an effective, ethical, and efficient manner.

American Thyroid Association
http://www.thyroid.org
The ATA is a worldwide organization dedicated to the advancement, understanding, prevention, diagnosis, and treatment of thyroid disorders and thyroid cancer. It is an international membership medical society with over 1,700 members from forty-three countries around the world.

Autoimmune Mom
http://www.autoimmunemom.com
Autoimmune Mom was born out of a frustration with a lack of online information about autoimmune conditions beyond the surface-level articles and blog posts, even on the top health websites. Founder Katie Cleary has Hashimoto's, reactive hypoglycemia, and pleva (a rare autoimmune skin condition).

Butterflies & Phoenixes
http://sarahjdowning.com
Sarah Downing was diagnosed with Hashimoto's thyroiditis. Her chronic illness blog *Butterflies & Phoenixes* spreads positivity and hope.

Dear Pharmacist
http://suzycohen.com/articles/
Pharmacist Suzy Cohen's syndicated column "Dear Pharmacist" reaches millions of readers each week. Suzy has spoken on such programs as *Good Morning America Health*, *The Dr. Oz Show*, *The 700 Club*, *The View*, and *The Doctors*. She is author of the book *Thyroid Healthy*.

Dear Thyroid
http://www.dearthyroid.com
A thyroid advocacy website where patients with thyroid disease and thyroid cancer feel safe writing about their diseases with the mission to support one another free of judgment.

The Endocrine Society
http://www.endocrine.org
A professional, international medical organization in the field of endocrinology and metabolism, founded in 1916.

EndocrineWeb
http://www.endocrineweb.com
EndocrineWeb provides patients with accurate and current information about endocrine disorders. In clear, straightforward language, it explains the causes and symptoms of these disorders and how they can be treated.

Girlfriends' Guide to Hashimoto's
https://www.facebook.com/groups/girlfriendsguidetohashimotos
Stacey Robbins is author of the book *You're Not Crazy and You're Not Alone: Losing the Victim, Finding Your Sense of Humor, and Learning to Love Yourself Through Hashimoto's*. Her Facebook group is designed to be like a big table where all the girlfriends gather and chat in an honest way about Hashimoto's.

Hashimoto's 411
http://hashimotos411.com
This website features well-researched Hashimoto's patients who are happy and eager to share their knowledge and experiences with others, whether newly diagnosed or seeking new ways to treat their autoimmune disease(s).

Hashimoto Happiness
https://www.facebook.com/groups/179205325602875/
Marissa Ravelo created a Facebook group called Hashimoto Happiness to support one another with laughter and positive thinking.

Healthy Thyroid Lady
http://www.healthythyroidlady.blogspot.com
Carol Gray was diagnosed with Graves' disease, then given RAI, which put her into hypothyroidism. She is author of the book *WOW, Your Mom Really Is CRAZY*, about coping with thyroid disease.

Lavt stofskifte (Hypothyroidism)
http://lavtstofskifte.info
Danish journalist Helle Sydendal advocates on behalf of thyroid patients in Denmark. She is author of the book *From Hypothyroid to Healthy*, which includes Dana Trentini's thyroid story.

National Academy on Hypothyroidism
http://www.nahypothyroidism.org
The NAH is a group of thyroidologists, headed by Kent Holtorf, MD, who are dedicated to the promotion of scientifically sound and medically validated concepts and information pertaining to the diagnosis and treatment of hypothyroidism.

Sick to Death!
http://sick2death.com
Sick to Death! Is a documentary-in-progress by award-winning filmmaker Maggie Hadleigh-West. It seeks to understand and change the corrupt medical practices around thyroid disease. Dana Trentini and Mary Shomon will be featured.

Society for Endocrinology
http://www.endocrinology.org
A UK-based membership organization representing a global community of scientists, clinicians, and nurses who work with hormones. Provides a list of patient support groups.

Thyroid Cancer Basics
http://www.thyca.org/download/document/350/TCBasics.pdf
An informative free guide that covers the thyroid cancer basics, helpful for newly diagnosed patients and their friends and family.

Thyroid Cancer Survivors' Association (ThyCa)
http://www.thyca.org
ThyCa is a nonprofit organization of thyroid cancer survivors, family members, and health-care professionals. The website maintains current information about thyroid cancer and support services available to people at any stage of testing, treatment, or lifelong monitoring for thyroid cancer, as well as their caregivers.

ThyroidChange
http://www.thyroidchange.org
ThyroidChange is a nonprofit organization dedicated to improving thyroid care worldwide. Patients, medical professionals, and other individuals comprise this collaborative network to address current guidelines regarding the treatment and diagnosis of thyroid hormone dysfunction.

Thyroid Disease Manager
http://www.thyroidmanager.org
Thyroid Disease Manager was developed by Leslie J. De Groot, MD, and a group of thyroid experts from around the world. It offers an up-to-date analysis of thyrotoxicosis, hypothyroidism, thyroid nodules, thyroid cancer, thyroiditis, and all aspects of human thyroid disease and thyroid physiology.

Thyroid Disease One Day at a Time
https://www.facebook.com/groups/392299214163296/
Thyroid Disease One Day at a Time is a Facebook group for those dealing with thyroid issues. Founder Beth Jones describes it well: "Some days I just need to talk/vent about my day, the good and the bad."

Thyroid Mom
http://www.thyroidmom.com
Blythe Clifford is a mother of two boys, both born with congenital hypothyroidism. Blythe was diagnosed with Hashimoto's and her husband with Graves' disease. Her blog *Thyroid Mom* raises awareness of congenital hypothyroidism.

Thyroid Nation
http://thyroidnation.com
Add the love of Zumba, a cascade of "health-driven" dominos leading Danna Bowman to adrenal fatigue and Hashimoto's . . . the dire need to heal and find support, ultimately inspiring and unifying the collective voice of thyroid thrivers everywhere.

Thyroid Petition Scotland
https://www.facebook.com/thyroidpetitionScotland

Lorraine Cleaver is a thyroid and hypoparathyroid patient. Together with Sandra Whyte and Marian Dyer, Lorraine petitioned the Scottish Parliament for better thyroid testing and treatment.

Thyroid Pharmacist

http://www.thyroidpharmacist.com

After two years of researching Hashimoto's, Izabella Wentz, PharmD, FASCP, decided to combine emerging knowledge with her pharmacy expertise to run rapid tests of change on herself that led her to discover the root cause of her condition. She is author of the book *Hashimoto's Thyroiditis: Lifestyle Interventions for Finding and Treating the Root Cause*.

Thyroid Sexy

https://www.facebook.com/thyroidsexy

Actress and model Gena Lee Nolin, who starred on the popular TV series *Baywatch*, has gone public with her struggle with Hashimoto's disease and hypothyroidism. Gena and Mary Shomon coauthored the book *Beautiful Inside and Out: Conquering Thyroid Disease with a Healthy, Happy, "Thyroid Sexy" Life*.

Thyroid Survivor Network

http://www.thyroidsurvivornetwork.com

The Thyroid Survivor Network is a patient advocacy group seeking to raise awareness and provide support for thyroid disease patients, including thyroid cancer survivors.

Thyroid UK

http://www.thyroiduk.org.uk/tuk/

Thyroid UK provides information and resources to promote effective diagnosis and appropriate treatment for people with thyroid disorders in the United Kingdom.

Zen Thyroid

https://twitter.com/ZenThyroid

After years of being misdiagnosed and developing a total distrust of the medical system, the thyroid patient who calls herself Zen Thyroid is grateful that her healing process has begun. On Twitter @ZenThyroid.

Finding Thyroid Experts

The American Academy of Anti-Aging Medicine Health-Care Professionals Directory

http://www.a4m.com

A nonprofit dedicated to the advancement of technology to detect, prevent, and treat aging-related disease and to promote research into methods to retard and optimize the human aging process. Click "Directory" in the top navigation bar for a worldwide antiaging directory to find antiaging physicians, clinics, medspas, products, and services.

American Association of Clinical Endocrinologists Database
https://www.aace.com
> Professional community of physicians specializing in endocrinology, diabetes, and metabolism. Click "Patients" in top navigation bar, then at the very bottom of the page you'll find under "Resources" the link "Find an Endocrinologist."

American Association of Endocrine Surgeons Membership List (PDF)
http://www.endocrinesurgery.org
> AAES is committed to providing surgical expertise in diseases of the thyroid, parathyroid, and adrenal glands as well as in neuroendocrine tumors of the pancreas and GI tract. Click "Find a Member" in the left sidebar to locate a physician in the United States, Canada, and internationally.

American Association of Integrative Medicine Find-a-Provider Directory
http://www.aaimedicine.com
> Website provides a directory by US state and specialties, including holistic medicine, integrative medicine, naturopathic medicine, women's health care, and hormone replacement therapy. Click "Find-a-Provider" on the homepage.

The American Association of Naturopathic Physicians Online Directory
http://www.naturopathic.org
> Website featuring information about naturopathy. Click "Find a Doctor" in the top navigation bar for a searchable directory of naturopathic doctors in the United States, with specialties that include adrenal fatigue/endocrinology and chronic fatigue/autoimmune disorders.

American Board of Integrative Holistic Medicine Physician Locator
http://www.abihm.org
> Click "Find an ABIHM Certified Physician" on the homepage, which provides a directory to locate ABIHM Certified Integrative Holistic Physicians by US state or Canadian province, with specialties that include bioidentical hormone therapy, endocrinology, environmental medicine, functional medicine, pain management, and pediatrics.

American College for Advancement in Medicine Physician+Link Directory
http://acam.site-ym.com
> A recognized leader in integrative medicine education and advancement. Click "Resources" in top navigation bar and select "Find a Provider with Physician+Link" to locate integrative medicine practitioners in the United States and internationally. The locator also includes the option to select specialties, including thyroid disease.

American Thyroid Association Thyroid Specialist Database
http://www.thyroid.org
> Organization devoted to thyroid biology and to the prevention and treatment of thyroid disease. Click "Find a Specialist" to find thyroid physicians and surgeons by US state and world location.

The Canadian Association of Naturopathic Doctors Locator
http://www.cand.ca/
> Information on naturopathic physicians in Canada. Click the top of the page for a directory of naturopathic doctors by province in Canada.

Hormone Health Network's Physician Referral Directory
http://www.hormone.org
> Directory comprised of over three thousand members of the Endocrine Society. Click "Contact a Health Professional" in the top navigation bar and select "Find an Endocrinologist."

The Institute for Functional Medicine Find a Practitioner Directory
https://www.functionalmedicine.org
> Functional medicine addresses the underlying causes of disease using a whole person approach. Click "Find a Practitioner" in the top navigation bar to find an international list of practitioners who have trained with IFM.

International College of Integrative Medicine Member Search
http://www.icimed.com
> ICIM provides a member search on its website to locate doctors by zip code and state in the United States, as well as an international member list. Click "Find a Practitioner" on the homepage.

NY Thyroid Center Surgeon Referral Service
Phone: 212-305-0442, e-mail: surgery@columbia.edu

ThyroidChange Doctor Lists
http://www.thyroidchange.org
> A nonprofit organization dedicated to improving thyroid care worldwide. Click "For Patients" in the top navigation bar and select "Find a Doctor," which provides lists of patient-recommended physicians in the United States, Australia, Canada, and internationally.

Thyroid Top Doctors Directory
http://www.thyroid-info.com
> Author of this book Mary Shomon provides a top thyroid doctors directory on her website with an extensive list of top doctors in the United States and internationally. The doctors listed are endocrinologists, thyroid specialists, thyroid surgeons, thyroidologists, integrative physicians, and other practitioners who have been highly recommended by patients. Click "Top Drs" on the homepage.

Women In Balance Institute Search Providers
http://womeninbalance.org
> Nonprofit organization born out of the desire to be a trusted health resource for women over age forty who are experiencing the natural hormonal transitions of perimenopause and menopause. Click "Our Health Provider Locator" that appears on the homepage to find a provider throughout the United States that specializes in bioidentical hormone replacement therapy and women's health.

Infertility, Fertility, Reproductive Medicine

About.com Fertility
http://infertility.about.com/
About.com Fertility offers authentic, engaging expertise from writers who are experts in their topic. Learn how to boost fertility, get pregnant, recognize infertility symptoms, and navigate fertility treatments.

About.com Miscarriage/Pregnancy Loss
http://miscarriage.about.com/
About.com Miscarriage/Pregnancy Loss offers credible advice for women and families undergoing the loss of a pregnancy, including coping tips, warning signs, and more.

American Society for Reproductive Medicine
http://www.asrm.org
ASRM is a nonprofit organization dedicated to advancing reproductive medicine through education, research, and advocacy. The website provides reproductive facts for patients. Click "Find a Healthcare Practitioner" in the right-hand column for a directory of physicians.

BabyCenter—Infertility
http://www.babycenter.com
BabyCenter reaches more than 45 million moms and dads monthly from around the world. Click "Getting Pregnant" in the top navigation bar to access trusted information on preparing to conceive, trying to conceive, and having trouble conceiving. BabyCenter offers many different online community groups to join.

DailyStrength Infertility Support Group
http://www.dailystrength.org
Click "Infertility" on the homepage for the Infertility Support Group at Daily-Strength.

Fertile Thoughts
http://www.fertilethoughts.com
Fertile Thoughts is a social networking site focused on fertility and infertility to provide support to women, men, couples, and singles who are building their families.

Fertility Friends—UK
http://www.fertilityfriends.co.uk
Fertility Friends is an infertility community in the United Kingdom with members at every stage of their journey. They provide an online forum on their website.

Infertility Resources
https://www.ihr.com
Detailed site with information on infertility, including specific lists of infertility providers, clinics, and more.

The International Council on Infertility Information Dissemination

http://www.inciid.org

> The nonprofit organization INCIID provides educational resources and a forum on its website.

Nurses' Professional Group

http://www.npg-asrm.org

> NPG is composed of nurse members of the American Society for Reproductive Medicine. Click "Members" in the top navigation bar and select "Find an NPG Member" to locate a reproductive nurse.

Path 2 Parenthood

http://www.path2parenthood.org

> The nonprofit organization P2P provides educational outreach events, an online library with HD videos, a daily blog, a resource directory available for download on mobile devices, telephone and in-person coaching, and a toll-free support line. Free of charge to consumers.

RESOLVE: The National Infertility Association

http://www.resolve.org

> RESOLVE is a nonprofit organization with a nationwide network to promote reproductive health and to ensure equal access to all family building options for men and women experiencing infertility or other reproductive disorders. RESOLVE provides educational material on the website as well as support groups and a help line.

Society for Reproductive Endocrinology and Infertility

http://www.socrei.org

> SREI membership requires certification by the American Board of Obstetrics and Gynecology in both obstetrics and gynecology and the subspecialty of reproductive endocrinology. Click "Publications" in the top navigation bar and select "For Patients" for resources, including a directory to find an SREI member.

Society of Reproductive Surgeons

http://www.reprodsurgery.org

> SRS serves as a forum for members of the American Society for Reproductive Medicine with special interest and competency in reproductive surgery. Click "Members" in the top navigation bar and select "Find an SRS Member."

Society for the Study of Reproduction (SSR)

https://www.ssr.org

> Founded in 1967, SSR promotes the study of reproduction by fostering interdisciplinary communication among scientists, holding conferences, and publishing meritorious studies. SSR publishes the journal *Biology of Reproduction*. Archive of all online issues is available by clicking "Biology of Reproduction" on the homepage.

Assisted Reproduction

CDC Division of Assisted Reproductive Technology
http://www.cdc.gov/art
> The Centers for Disease Control and Prevention (CDC) provides patient resources on assisted reproductive technologies (ART).

Society for Assisted Reproductive Technology (SART)
http://www.sart.org
> SART is a US organization of professionals dedicated to the practice of assisted reproductive technologies (ART). Its website provides patient resources and latest news. Click "IVF Success" in the top navigation bar to find a SART-member clinic.

Pregnancy/Childbirth

About.com Pregnancy & Childbirth
http://pregnancy.about.com
> About.com Pregnancy and Childbirth offers credible pregnancy advice, including pregnancy health, ovulation calculators, ultrasound information, due date calendars, and more.

American College of Obstetricians and Gynecologists Physician Finder
http://www.acog.org
> ACOG is the United States' leading group of professionals providing health care for women. Click "For Patients" for information from leading experts in women's health care. Click "ACOG" for "Find an Ob-Gyn."

BabyCenter
http://www.babycenter.com
> BabyCenter reaches more than 45 million moms and dads monthly from around the world. Click "Getting Pregnant" in the top navigation bar to access trusted information on pregnancy. It offers many different online community groups to join.

Fetal Health Foundation
http://www.fetalhealthfoundation.org
> The mission of Fetal Health Foundation is to provide support, provide information, fund research, increase awareness, and be an outlet for leading medical information pertaining to fetal distresses and syndromes.

Hand to Hold
http://handtohold.org
> Hand to Hold is a nonprofit organization that matches seasoned parents of preemies (Helping Hands) with parents in need of support. Services provided directly to parents are done free of charge.

Hope for Two . . . Pregnant with Cancer
http://www.hopefortwo.org

The Hope for Two . . . Pregnant with Cancer network offers free support for women diagnosed with cancer while pregnant. It connects women who are currently pregnant with cancer with other women who have experienced a similar cancer diagnosis.

National Advocates for Pregnant Women
http://www.advocatesforpregnantwomen.org
The nonprofit NAPW works to secure the human and civil rights, health, and welfare of all women, focusing particularly on pregnant and parenting women, and those who are most vulnerable to state control and punishment—low income women, women of color, and drug-using women.

Our Bodies Ourselves
http://www.ourbodiesourselves.org
OBOS is a nonprofit organization that develops and promotes evidence-based information on girls' and women's reproductive health and sexuality. Click "Infertility" and/or "Pregnancy & Birth" on the homepage for information.

Parents
http://www.parents.com/pregnancy
Parents magazine provides information covering pregnancy, children, health, safety, food, and parenting related topics. It is also the online home of *Parents*, *FamilyFun*, *American Baby*, and *Parents Latina* magazines.

Preeclampsia Foundation
http://www.preeclampsia.org
The Preeclampsia Foundation is a US-based patient advocacy organization that provides education and support for those impacted by preeclampsia and other hypertensive disorders of pregnancy. Educational materials vetted by a medical board of experts are available in print, DVD, and online. An online forum provides 24/7 information and support to visitors across the globe.

Pregnancy.com
http://www.pregnancy.com
Pregnancy.com, powered by BabyCenter, provides information on all things related to pregnancy.

Society for Maternal-Fetal Medicine (SMFM)
https://www.smfm.org
Maternal-Fetal physicians are obstetricians with additional training in the area of high-risk, complicated pregnancies. Click "Find an MFM" in the top navigation bar to find a specialist.

To Labor
http://tolabor.com/
An organization of labor assistants and doulas. Click "Find A Doula" in the top navigation bar, for a searchable directory of professional birth doulas.

What to Expect

http://www.whattoexpect.com

> Home page for the popular book *What to Expect When You're Expecting*.

Your Pregnancy Week by Week

www.yourpregnancybook.com

> Home page for the popular book *Your Pregnancy Week by Week*

Postpartum Health

Mayo Clinic

http://www.mayoclinic.org

> The Mayo Clinic offers information about postpartum care. Click "Patient Care and Health Information" in top navigation bar, then select "Healthy Lifestyle," "Labor and delivery, postpartum care."

Online PPMD Support Group

http://www.ppdsupportpage.com

> The Online PPMD Support Group provides online resources and discussion forums regarding postpartum mood disorders. Click "Communicate" in top navigation bar, then "Discussion Forum."

Postpartum Progress

http://postpartumprogress.org

> Postpartum Progress is a peer-to-peer organization that works to create an atmosphere in which women can recognize when they need help for maternal mental illness and feel safe reaching out for help. Click "Find Help" to join its free private Warrior Mom Forum.

Postpartum Support International

http://www.postpartum.net

> PSI is a nonprofit organization dedicated to increasing awareness among public and professional communities about the emotional changes that women experience during pregnancy and postpartum. It offers emergency help, online support meetings, and resources. Click "Get Help" and select "Get Help" to find area volunteers.

Breastfeeding

About.com Breastfeeding

http://breastfeeding.about.com/

> About.com Breastfeeding offers answers, advice, tips, and solutions to common breastfeeding issues.

La Leche League International

http://www.lalecheleague.org

> La Leche League International is a nonprofit organization that distributes information on and promotes breastfeeding. Leaders accredited by LLL are available

around the world to help mothers who wish to breastfeed their babies. Click "Find a Leader" in the top navigation bar.

National Alliance for Breastfeeding Advocacy
http://www.naba-breastfeeding.org
    NABA is dedicated to the protection, promotion, and support of breastfeeding. Their mission is to coordinate efforts for breastfeeding reform in the United States.

Perimenopause and Menopause

North American Menopause Society
http://www.menopause.org
    NAMS is a nonprofit organization dedicated to promoting the health and quality of life of all women through perimenopause and beyond. Click "For Women" in the top navigation bar, then "Find a Menopause Practitioner."

Diet and Nutrition

Anti-Inflammatory Diet—Andrew Weil, MD
http://www.drweil.com/drw/u/ART02012/anti-inflammatory-diet
http://www.drweil.com/drw/u/ART02995/Dr-Weil-Anti-Inflammatory-Food-Pyramid.html
    Provides an overview of this leading integrative physician's diet recommendations, and his recommended food pyramid.

Autoimmune Paleo
http://autoimmune-paleo.com
    Book and site focusing on the benefits of an "autoimmune paleo" diet for autoimmune diseases.

Autoimmune Protocol Diet—Dr. Sarah Ballantyne's Paleo Mom
http://www.thepaleomom.com/autoimmunity/the-autoimmune-protocol
    A quick overview of the autoimmune protocol developed by Dr. Ballantyne as part of her paleo diet approach.

GAPS Diet
http://www.gapsdiet.com
    The GAPS diet was derived from the specific carbohydrate diet (SCD) created by Dr. Sidney Valentine Haas to naturally treat chronic inflammatory conditions in the digestive tract as a result of a damaged gut lining.

The Paleo Diet—Dr. Loren Cordain
http://thepaleodiet.com/
    Dr. Loren Cordain is one of the world's leading experts on the natural human diet of our Stone Age ancestors, the paleo diet. His book and website focus on the benefits and implementation of a paleo-style diet approach.

Specific Carbohydrate Diet (SCD)—Breaking the Vicious Cycle
http://www.breakingtheviciouscycle.info
> Website and book featuring information about the specific carbohydrate diet, with sample menus, a food list, and more.

Thyroid Drug Manufacturers

Abbott Laboratories/AbbVie
http://www.abbott.com
100 Abbott Park Road, Abbott Park, IL 60064-3500, 800-255-5162, Manufactures: Synthroid (levothyroxine) www.synthroid.com

Akrimax/Tirosint
http://www.akrimax.com
11 Commerce Drive, 1st Floor, Cranford, NJ 07016, 908-372-0506
Tirosint-www.tirosint.com

Erfa
http://www.thyroid.erfa.net
Canadian maker of prescription natural thyroid

Forest Pharmaceuticals
13600 Shoreline Drive, St. Louis, MO 63045, 800-678-1605, Fax: 314-493-7457, http://www.forestpharm.com, Manufactures: Armour Thyroid (natural desiccated thyroid) Armour Thyroid: www.armourthyroid.com

Genzyme Therapeutics
500 Kendall Street, Cambridge, MA 02142, 800-745-4447, 617-768-9000, http://www.genzyme.com, Manufactures: Thyrogen (thyrotropin alfa/recombinant TSH)

Jones Pharma Incorporated, Subsidiary of Pfizer
501 Fifth Street, Bristol, TN 37620, 888-840-5370, 800-776-3637 Fax: 866-990-0545, http://www.kingpharm.com, Manufactures: Levoxyl (levothyroxine) Levoxyl—www.levoxyl.com—866-LEVOXYL (538-6995), Cytomel (liothyronine), Tapazole (methimazole)

Lannett Pharmaceuticals
9000 State Road, Philadelphia, PA 19136, 800-325-9994, 215-333-9000, http://www.lannett.com, Manufactures: Unithroid (distributes for manufacturer Jerome Stevens) (levothyroxine)

RLC Laboratories
28248 N. Tatum Boulevard, Suite B1-629, Cave Creek, AZ 85331, 623-879-8537, Fax: 623-879-8683, Toll-free: 877-797-7997, http://www.rlclabs.com, Manufactures: WP Thyroid and Nature-Throid
Nature-Throid—www.nature-throid.com
WP Thyroid—www.wpthyroid.com

Other Recommended Books

The Autoimmune Solution, by Amy Myers, MD
The Blood Sugar Solution 10-Day Detox Diet, by Mark Hyman, MD
Fit and Fabulous in 15 Minutes, by Teresa Tapp
From Fatigued to Fantastic, by Jacob Teitelbaum, MD
Graves' Disease: A Practical Guide, by Elaine Moore and Lisa Moore
Hashimoto's Thyroiditis: Lifestyle Interventions for Finding and Treating the Root Cause,
     by Izabella Wentz, PharmD, FASCP
The Hormone Cure, by Sara Gottfried, MD
Listening to Your Hormones, by Gillian Ford
Making Babies: A Proven 3-Month Program for Maximum Fertility, by Sami S. David,
     MD, and Jill Blakeway, LAc
Overcoming Thyroid Disorders, and *Iodine: Why You Need It, Why You Can't Live
     Without It*, by David Brownstein, MD
Taking Charge of Your Fertility, by Toni Wechsler
Thyroid Healthy, Lose Weight, Look Beautiful and Live the Life You Imagine, by Suzy
     Cohen, RPh
Thyroid Power, Thyroid Mind Power, and Feeling Fat, Fuzzy or Frazzled?, by Richard
     Shames, MD, and Karilee Shames, RN, PhD

Appendix B
Experts Featured in the Book

David Borenstein, MD

Integrative physician David Borenstein is the founder of Manhattan Integrative Medicine and the New York Stem Cell Treatment Center. He obtained his medical degree from the Technion Faculty of Medicine in Haifa, Israel. During the course of his career he has attended numerous specialized training courses in order to expand the scope of his medical expertise. He is board certified in physical medicine and rehabilitation, certified in medical acupuncture, and is a member of numerous professional societies.

Manhattan Integrative Medicine
1841 Broadway, Suite 1012
New York, NY 10023
212-262-2412
http://www.davidborensteinmd.com
http://www.nystemcellcenter.com
Facebook: https://www.facebook.com/ManhattanIntegrativeMedicine
Twitter: https://twitter.com/BorensteinMD

Laurie Borenstein

Laurie Borenstein is a certified health and nutrition coach, with certification from the Institute for Integrative Nutrition in New York City. She is the founder of Life Intake, an integrative nutrition practice where she works with clients by telephone to help create and implement an integrative nutritional plan for optimal health. She specializes in integrative nutrition treatments for a variety of health issues and disorders, including hormonal imbalance, thyroid issues, candida, adrenal fatigue, metabolic syndrome, irritable bowel syndrome, among others. Laurie also provides weight management counseling and wellness coaching in both individual and group settings.

Life Intake
Integrative Nutrition

http://laurie-bittan-borenstein.healthcoach1.integrativenutrition.com
Facebook: https://www.facebook.com/pages/Life-Intake/165858020130268?pn
ref=about.overview
Twitter: https://twitter.com/LifeIntake

Phil Boyle, MD, CFCMC

Phil Boyle has been the director of NaPro FertilityCare Ireland since 1998, when he opened the first European clinic. He graduated with a degree in medicine from Galway University in 1992 and is a member of both the Irish (MICGP) and Royal (MRCGP) College of General Practitioners. Dr. Boyle is a member of the American Academy of FertilityCare professionals (AAFCP) and is a Certified FertilityCare Medical Consultant (CFCMC). He is a member of the Irish Fertility Society and president of the International Institute for Restorative Reproductive Medicine.

Phil Boyle, MD, CFCMC
NaPro Fertility Clinic
Dublin, Ireland
(01) 2933816
http://naprofertility.ie

David Brownstein, MD

David Brownstein is a board-certified family physician who utilizes the best of conventional and alternative therapies. He is the medical director for the Center for Holistic Medicine in West Bloomfield, Michigan. He is a member of the American Academy of Family Physicians and the International College of Integrative Medicine (ICIM). Dr. Brownstein has lectured internationally about his success using natural items and has authored thirteen books: *Iodine: Why You Need It, Why You Can't Live Without It*; *Vitamin B12 for Health*; *Drugs That Don't Work and Natural Therapies That Do*; *The Miracle of Natural Hormones*; *Overcoming Thyroid Disorders*; *Overcoming Arthritis*; *Salt Your Way to Health*; *The Guide to Healthy Eating*; *The Guide to a Gluten-Free Diet*; *The Guide to a Dairy-Free Diet*; *The Soy Deception*; *The Skinny on Fats*; and *The Statin Disaster*.

Center for Holistic Medicine
6089 West Maple Road, Suite 200
West Bloomfield, MI 48322
248-851-1600
http://www.centerforholisticmedicine.com/officeInfo.htm
http://www.drbrownstein.com
Facebook: https://www.facebook.com/drdavidbrownstein
Twitter: https://twitter.com/drbrownstein

Jill Carnahan, MD

Jill Carnahan is dually board-certified in family medicine and integrative holistic medicine. Dr. Carnahan completed her residency at the University of Illinois Program in Family Medicine at Methodist Medical Center. In 2006 she was voted by faculty to receive the Resident Teacher of the Year award and elected to Central Illinois 40 Leaders Under 40. She was also part of the first one hundred health-care practitioners to be certified in functional medicine through the Institute of Functional Medicine. In 2010, she founded Flatiron Functional Medicine in Boulder, Colorado, where she practices functional medicine with medical partner Dr. Robert Rountree. Dr. Carnahan is also a thirteen-year survivor of breast cancer and Crohn's disease and passionate about teaching patients how to "live well" and thrive in the midst of complex and chronic illness. She is also committed to teaching other physicians how to address underlying cause of illness through the principles of functional medicine rather than just treating symptoms.

Flatiron Functional Medicine
400 S. McCaslin Boulevard, Suite 210
Louisville, CO 80027
303-993-7910
http://www.jillcarnahan.com
Facebook: https://www.facebook.com/flatironfunctionalmedicine
Twitter: https://twitter.com/DocCarnahan

Suzy Cohen, RPH

"America's Pharmacist" Suzy Cohen has been a health writer for over fifteen years and has dedicated her life to researching an immense variety of health topics. Her syndicated column, "Dear Pharmacist," reaches millions of readers each week. She has spoken on such programs as *Good Morning America Health*, *The Dr. Oz Show*, *The 700 Club*, *The View*, and *The Doctors*. Suzy is author of the books *Thyroid Healthy*, *Drug Muggers*, and *Headache Free*. She created a supplement line that includes Thyro-Script, a synergistic blend of herbs, nutrients, and digestive enzymes for healthy thyroid function.

http://suzycohen.com
http://scriptessentials.com
Facebook: https://www.facebook.com/SuzyCohenRPh
Twitter: https://twitter.com/SuzyCohen

Adrienne Clamp, MD

Adrienne Clamp graduated from the University of Kansas School of Medicine, did a residency in family medicine, and her professional life included obstetrics. She became interested in thyroid disease after becoming hypothyroid herself and finding she did not feel well with the standard approach to thyroid replacement. Dr. Clamp has an interest in alternative medicine and is trained in acupuncture and Chinese Traditional Medicine as well as traditional Western medicine. She is also studying at Virginia Theological Seminary for a doctorate of ministry. She is an integrative physician in practice at Well Being Being Well.

Well Being Being Well
6862 Elm Street, #720

McLean, VA 22101
703-635-2158
http://www.dradrienneclamp.com

Suzanne Connole, MSTOM, LAc

Suzanne Connole is a New York State–licensed acupuncturist and Chinese herbalist with an MS in traditional Oriental medicine. Suzanne has focused her practice on women's health, including treatment and support for infertility issues. She also has had training as a doula and is a faculty member at both Tri-State College of Acupuncture and Pacific College of Oriental Medicine.

Five Seasons Healing
80 East 11th Street, Suite 211
New York, NY 10003
917-538-5755
suzconnole@gmail.com
http://fiveseasonshealing.com
http://www.suzanneconnole.com

Kent Holtorf, MD

Kent Holtorf is the founder and medical director of the Holtorf Medical Group and the nationwide Holtorf Medical Group Affiliate Centers. He is also founder and director of the nonprofit National Academy of Hypothyroidism (NAH), which is dedicated to dissemination of new information to doctors and patients on the diagnosis and treatment of hypothyroidism. He has personally trained numerous physicians across the country in the use of bioidentical hormones, hypothyroidism, complex endocrine dysfunction, and innovative treatments of chronic fatigue syndrome, fibromyalgia, and chronic infectious diseases, including Lyme disease. He is a fellowship lecturer for the American Board of Anti-Aging Medicine, the endocrinology expert for AOL Health, and is a guest editor and peer reviewer for a number of medical journals, including *Endocrine*, *Postgraduate Medicine*, and *Pharmacy Practice*. Dr. Holtorf has published a number of peer-reviewed endocrine reviews, including on the safety and efficacy of bioidentical hormones, and the inaccuracies of standard thyroid testing.

Holtorf Medical Group
Locations in Torrance, CA; Atlanta, GA; Foster City, CA; Philadelphia, PA
877-508-1177
http://www.holtorfmed.com
Facebook: https://www.facebook.com/holtorfmed
Twitter: https://twitter.com/holtorfmed

Mark Hyman, MD

Mark Hyman is a practicing family physician, a nine-time *New York Times* best-selling author, and an internationally recognized leader, speaker, educator, and advocate in his field. Dr. Hyman is the director of the Cleveland Clinic Center for Functional

Medicine. He is also the founder and medical director of the UltraWellness Center, chairman of the board of the Institute for Functional Medicine, a medical editor of *The Huffington Post*, and has been a regular medical contributor on many television shows, including *CBS This Morning*, the *Today Show*, *The View*, the *Katie Couric Show*, *The Dr. Oz Show*, and CNN. His books include *Eat Fat, Get Thin* and *The Blood Sugar Solution 10-Day Detox Diet*.

The UltraWellness Center
55 Pittsfield Road, Suite 9
Lenox Commons
Lenox, MA 01240
413-637-9991
http://www.ultrawellnesscenter.com
http://drhyman.com
Facebook: https://www.facebook.com/drmarkhyman
Twitter: https://twitter.com/markhymanmd

Jochen H. Lorch, MD, MS

Jochen Lorch is a medical oncologist whose interests are head and neck oncology and thyroid cancer at the Dana-Farber Cancer Institute in Boston, Massachusetts. He graduated from medical school in Regensburg, Germany. He completed his residency in internal medicine at the University of Pennsylvania/Presbyterian Medical Center and a fellowship in hematology and oncology at Northwestern University. He is board certified in hematology, internal medicine, and medical oncology. Dr. Lorch is an assistant professor of medicine at Harvard Medical School and director of the Thyroid Center at Dana-Farber Cancer Institute.

Dana-Farber Cancer Institute
Head and Neck Cancer
450 Brookline Avenue
Boston, MA 02215
877-332-4294

Fiona McCulloch, ND

Fiona McCulloch earned her doctor of naturopathic medicine (ND) degree from the Canadian College of Naturopathic Medicine in 2001. In Toronto, she owns a multipractitioner clinic called White Lotus Naturopathic Clinic and Integrated Health. Dr. McCulloch's first book, *7 Steps to Reverse Your PCOS: Your Formula for Fertility, Femininity and Fat Loss*, will be published in 2016. A dedicated author, researcher, and teacher, she publishes articles in *Naturopathic Doctor News Review*, *Naturopathic Currents*, and peer-reviews for *Natural Standard*, an evidence-based natural medicine database. She lectures annually to students at the Canadian College of Naturopathic Medicine on advanced topics in infertility care, as well as to licensed healthcare practitioners through a variety of events and symposiums. Dr. McCulloch is also the subject matter expert for thyroid conditions for the Certification Board for Nutrition Specialists (CNS).

White Lotus Naturopathic Clinic and Integrated Health
18 Greenfield Avenue, Suite 201
Toronto, Ontario M2N 3C8
Canada
416-730-8218
http://www.whitelotusclinic.ca
Facebook: https://www.facebook.com/drfionand
Twitter: https://twitter.com/DrFionaND

Hugh Melnick, MD, FACOG

Hugh Melnick, a reproductive endocrinologist, has been treating infertile couples since 1976, and is considered a pioneer in the field of outpatient IVF treatment. Dr. Melnick is a graduate of the University of Pennsylvania and Temple University School of Medicine. He completed his residency training at Lenox Hill Hospital in New York City, where he later served as director of both the endocrinology clinic and the postgraduate medical course on human endocrinology. Dr. Melnick served as a research fellow in the Department of Experimental Pathology at the University of Birmingham in England and spent two years as an attending physician at the New York Fertility Research Foundation. He has published many scientific articles in medical journals and textbooks, and wrote *The Pregnancy Prescription*, for couples experiencing infertility problems. Dr. Melnick has lectured on topics related to infertility and reproductive endocrinology. In 1983, he founded Advanced Fertility Services, the first private, freestanding in vitro fertilization center in the NY tristate area and has been its director since.

Advanced Fertility Institute
1625 Third Avenue
New York, NY 10128
212-369-8700
http://www.infertilityny.com
http://www.mythyroidmd.com
Facebook: https://www.facebook.com/afsivf
Twitter: https://twitter.com/afsivf

Thomas Moraczewski, MD

Thomas Moraczewski is a physician board-certified in both obstetrics-gynecology and antiaging and regenerative medicine, with over thirty-five years' experience. He has delivered approximately six thousand babies in addition to having performed thousands of major and minor surgeries. He underwent further training in the hormonal area doing fellowships in antiaging medicine as well as advanced metabolic endocrinology. He currently practices hormonal medicine at the Center for Natural & Integrative Medicine in Orlando, Florida. He provides consultations regarding male and female hormonal issues, including PCOS, breast cancer prevention, menopause, alternative methods to treat uterine fibroids and cervical dysplasia, preconception counseling, and autoimmune disorders, particularly Hashimoto's.

The Center for Natural & Integrative Medicine
6651 Vineland Road, Suite 150
Orlando, FL 32819
407-355-9246
http://www.drkalidas.com/index.php
Facebook: https://www.facebook.com/CNIMedicine

Amy Myers, MD

Amy Myers is a renowned leader in functional medicine and *New York Times* best-selling author of *The Autoimmune Solution*. She received her medical degree from LSU Health Sciences Center and spent five years working in emergency medicine before training with the Institute of Functional Medicine. She is author of the *New York Times* best-seller *The Autoimmune Solution: Prevent and Reverse the Full Spectrum of Inflammatory Symptoms and Diseases*. Dr. Myers is the medical director of Austin UltraHealth in Austin, Texas.

Austin UltraHealth
5656 Bee Cave Road, Suite D 203
Austin, TX 78746
512-383-5343
http://www.amymyersmd.com
Facebook: https://www.facebook.com/AmyMyersMD
Twitter: https://twitter.com/AmyMyersMD

Roberto Negro, MD, FACE

Roberto Negro is senior assistant physician at the Endocrine Unit of Vito Fazzi Hospital in Lecce, Italy, since 2005. He has been professor of endocrinology at University of Parma, Italy (2007–2009); reviewing editor of the *Journal of Endocrinological Investigations* (2009–2012); a fellow at the American College of Endocrinology (2011); and reviewing editor of the *Journal of Clinical Endocrinology & Metabolism* (since 2012). He is author and coauthor of more than forty published papers, with thyroid and pregnancy as his main field of interest. He has been part of the panel of experts appointed by the American Thyroid Association for the compilation of its "Guidelines of the American Thyroid Association for the Diagnosis and Management of Thyroid Disease During Pregnancy and Postpartum" and by the European Thyroid Association for the compilation of its "Guidelines for Subclinical Hypothyroidism in Pregnancy and Childhood." Awards and honors include, in 2007 and again in 2008, the Endocrine Society and Pfizer, Inc. International Award for Excellence in Published Clinical Research in the *Journal of Clinical Endocrinology & Metabolism*.

Vito Fazzi Hospital
Piazzetta Muratore
73100 Lecce, Italy
+39 0832 661111

Kevin Passero, ND

Kevin Passero is a licensed naturopathic doctor who graduated from one of only eight accredited naturopathic medical schools in North America. His mission is to provide cutting-edge natural and holistic therapies. Dr. Passero completed four years of postgraduate naturopathic medical education at the National College of Naturopathic Medicine (NCNM) in Portland, Oregon, after receiving a bachelor's degree in environmental biology from the University of Colorado. He is a former president of the Maryland Naturopathic Doctors Association and is an active member of the American Association of Naturopathic Physicians. He is author of *The Drug-Free Acid Reflux Solution* and *Save Your Brain from Alzheimer's & Dementia*, and hosts a health-radio show in the Washington, DC, area.

Green Healing Wellness
130 Lubrano Drive, Suite L15
Annapolis, MD 21401
443-433-5540

1330 New Hampshire Ave NW
Washington, DC 20036
202-670-2173

http://www.greenhealingnow.com/
Facebook: https://www.facebook.com/GreenHealingWellness
Twitter: https://twitter.com/drpassero

Scot C. Remick, MD, FACP

Scot Remick serves as physician leader, oncology services at Maine Health System and chief of oncology service at Maine Medical Center in Portland, Maine, and on the faculty at Tufts University School of Medicine. He is a graduate of New York Medical College. He completed his internal medicine residency training on the Osler Medical Service of the Johns Hopkins Hospital and medical oncology fellowship training at the University of Wisconsin. He has held numerous faculty and leadership positions throughout his career at Albany Medical College, Case Western Reserve University, and West Virginia University. Dr. Remick is an expert in anticancer drug development and AIDS-related malignancies. He has developed novel therapeutic approaches to anaplastic thyroid cancer, having published extensively and led numerous clinical trials on this highly lethal disease.

Main Medical Center
22 Bramhall Street
Portland, ME 04102
207-662-0111
http://www.mmc.org/mmchomepage

John A. Robinson, NMD

John A. Robinson is a board-certified naturopathic medical doctor, hormone and thyroid disease expert, and advocate. He is the chief medical officer of the medical practice the Hormone Zone, also the title of his book, and creator of the unique thyroid system ThyroZone. Since 2006, he has been privileged to serve thousands of patients, optimizing their hormone balance, boldly "answering the unanswered questions" for their thyroid condition, and leading them toward true wellness. Both he and his wife, Yale-trained naturopathic physician Cristina Romero-Bosch, practice in Scottsdale, Arizona.

> The Hormone Zone
> 8060 East Gelding Drive, Suite 106
> Scottsdale, AZ 85260
> 480-338-8070
> http://www.drjohnarobinson.com
> Facebook: https://www.facebook.com/pages/Dr-John-Robinson-NMD/175079794970
> Twitter: https://twitter.com/DrRobinsonNMD

Aviva Romm, MD

Aviva Romm is a Yale-trained physician specializing in integrative medicine for women and children, a midwife, an herbalist, an award-winning author, and the creator/owner of WomanWise, online courses dedicated to vitality and optimal health for women and children. She is the recent past president of the American Herbalists Guild, a founder of the Yale Integrative Medicine program, and the author of seven books on natural medicine for women and children: *Botanical Medicine for Women's Health*; *The Natural Pregnancy Book*; *Naturally Healthy Babies and Children*; *Natural Health after Birth*; *Vaccinations: A Thoughtful Parent's Guide*; *ADHD Alternatives* (with her husband, Tracy Romm, EdD); and *The Pocket Guide to Midwifery Care*.

> Aviva Romm, MD
> PO Box 216
> Monterey, MA 01245
> http://avivaromm.com
> http://healthiestkids.com
> Facebook: https://www.facebook.com/AvivaRommMD
> Twitter: https://twitter.com/avivaromm

Julia Schopick

Julia Schopick is the author of the book *Honest Medicine* and creator of the award-winning blog *HonestMedicine.com*, and has been a published writer and a public relations consultant for more than thirty years. She has been published in the *American Medical News* (the AMA publication), *ADVANCE* (the professional publication for physical therapists), *SEARCH* (the newsletter of the National Brain Tumor Foundation), and *Alternative and Complementary Therapies*. In addition, her work and essays have been featured in the *British Medical Journal*, *Modern Maturity*, and

Chicago Sun-Times. She runs workshops and seminars on patient advocacy, LDN, and other therapies that are overlooked by mainstream medicine.

Julia Schopick
Oak Park, IL 60302
708-848-4788
http://www.honestmedicine.com
Julia@HonestMedicine.com
Facebook: https://www.facebook.com/pages/Julia-Schopick-Presents-Honest-Medicine
/145402085476798

Kim Schuette, CN

Kim Schuette has worked in the field of nutrition since 1999. In 2002 she established Biodynamic Wellness, where she practices with a team of four other nutritionists. Kim introduced the GAPS diet to clients in 2006 and in 2011 became a certified GAPS practitioner. Additionally she has been trained in hair mineral analysis, salivary hormone balancing, and blood chemistry assessment. Kim teaches workshops on children's health, mindful preconception, hormone balancing, transitioning to real food, and detoxification. She is an award-winning activist for her work in children's nutrition and preconception nutrition. She serves on the board of directors of the Weston A. Price Foundation.

Biodynamic Wellness
107 N. Acacia Avenue
Solana Beach, CA 92075
858-259-6000
http://www.biodynamicwellness.com
Facebook: https://www.facebook.com/biodynamicwellness
Instagram: https://instagram.com/biodynamicwellness/?ref=badge

Richard Shames, MD

Harvard-educated integrative physician Richard Shames is coauthor of several books on thyroid disease, including *Thyroid Mind Power, Thyroid Power,* and *Feeling Fat, Fuzzy or Frazzled?* and is in practice in San Rafael, California, in addition to providing telephone health coaching to people with thyroid and hormonal imbalance.

Shames Family Services
25 Mitchell Blvd., #8
San Rafael, CA 94903
415-472-2343
http://thyroidpower.com
Facebook: https://www.facebook.com/pages/Shames-Family-Services/2045440229
00098
Twitter: https://twitter.com/ThyroidPower

Jennifer Sipos, MD

Jennifer A. Sipos is an associate professor of medicine and director of the Benign Thyroid Disorders Program at the Ohio State University. Dr. Sipos has developed an interest in the use of ultrasonography for the diagnosis and management of thyroid cancer. She is codirector of the Introductory Ultrasound Course for the Endocrine Society and is also teaching at the Endocrine Society's Continuing Endocrine Update and American Thyroid Association meetings. She has taught ultrasound courses internationally, at meetings for the European Thyroid Association, the Asia and Oceania Thyroid Association, and the Indian Endocrine Society. Additionally, she is involved in clinical research with a particular interest in factors involved in the development of salivary damage after radioiodine therapy. She also participates in clinical trials for targeted molecular therapies in refractory thyroid cancer and the diagnostic use of molecular markers in thyroid nodules.

The Ohio State University
Wexner Medical Center
Division of Endocrinology, Diabetes and Metabolism
577 McCampbell Hall
1581 Dodd Drive
Columbus, OH 43210
614-685-3333

Izabella Wentz, PharmD, FASCP

Izabella Wentz is a pharmacist who has dedicated herself to addressing the root causes of autoimmune thyroid disease after being diagnosed with Hashimoto's thyroiditis in 2009. She is the author of the *New York Times* best-selling book *Hashimoto's Thyroiditis: Lifestyle Interventions for Finding and Treating the Root Cause* and is an ardent champion of incorporating lifestyle change into the treatment of autoimmune disease.

Thyroid Pharmacist
http://www.thyroidpharmacist.com
Facebook: https://www.facebook.com/ThyroidLifestyle

Toni Weschler, MPH

Toni Weschler has a master's degree in public health and is a nationally respected women's health educator and speaker. She is the author of *Taking Charge of Your Fertility*, the groundbreaking book that introduced the Fertility Awareness Method to the mainstream. For two decades, *Taking Charge of Your Fertility* has helped literally hundreds of thousands of women avoid pregnancy naturally, maximize their chances of getting pregnant, or simply gain better control of their gynecological and sexual health. Toni is also the author of *Cycle Savvy*, a book for teenage girls about their body. A frequent guest on television, radio shows, and the Internet, she lives in Seattle, Washington.

Taking Charge of Your Fertility
http://www.tcoyf.com

Jonathan V. Wright, MD

A Harvard University and University of Michigan Medical School graduate, Jonathan V. Wright also received an honorary naturopathic doctor (ND) degree from Baster University. He is a pioneer in research and application of natural treatments for health problems not requiring surgery. He has authored/coauthored fourteen books, selling over 1.5 million copies, with two texts achieving best-selling status, as well as numbers of medical articles on the efficacy of natural substances. A sought-after speaker, Dr. Wright has educated thousands of physicians in his natural techniques and protocols. In 1973 he founded Tahoma Clinic, where he practices medicine and serves as medical director. In the early 1980s he wrote the first prescription for bi-oidentical estrogen, based on his research. Dr. Wright was inducted into the Orthomolecular Medicine Hall of Fame in 2012.

Tahoma Clinic
6839 Fort Dent Way, #134
Tukwila, WA 98188
206-812-9988
http://tahomaclinic.com
Facebook: https://www.facebook.com/TahomaClinic
Twitter: https://twitter.com/tahomaclinic

Appendix C
Top Infertility Centers

Alabama
The Center for Reproductive Medicine
http://www.infertilityalabama.com
251-438-4200

Arkansas
Arkansas Fertility and Gynecological Associates
http://www.arkansasfertility.com
877-801-5353

Arizona
Arizona Reproductive Medicine Specialists ARMS
https://arizonafertility.com
602-351-5327

California
Fertility Miracles
http://www.fertilitymiracles.com
888-898-8123

Growing Generations
http://www.growinggenerations.com
323-965-7500

Southern California Reproductive Center
http://www.scrcivf.com
877-819-6515

Colorado
Colorado Center for Reproductive Medicine, Englewood
http://www.colocrm.com
303-586-3407

Conceptions Reproductive Associates of Colorado
http://www.conceptionsrepro.com
303-720-7887

Connecticut
Reproductive Medicine Associates of CT
http://www.rmact.com
800-865-5431

Delaware
Reproductive Associates of Delaware
https://ivf-de.org
302-602-8822

Florida
Florida Institute for Reproductive Medicine
http://www.fertilityjacksonville.com
800-556-5620

NewLIFE
https://fertilityleaders.com
850-857-3733

Georgia
Reproductive Biology Associates
http://rba-online.com
404-257-1900

Hawaii
Advanced Reproductive Medicine & Gynecology of Hawaii
http://www.armghawaii.com
808-262-0544

Illinois
Fertility Centers of Illinois
http://fcionline.com

Sher Institute Fertility Clinic
http://haveababy.com/fertility-clinics/central-illinois-fertility-clinic

Massachusetts
Baystate Reproductive Medicine
http://www.baystatehealth.org/
413-794-0000

Missouri
The Infertility Center of St. Louis
http://www.infertile.com
314-576-1400

New Mexico
Center for Reproductive Medicine
http://www.infertility-ivf.com
888-990-2727

Nevada
The Fertility Center of Las Vegas
http://fertilitycenterlv.com
702-254-1777

The Nevada Center for Reproductive Medicine
http://www.nevadafertility.com/nevada
775-828-1200

New York
Advanced Fertility Services
http://www.infertilityny.com
212-369-8700

Center for Reproductive Medicine of Weill Cornell Medical College
http://www.ivf.org
646-962-2764

5th Avenue Fertility
http://www.drsamidavidmd.com
212-831-0430

New Hope Fertility Center
http://www.newhopefertility.com
212-969-7422

NYU Langone Medical Center
http://nyulangone.org/locations/fertility-center
212-263-8990

RMA of New York
http://rmany.com
212-756-5777

North Carolina
UNC Fertility
http://uncfertility.com
919-908-0000

Ohio
Institute for Reproductive Health
http://www.cincinnatifertility.com/
513-924-5550

Oregon
Oregon Health & Science University Center for Women's Health
http://www.ohsu.edu/xd/health/services/women
503-418-4500

Texas
Texas Health Presbyterian Hospital Plano–ARTS Program
http://www.texasivf.com
866-IVF-TEXAS

Virginia
Dominion Fertility
https://www.dominionfertility.com
703-920-3890

OUTSIDE THE UNITED STATES
Canada
https://www.cfas.ca
Click "Public Affairs & News," "For the Public," and "IVF Clinics" for a directory of clinics in Canada.

United Kingdom
http://guide.hfea.gov.uk
Provides directory to locate fertility clinics in the United Kingdom

Australia
http://www.fertilitysociety.com.au
The Fertility Society of Australia provides listings of accredited ART units in Australia. Click "Patient Information."

Appendix D
Sample Fertility Chart

Thanks to Toni Weschler, author of the book *Taking Charge of Your Fertility*, for providing free access to this blank fertility chart. You can download a variety of other fertility charts from her website, http://www.tcoyf.com/downloadable-charts.

Month _____ Year _____ Age _____ Fertility Cycle _____

Last 12 Cycles: Shortest _____ Longest _____ This Luteal Phase Length _____ This Cycle Length _____

Cycle Day: 1–40

Row labels:
- Cycle Day
- Date
- Day of Week
- Time Temp Taken
- Temps & Luteal Phase
- Peak Day
- WAKING TEMPERATURES (99 / 98 / 97 scale)
- Pregnancy Test
- Artificial Insemination or IVF
- Circle Intercourse on Cycle Day
- Eggwhite
- Creamy
- PERIOD, Spotting, Dry, or Sticky
- Fertile Phase and PEAK DAY
- Vaginal Sensation
- Dry Sticky Moist Wet Lube
- Cervix (O / F M S)
- Ovulatory Pain

May be slippery, gushing and watery.
May be a thin or thick stretch to 1".
Clear, cloudy, streaked or red-tinged.
Wet or lubricative vaginal sensation.

CREAMY
Wet—and may be creamy, lotiony, milky, clumpy
gummy/wet or springy/wet. Breaks easily.
May form wet mounds or stretch to 3/4".
Usually opaque.
Wet, moist or cold vaginal sensation.

STICKY
Sticky—and may be thick, tacky, pasty, crumbly,
gummy/dry or springy/dry.
May form thick peaks or stretch to 1/4".
White, yellow, or cloudy.
Dry or sticky vaginal sensation.

	1	2	3	4	5	6	7	8	9	10	11	12	13	14	15	16	17	18	19	20	21	22	23	24	25	26	27	28	29	30	31	32	33	34	35	36	37	38	39	40
Ovulation Predictor Kit																																								
Fertility Monitor																																								
Diagnostic Tests and Procedures																																								
Medications or Injections																																								
Accupuncture or Other Treatments																																								
Herbs, Vitamins, and Supplements																																								
Exercise																																								
Notes							BSE																																	

Travel
PMS
Illness
Stress
Moodiness
Special Event
Annual Exam
Breast Self-Exam

tcoyf.com

Pregnancy with examples

References

Abalovich, Marcos, Nobuyuki Amino, Linda A. Barbour, Rhoda H. Cobin, Leslie J. De Groot, Daniel Glinoer, Susan J. Mandel, and Alex. Stagnaro-Green. 2007. "Management of Thyroid Dysfunction During Pregnancy and Postpartum: An Endocrine Society Clinical Practice Guideline." *Journal of Clinical Endocrinology & Metabolism* 92 (8) (Supplement): S1–S47. doi: 10.1210/jc.2007-0141.

Abalovich, Marcos, Laura Mitelberg, Carlos Allami, Silvia Gutierrez, Graciela Alcaraz, Patricia Otero, and Oscar Levalle. 2007. "Subclinical Hypothyroidism and Thyroid Autoimmunity in Women with Infertility." *Gynecological Endocrinology* 23 (5) (May): 279–83. doi: 10.1080/09513590701259542.

Akhter, S., Z. U. Nahar, S. Parvin, A. Alam, S. Sharmin, and M. I. Arslan. 2012. "Thyroid Status in Patients with Low Serum Ferritin Level." *Bangladesh Journal of Medical Biochemistry* 5 (1): 5–11. doi.org/10.3329/bjmb.v5i1.13424.

American College of Obstetricians and Gynecologists. 2002. "Guideline: Thyroid Disease in Pregnancy." *Practice Bulletin No. 37* 100 (2) (August): 387–96. http://journals.lww.com/greenjournal/Fulltext/2002/08000/ACOG_Practice_Bulletin_No_37_Thyroid_Disease_in.47.aspx.

American Thyroid Association. 2013. "The Case for Universal Thyroid Screening in Pregnancy." (October). http://www.thyroid.org/the-case-for-universal-thyroid-screening-in-pregnancy.

Auf'mkolk, Michael, Jonathan C. Ingbar, Ken Kubota, Syed M. Amir, and Sidney H. Ingbar. 1985. "Extracts and Auto-Oxidized Constituents of Certain Plants Inhibit the Receptor-Binding and the Biological Activity of Graves' Immunoglobulins." *Endocrinology* 116 (5) (May): 1687–93. http://www.ncbi.nlm.nih.gov/pubmed/2985357.

Balasch, Juan, and Eduard Gratacos. 2012. "Delayed Childbearing: Effects on Fertility and the Outcome of Pregnancy." *Current Opinion in Obstetrics and Gynecology* 24 (3) (June): 187–93. doi: 10.1097/GCO.0b013e3283517908.

Baral, Matthew. 2010. "Probiotics and Pregnant Women: Study Regards Safety of Maternal Probiotic Supplementation During the First Trimester." *Natural Medicine Journal* 2 (4) (April). http://naturalmedicinejournal.com/journal/2010-04/probiotics-and-pregnant-women.

Battaglia, Cesare, Michela Salvatori, Nicoletta Maxia, Felice Petraglia, Fabio Facchinetti, and Annibale Volpe. 1999. "Adjuvant L-arginine Treatment for In-Vitro Fertilization in Poor Responder Patients." *Human Reproduction* 14 (7) (July): 1690–97. http://www.ncbi.nlm.nih.gov/pubmed/10402369.

Ben-Meir, Assaf, Eliezer Burstein, Aluet Borrego-Alvarez, Jasmine Chong, Ellen Wong, Tetyana Yavorska, Taline Naranian, Maggie Chi, Ying Wang, Yaakov Bentov, Jennifer Alexis, James Meriano, Hoon-Ki Sung, David L Gasser, Kelle H. Moley, Siegfried Hekimi, Robert F. Casper, and Andrea Jurisicova. 2015. "Coenzyme Q10 Restores Oocyte Mitochondrial Function and Fertility During Reproductive Aging." *Aging Cell* 14 (5) (October): 887–95. doi: 10.1111/acel.12368.

Benvenga, Salvatore, Luigi Bartolone, Maria Angela Pappalardo, Antonia Russo, Daniela Lapa, Grazia Giorgianni, Giovanna Saraceno, and Francesco Trimarchi. 2008. "Altered Intestinal Absorption of L-Thyroxine Caused by Coffee." *Thyroid* 18 (3) (March): 293–301. doi: 10.1089/thy.2007.0222.

Blackwell, J. 2004. "Evaluation and Treatment of Hyperthyroidism and Hypothyroidism." *American Academy of Nurse Practitioners* 16 (10) (October): 422–25. http://www.ncbi.nlm.nih.gov/pubmed/15543918.

Boehm, T. M., K. D. Burman, S. Barnes, and L. Wartofsky. 1980. "Lithium and Iodine Combination Therapy for Thyrotoxicosis." *Acta Endocrinologica* 94 (2) (June): 174–83. http://www.ncbi.nlm.nih.gov/pubmed/7415757.

Bolk, Nienke, Theo J. Visser, Judy Nijman, Ineke J. Jongste, Jan G. P. Tijssen, and Arie Berghout. 2010. "Effects of Evening vs Morning Levothyroxine Intake: A Randomized Double-blind Crossover Trial." *Archives of Internal Medicine* 170 (22) (December): 1996–2003. doi: 10.1001/archinternmed.2010.436.

Borenstein, David. Telephone interview by Mary Shomon, August 21, 2015.

Borenstein, Laurie. E-mail to Mary Shomon, August 25, 2015.

Boyle, Phil. E-mail to Julia Schopick, August 28, 2015.

Braverman, Lewis E., and Robert D. Utiger. 2005. *Werner and Ingbar's The Thyroid: A Fundamental and Clinical Text*, 9th ed. Philadelphia: Lippincott Williams & Wilkins.

Brownstein, David. E-mail to Dana Trentini, August 2, 2015.

Burch, Henry B. Presentation at the annual meeting of the American Association of Clinical Endocrinologists and Clinical Congress, 2000.

Burrow, Gerard N., Delbert A. Fisher, and P. Reed Larsen. 1994. "Maternal and Fetal Thyroid Function." *New England Journal of Medicine* 331 (October): 1072–78. doi: 10.1056/NEJM 199410203311608.

Carnahan, Jill. E-mail to Dana Trentini, August 15, 2015.

Carp, H. J., C. Selmi, and Y. Shoenfeld. 2012. "The Autoimmune Bases of Infertility and Pregnancy Loss." *Journal of Autoimmunity* 38 (2–3) (May): J266–J274. doi: 10.1016/j.jaut.2011.11.016.

Chang, Donny L. F., and Elizabeth N. Pearce. 2013. "Screening for Maternal Thyroid Dysfunction in Pregnancy: A Review of the Clinical Evidence and Current Guidelines." *Journal of Thyroid Research*. doi.org/10.1155/2013/851326.

Christensen, S. Borup, U. B. Ericsson, L. Janzon, S. Tibblin, and A. Melander. 1984. "Influence of Cigarette Smoking on Goiter Formation, Thyroglobulin and Thyroid

Hormone Levels in Women." *Clinical Endocrinology and Metabolism* 58 (4) (April): 615–18. http://www.ncbi.nlm.nih.gov/pubmed/6699129.

Clamp, Adrienne. E-mail to Dana Trentini, August 30, 2015.

Clark, J. O., and G. E. Mullin. 2008. "A Review of Complementary and Alternative Approaches to Immunomodulation." *Nutrition in Clinical Practice* 23 (1) (February): 49–62. http://www.ncbi.nlm.nih.gov/pubmed/18203964.

Cohen, Suzy. E-mail to Dana Trentini, August 24, 2015.

Connole, Suzanne. E-mail to Dana Trentini, August 14, 2015.

Contempré, Bernard, Eric Jauniaux, Rosa Calvo, Davor Jurkovic, Stuart Campbell, and Gabriella Morreale de Escobar. 1993. "Detection of Thyroid Hormones in Human Embryonic Cavities During the First Trimester of Pregnancy." *Journal of Clinical Endocrinology and Metabolism* 77 (6) (December): 1719–22. http://www. ncbi.nlm.nih.gov/pubmed/8263162.

De Groot, Leslie, Marcos Abalovich, Erik K. Alexander, Nobuyuki Amino, Linda Barbour, Rhoda H. Cobin, Creswell J. Eastman, John H. Lazarus, Dominique Luton, Susan J. Mandel, Jorge Mestman, Joanne Rovet, and Scott Sullivan. 2012. "Management of Thyroid Dysfunction During Pregnancy and Postpartum: An Endocrine Society Clinical Practice Guideline." *Journal of Clinical Endocrinology & Metabolism* 97 (8) (August): 2543–65. doi: 10.1210/jc.2011-2803.

De Vivo, Antonio, Alfredo Mancuso, Annamaria Giacobbe, and Francesco Vermiglio. 2010. "Thyroid Function in Women Found to Have Early Pregnancy Loss." *Thyroid* 20 (6) (June): 633–37. doi: 10.1089/thy.2009.0323.

Ehlers, Margaret, Annette Thiel, Christian Bernecker, and Matthias Schott. 2012. "Evidence of a Combined Cytotoxic Thyroglobulin and Thyroperoxidase Epitope-Specific Cellular Immunity in Hashimoto's Thyroiditis." *Journal of Clinical Endocrinology and Metabolism* 97 (4) (April): 1347–54. doi: 10.1210/jc.2011-2178.

Endocrine Society. 2015. "Endocrine Facts and Figures: Thyroid." http://endocrine facts.org/health-conditions/thyroid.

Erbil, Y., U. Barbaros, H. Işsever, I. Borucu, A. Salmaslioğlu, Ö. Mete, A. Bozbora, and S. Özarmağan. 2007. "Predictive Factors for Recurrent Laryngeal Nerve Palsy and Hypoparathyroidism after Thyroid Surgery." *Clinical Otolaryngology* 32 (1) (February): 32–37. http://www.ncbi.nlm.nih.gov/pubmed/17298308.

Erbil, Y., U. Barbaros, A. Salmaslioğlu, B. Tulumoğlu Yanik, A. Bozbora, and S. Özarmağan. 2006. "The Advantage of Near-Total Thyroidectomy to Avoid Postoperative Hypoparathyroidism in Benign Multinodular Goiter." *Langenbeck's Archives of Surgery* 391 (6) (November): 567–73. http://www.ncbi.nlm.nih.gov/pubmed/17021791.

Fouany, M. R., and F. I. Harara. 2013. "Is There a Role for DHEA Supplementation in Women with Diminished Ovarian Reserve?" *Assisted Reproduction and Genetics* 30 (9) (September): 1239–44. doi: 10.1007/s10815-013-0018-x.

Garber, Jeffrey R., Rhoda H. Cobin, Hossein Gharib, James V. Hennessey, Irwin Klein, Jeffrey I. Mechanick, Rachel Pessah-Pollack, Peter A. Singer, and Kenneth A. Woeber. 2012. "Clinical Practice Guidelines for Hypothyroidism in Adults: Co-sponsored by the American Association of Clinical Endocrinologists and the American Thyroid Association." *Endocrine Practice* 18 (6) (November): 988–1028. https://www.aace.com/files/final-file-hypo-guidelines.pdf.

Gaujoux, S., L. Leenhardt, C. Trésallet, A. Rouxel, C. Hoang, C. Jublanc, J. P. Chigot, and F. Menegaux. 2006. "Extensive Thyroidectomy in Graves' Disease." *American College of Surgeons* 202 (6) (June): 868–73. http://www.ncbi.nlm.nih.gov/pubmed/16735199.

Gharib, Hossein. 2014. "Emergent Management of Thyroid Disorders." *Endocrine Society* (June). doi: http://dx.doi.org/10.1210/EME.9781936704811.part4.

Gharib H., and E. Papini. (2007) "Thyroid Nodules: Clinical Importance, Assessment, and Treatment." *Endocrinology and Metabolism Clinics of North America* (36 (3) (September): 707–35. http://www.ncbi.nlm.nih.gov/pubmed/17673125.

Gohel, Mukesh G., Aashka M. Shah, Akash M. Shah, and Jemil S. Makadia. 2014. "A Study of Serum Calcium, Magnesium and Phosphorus Level in Hypothyroidism Patients." *International Journal of Medical and Health Sciences* 3 (4) (October): 308–12. http://www.ijmhs.net/journals-aid-229.html.

Greenberg, James, and Stacey Bell. 2011. "Multivitamin Supplementation During Pregnancy: Emphasis on Folic Acid and L-Methylfolate." *Reviews in Obstetrics & Gynecology* 4 (3–4): 126–27. http://www.ncbi.nlm.nih.gov/pmc/articles/PMC3250974.

Greenberg, James A., Stacey J. Bell, and Wendy Van Ausdal. 2008. "Omega-3 Fatty Acid Supplementation During Pregnancy." *Reviews in Obstetrics and Gynecology* 1 (4) (Fall): 162–69. http://www.ncbi.nlm.nih.gov/pmc/articles/PMC2621042.

Hackmon, Rinat, Monica Blichowski, and Gideon Koren. 2012. "The Safety of Methimazole and Propylthiouracil in Pregnancy: A Systematic Review." *Obstetrics and Gynaecology Canada* 34 (11) (November): 1077–86. http://www.ncbi.nlm.nih.gov/pubmed/23231846.

Haddow, James E., Glenn E. Palomaki, Walter C. Allan, Josephine R. Williams, George J. Knight, June Gagnon, Cheryl E. O'Heir, Marvin L. Mitchell, Rosalie J. Hermos, Susan E. Waisbren, James D. Faix, and Robert Z. Klein. 1999. "Maternal Thyroid Deficiency During Pregnancy and Subsequent Neuropsychological Development of the Child." *New England Journal of Medicine* 341 (August): 549–55. doi: 10.1056/NEJM199908193410801.

Harness, Jay K., Lit Fung, Norman W. Thompson, Richard E. Burney, and Michael K. McLeod. 1986. "Total Thyroidectomy: Complications and Technique." *World Journal of Surgery* (5) (October): 781–86. http://www.ncbi.nlm.nih.gov/pubmed/3776215.

Hassan, M. A., and S. R. Killick. 2004. "Negative Lifestyle Is Associated with a Significant Reduction in Fecundity." *Fertility and Sterility* 81 (2) (February): 384–92. http://www.ncbi.nlm.nih.gov/pubmed/14967378.

Haymart, Megan. 2010. "The Role of Clinical Guidelines in Patient Care: Thyroid Hormone Replacement in Women of Reproductive Age." *Thyroid* 20 (3) (March): 301–7. doi: 10.1089/thy.2009.0321.

Haymart, Megan R., Max A. Cayo, and Herbert Chen. 2010. "Thyroid Hormone Replacement in Women of Reproductive Age: Is Surgeon Knowledge Related to Operative Volume?" *Thyroid* 20 (6) (June): 627–31. doi: 10.1089/thy.2009.0320.

Holtorf, Kent. "The Optimal Treatment for Hypothyroidism: Kent Holtorf, MD." Interview by Mary J. Shomon, updated July 30, 2015. http://thyroid.about.com

/od/hypothyroidismhashimotos/a/The-Optimal-Treatment-For-Hypothyroidism
.htm.

Hussain, Munawar, Elsamawal El Hakim, and David J. Cahill. 2012. "Progesterone Supplementation in Women with Otherwise Unexplained Recurrent Miscarriages." *Human Reproductive Sciences* 5 (3) (September): 248–51. doi: 10.4103/0974-1208 .106335.

Hyman, Mark. Telephone interview by Dana Trentini, August 8, 2015.

Inoue, Miho, Naoko Arata, Gideon Koren, and Shinya Ito. 2009. "Hyperthyroidism During Pregnancy." *Canadian Family Physician* 55 (7) (July): 701–3. http://www .ncbi.nlm.nih.gov/pmc/articles/PMC2718594.

Jabbar, Abdul, Aasma Yawar, Sabiha Waseem, and Jaweed Akhter. 2008. "Vitamin B12 Deficiency Common in Primary Hypothyroidism." *Journal of Pakistan Medical Association* 58 (5) (May): 258–61. http://www.ncbi.nlm.nih.gov/pubmed /18655403.

Jadali, Zohreh. 2013. "Autoimmune Thyroid Disorders in Hepatitis C Virus Infection: Effect of Interferon Therapy." *Indian Journal of Endocrinology and Metabolism* 17 (1) (January): 69–75. doi: 10.4103/2230-8210.107856.

Janegova, Andrea, Pavol Janega, Boris Rychly, Kristina Kuracinova, and Pavel Babal. 2015. "The Role of Epstein-Barr Virus Infection in the Development of Autoimmune Thyroid Diseases." *Endokrynologia Polska* 66 (2): 132–36. doi: 10.5603 /EP.2015.0020.

Janssen, Onno E., Nadine Mehlmauer, Susanne Hahn, Alexandra H. Öffner, and Roland Gärtner. 2004. "High Prevalence of Autoimmune Thyroiditis in Patients in Polycystic Ovary Syndrome." *European Journal of Endocrinology* 150 (3) (March): 363–69. http://www.ncbi.nlm.nih.gov/pubmed/15012623.

Karras, Spiros, and Gerasimos E. Krassas. 2012. "Breastfeeding and Antithyroid Drugs: A View from Within." *European Thyroid Journal* 1 (1) (April): 30–33. doi: 10.1159/000336595.

Kim, Dong Wook, Myung Ho Rho, Hak Jin Kim, Jae Su Kwon, Young Sun Sung, and Sang Wook Lee. 2005. "Percutaneous Ethanol Injection for Benign Cystic Thyroid Nodules: Is Aspiration of Ethanol-Mixed Fluid Advantageous?" *American Journal of Neuroradiology* 26: 2122–27. http://www.ajnr.org/content/26/8/2122.full.

Krassas, G. E., K. Poppe, and D. Glinoer. 2010. "Thyroid Function and Human Reproductive Health." *Endocrine Reviews* 31 (5) (October): 702–55. doi: 10.1210 /er.2009-0041.

Kung, Annie W. C., M. T. Chau, Terence T. Lao, and L. C. K. Low. 2002. "The Effect of Pregnancy on Thyroid Nodule Formation." *Clinical Endocrinology & Metabolism* no. 87 (3) (March): 1010–14. http://www.ncbi.nlm.nih.gov/pubmed/11889153.

Ku, Chun-Fan, Chung-Yau Lo, Wai-Fan Chan, Annie W. C. Kung, and Karen S. L. Lam. 2005. "Total Thyroidectomy Replaces Subtotal Thyroidectomy as the Preferred Surgical Treatment for Graves' Disease." *Royal Australasian College of Surgeons* 75 (7) (July): 528–31. http://www.ncbi.nlm.nih.gov/pubmed/15972039.

Lacka, K., and A. Szeliga. 2015. "Significance of Selenium in Thyroid Physiology and Pathology." *Pol Merkur Lekarski* 38 (228) (June): 348–53. http://www.ncbi.nlm .nih.gov/pubmed/26098657.

Lal, Geeta, et al. 2005. "Should Total Thyroidectomy Become the Preferred Procedure for Surgical Management of Graves' Disease?" *Thyroid* 15 (6) (June): 569–74. http://www.ncbi.nlm.nih.gov/pubmed/16029123.

Laurberg, P., and S. L. Andersen. 2014. "Therapy of Endocrine Disease: Antithyroid Drug Use in Early Pregnancy and Birth Defects: Time Windows of Relative Safety and High Risk?" *European Journal of Endocrinology* 171 (1) (July): R13–R20. doi: 10.1530/EJE-14-0135.

Lauritano, Ernesto Cristiano, Anna Lisa Bilotta, Maurizio Gabrielli, Emidio Scarpellini, Andrea Lupascu, Antonio Laginestra, Marialuisa Novi, Sandra Sottili, Michele Serricchio, Giovanni Cammarota, Giovanni Gasbarrini, Alfredo Pontecorvi, and Antonio Gasbarrini. 2007. "Association Between Hypothyroidism and Small Intestinal Bacterial Overgrowth." *Clinical Endocrinology and Metabolism* 92 (11) (November): 4180–84. http://www.ncbi.nlm.nih.gov/pubmed/17698907.

Lazarus, J. H. 2005. "Thyroid Disorders Associated with Pregnancy: Etiology, Diagnosis, and Management." *Treatments in Endocrinology* 4 (1): 31–41. http://www.ncbi.nlm.nih.gov/pubmed/15649099.

Leung, Angela M., Elizabeth N. Pearce, and Lewis E. Braverman. 2011. "Iodine Nutrition in Pregnancy and Lactation." *Endocrinology and Metabolism Clinics of North America* 40 (4) (December): 765–77. doi: 10.1016/j.ecl.2011.08.001.

Leung, Angela M., Elizabeth N. Pearce, and Lewis E. Braverman. 2009. "Iodine Content of Prenatal Multivitamins in the United States." *New England Journal of Medicine* 360 (February): 939–40. doi: 10.1056/NEJMc0807851.

Llorente, Pablo Moreno, José M. Gómez, Núria Gómez, José M. Francos, Emilio Ramos, and Antonio Rafecas. 2006. "Subtotal Thyroidectomy: A Reliable Method to Achieve Euthyroidism in Graves' Disease. Prognostic Factors." *World Journal of Surgery* 30 (11) (November): 1950–56. http://www.ncbi.nlm.nih.gov/pubmed/17006611.

Lorch, Jochen. Telephone interview by Dana Trentini, August 18, 2015.

Mackawy, Amal Mohammed Husein, Bushra Mohammed Al-ayed, and Bashayer Mater Al-rashidi. 2013. "Vitamin D Deficiency and Its Association with Thyroid Disease." *International Journal of Health Sciences* 7 (3) (November): 267–75. http://www.ncbi.nlm.nih.gov/pmc/articles/PMC3921055.

MacKay, Douglas, Andrea Wong, and Haiuyen Nguyen. 2015. "Iodine Supplementation During Pregnancy and Lactation. A Collaborative Public Health Initiative in the United States." *Natural Medicine Journal* 7 (7) (July). http://naturalmedicinejournal.com/journal/2015-07/iodine-supplementation-during-pregnancy-and-lactation.

Matalon, S. T., M. Blank, A. Ornoy, and Y. Shoenfeld. 2001. "The Association Between Anti-Thyroid Antibodies and Pregnancy Loss." *American Journal of Reproductive Immunology* 45 (2) (February): 72–77. http://www.ncbi.nlm.nih.gov/pubmed/11216877.

Mazzaferri, Ernest. 2008. "Thyroid Hormone Therapy," *Clinical Thyroidology for Patients: Summaries for Patients from Clinical Thyroidology* 1 (1) (August).

McCulloch, Fiona. E-mail to Dana Trentini, August 17, 20, and 22, 2015.

McDermott, M. T. 2004. "Thyroid Disease and Reproductive Health." *Thyroid* 14 (1): S1–S3. http://www.ncbi.nlm.nih.gov/pubmed/15142371.

Medici, Marco, Tim I. M. Korevaar, Sarah Schalekamp-Timmermans, Romy Gaillard, Yolanda B. de Rijke, and W. Edward Visser. 2014. "Maternal Early-Pregnancy Thyroid Function is Associated with Subsequent Hypertensive Disorders of Pregnancy: The Generation R Study." *Clinical Endocrinology and Metabolism* 99 (12) (December): E2591–E2598. doi: 10.1210/jc.2014-1505.

Melnick, Hugh. E-mail to Dana Trentini, August 25, 28, 29, and 31, 2015.

Modesto, Thiago, Henning Tiemeler, Robin P. Peeters, Vincent Jaddoe, Albert Hofman, and Frank C. Verhulst. 2015. "Maternal Mild Thyroid Hormone Insufficiency in Early Pregnancy and Attention-Deficit/Hyperactivity Disorder Symptoms in Children." *Journal of American Medical Association Pediatrics* 169 (9) (September): 838–45. doi: 10.1001/jamapediatrics.2015.0498.

Momotani, N., T. Hisaoka, J. Noh, N. Ishikawa, and K. Ito. 1992. "Effects of Iodine on Thyroid Status of Fetus versus Mother in Treatment of Graves' Disease Complicated by Pregnancy." *Clinical Endocrinology and Metabolism* 75 (3) (September): 738–44. http://www.ncbi.nlm.nih.gov/pubmed/1517362.

Monahan, Mark, Kristien Boelaert, Kate Jolly, Shiao Chan, Pelham Barton, and Tracy E. Roberts. 2015. "Costs and Benefits of Iodine Supplementation for Pregnant Women in a Mildly to Moderately Iodine-Deficient Population: A Modelling Analysis." *Lancet Diabetes & Endocrinology* 3 (9) (August): 715–22. doi: http://dx.doi.org/10.1016/S2213-8587(15)00212-0.

Monk, Catherine, Julie Spicer, and Frances A. Champagne. 2012. "Linking Prenatal Maternal Adversity to Developmental Outcomes in Infants: The Role of Epigenetic Pathways." *Development and Psychopathology* 24 (4) (November): 1361–76. doi: 10.1017/S0954579412000764.

Monteleone, P., et al. 2011. "Female Infertility Related to Thyroid Autoimmunity: The Ovarian Follicle Hypothesis." *American Journal of Reproductive Immunology* no. 66 (2) (August): 108–14. doi: 10.1111/j.1600-0897.2010.00961.x.

Moraczewski, Thomas. E-mail to Dana Trentini, August 11, 12, 13, and 16, 2015.

Mowat, Alex, Cora Newton, Clare Boothroyd, Kristy Demmers, and Steven Fleming. 2014. "The Effects of Vaginal Lubricants on Sperm Function: An In Vitro Analysis." *Assist Reproduction and Genetics* 31 (3) (March): 333–39. doi: 10.1007/s10815–013–0168-x.

Muter, Joanne, Emma S. Lucas, Yi-Wah Chan, Paul J. Brighton, Jonathan D. Moore, Lauren Lacey, Siobhan Quenby, Eric W. F. Lam, and Jan J. Brosens. 2015. "The Clock Protein Period 2 Synchronizes Mitotic Expansion and Decidual Transformation of Human Endometrial Stromal Cells." *Federation of American Societies for Experimental Biology* 29 (4) (April): 1603–14. doi: 10.1096/fj.14-267195.

Myers, Amy. Telephone interview by Dana Trentini, August 16, 2015.

Na, Dong Gyu, Jeong Hyun Lee, So Lyung Jung, Ji-hoon Kim, Jin Yong Sung, Jung Hee Shin, Eun-Kyung Kim, Joon Hyung Lee, Dong Wook Kim, Jeong Seon Park, Kyu Sun Kim, Seon Mi Baek, Younghen Lee, Semin Chong, Jung Suk Sim, Jung Yin Huh, Jae-Ik Bae, Kyung Tae Kim, Song Yee Han, Min Young Bae, Yoon Suk

Kim, and Jung Hwan Baek. 2012. "Radiofrequency Ablation of Benign Thyroid Nodules and Recurrent Thyroid Cancers: Consensus Statement and Recommendations." *Korean Journal of Radiology* 13 (2) (March): 117–25. doi.org/10.3348 /kjr.2012.13.2.117.

Nagaria, Tripti, P. K. Patra, and Jai Prakash Sahu. 2011. "Evaluation of Serum Anti-sperm Antibodies in Infertility." *Obstetrics and Gynecology of India* 61 (3) (June): 307–16. doi: 10.1007/s13224-011-0034-7.

National Institute of Diabetes and Digestive and Kidney Diseases, National Institutes of Health. 2014. Fact Sheet on Lactose Intolerance." http://digestive.niddk.nih .gov/ddiseases/pubs/lactoseintolerance.

Negro, Roberto, G. Formoso, L. Coppola, G. Presicce, T. Mangieri, A. Pezzarossa, and D. Dazzi. 2007. "Euthyroid Women with Autoimmune Disease Undergoing Assisted Reproduction Technologies: The Role of Autoimmunity and Thyroid Function." *Endocrinological Investigation* 30 (1) (January): 3–8. http://www.ncbi.nlm .nih.gov/pubmed/17318015.

Negro, Roberto, Alan Schwartz, Riccardo Gismondi, Andrea Tinelli, Tiziana Mangieri, and Alex Stagnaro-Green. 2010. "Increased Pregnancy Loss Rate in Thyroid Antibody Negative Women with TSH Levels Between 2.5 and 5.0 in the First Trimester of Pregnancy." *Clinical Endocrinology and Metabolism* 95 (9) (September): E44–E48. doi: 10.1210/jc.2010–0340.

Negro, Roberto, Gabriele Greco, Tiziana Mangieri, Antonio Pezzarossa, Davide Dazzi, and Haslinda Hassan. 2007. "The Influence of Selenium Supplementation on Postpartum Thyroid Status in Pregnant Women with Thyroid Peroxidase Antibodies." *Clinical Endocrinology and Metabolism* 92 (4) (April): 1263–68. http://www.ncbi .nlm.nih.gov/pubmed/17284630.

Negro, Roberto. E-mail to Dana Trentini, August 6, 2015.

Ozkan, Sebiha, Sangita Jindal, Keri Greenseid, Jun Shu, Gohar Zeitlian, Cheryl Hickmon, and Lubna Pal. 2010. "Replete Vitamin D Stores Predict Reproductive Success Following In Vitro Fertilization." *Fertility Sterility* 94 (4) (September): 1314–19. doi: 10.1016/j.fertnstert.2009.05.019.

Pandey, Shilpi, Suruchi Pandey, Abha Maheshwari, and Siladitya Bhattacharya. 2010. "The Impact of Female Obesity on the Outcome of Fertility Treatment." *Human Reproductive Sciences* 3 (2) (May): 62–67. doi: 10.4103/0974-1208.69332.

Passero, Kevin. Telephone interview by Mary Shomon, August 26, 2015.

Paulmyer-Lacroix, Odile, Laura Despierres, Blandine Courbiere, and Nathalie Bardin. 2014. "Antiphospholipid Antibodies in Women Undergoing In Vitro Fertilization Treatment: Clinical Value of IgA Anti-β2glycoprotein I Antibodies Determination." *BioMed Research International.* doi: 10.1155/2014/314704.

Paulus, Wolfgang E., Mingmin Zhang, Erwin Strehler, Imam El-Danasouri, and Karl Sterzik. 2002. "Influence of Acupuncture on the Pregnancy Rate in Patients Who Undergo Assisted Reproduction Therapy." *Fertility and Sterility* 77 (4) (April): 721–24. http://www.ncbi.nlm.nih.gov/pubmed/11937123.

Pearce, Elizabeth N., G. C. Roman, A. Ghassabian, J. J. Bongers-Schokking, V. W. Jaddoe, A. Hofman, Y. B. de Rijke, F. C. Verhulst, and H. Tiemeier. 2013. "Severe Maternal Hypothyroxinemia Is Associated with Probable Autism in Offspring."

Clinical Thyroidology 25 (August): 252–53. http://www.thyroid.org/wp-content/uploads/publications/clinthy/volume25/issue11/clinthy_v2511_252_253.pdf.

Pires, Eusebio S., Firuza R. Parikh, Purvi V. Mande, Shonali A. Uttamchandani, Sujata Savkar, and Vrinda V. Khole. 2001. "Can Anti-Ovarian Antibody Testing Be Useful in an IVF-ET Clinic?" *Assisted Reproduction and Genetics* 28 (1) (January): 55–64. doi: 10.1007/s10815-010-9488-2.

Poppe, Kris, Daniel Glinoer, Andre Van Steirteghem, Herman Tournaye, Paul Devroey, Johan Schiettecatte, and Brigitte Velkeniers. 2002. "Thyroid Dysfunction and Autoimmunity in Infertile Women." *Thyroid* 12 (11) (November): 997–1001. http://www.ncbi.nlm.nih.gov/pubmed/12490077.

Poppe, Kris, Brigitte Velkeniers, and Daniel Glinoer. 2007. "Thyroid Disease and Female Reproduction." *Clinical Endocrinology* 66 (3) (January): 309–21. doi: 10.1111/j.1365-2265.2007.02752.x.

Poppe, Kris, Daniel Glinoer, Herman Tournaye, Paul Devroey, Andre Van Steirteghem, Leonard Kaufman, and Brigitte Velkeniers. 2003. "Assisted Reproduction and Thyroid Autoimmunity: An Unfortunate Combination?" *Clinical Endocrinology and Metabolism* 88 (9) (September): 4149–52. http://www.ncbi.nlm.nih.gov/pubmed/12970279.

Prema, Sejekan. 2010. "Thyroid Screening in Pregnancy—A Study of 82 Women." *Journal of Obstetrics and Gynecology of India* 60 (3) (May): 232–37. doi: 10.1007/s13224-010-0031-2.

Prummel, M. F., and W. M. Wiersinga. 1993. "Smoking and Risk of Graves' Disease." *Journal of American Medical Association* 269 (4) (January): 479–82. http://www.ncbi.nlm.nih.gov/pubmed/8419666.

Quintino Moro, Alessandra, Denise E. Zantut-Wittmann, Marcos Tambascia, Helymar da Costa Machado, and Arlete Fernandes. 2014. "High Prevalence of Infertility Among Women with Graves' Disease and Hashimoto's Thyroiditis." *International Journal of Endocrinology*. doi.org/10.1155/2014/982705.

Razack, Mohamed S., John M. Lore Jr., Howard A. Lippes, Daniel P. Schaefer, and Hadi Rassael. 1997. "Total Thyroidectomy for Graves' Disease." *Head and Neck* 19 (5) (August): 378–83. http://www.ncbi.nlm.nih.gov/pubmed/9243264.

Remick, Scot C. Telephone interview by Dana Trentini, August 18, 2015.

Robinson, John A. E-mail to Dana Trentini, August 18, 2015.

Román, Gustavo, Akhgar Ghassabian, Jacoba J. Bongers-Schokking, Vincent W. V. Jaddoe, Albert Hofman, Yolanda B. de Rijke, Frank C. Verhulst, and Henning Tiemeier. 2013. "Association of Gestational Maternal Hypothyroxinemia and Increased Autism Risk." *Annals of Neurology* 74 (5) (November): 733–42. doi: 10.1002/ana.23976.

Romm, Aviva. Telephone interview by Dana Trentini, August 26, 2015.

Rosato, L., N. Avenia, M. De Palma, G. Gulino, P. G. Nasi, and L. Pezzulio. 2002. "Complications of Total Thyroidectomy: Incidence, Prevention and Treatment." *Chirurgia italiana* 54 (5) (September): 635–42. http://www.ncbi.nlm.nih.gov/pubmed/12469460.

Sategna-Guidetti, C., Umberto Volta, Carolina Ciacci, and C. Brossa. 2001. "Prevalence of Thyroid Disorders in Untreated Adult Celiac Disease Patients and Effect of Gluten Withdrawal: An Italian Multicenter Study." *American Journal of Gastroen-*

terology 96 (3) (March): 751–57. http://www.ncbi.nlm.nih.gov/pubmed /11280546.

Schisterman, Enrique F., Robert M. Silver, Laurie L. Lesher, David Faraggi, Jean Wactawski-Wende, Janet M. Townsend, Anne M. Lynch, Neil J. Perkins, Sunni L. Mumford, and Noya Galai. 2014. "Preconception Low-Dose Aspirin and Pregnancy Outcomes: Results from the EAGeR Randomised Trial." *The Lancet* 384 (9937) (July): 29–36. doi: http://dx.doi.org/10.1016/S0140-6736(14)60157-4.

Schopick, Julia. E-mail to Mary Shomon, August 27, 2015.

Schuette, Kim. E-mail to Dana Trentini, August 23, 2015.

Schwartz, D., and M. J. Mayaux. 1982. "Female Fecundity as a Function of Age. Results of Artificial Insemination in 2193 Nulliparous Women with Azoospermic Husbands." *The New England Journal of Medicine* 306 (7) (February): 404–6. http://www.ncbi.nlm.nih.gov/pubmed/7057832.

Scoccia, Bert, Habibe Demir, Yuna Kang, Michelle A. Fierro, and Nicola J. Winston. 2012. "In Vitro Fertilization Pregnancy Rates in Levothyroxine-Treated Women with Hypothyroidism Compared to Women Without Thyroid Dysfunction Disorders." *Thyroid* 22 (6) (June): 631–36. doi: 10.1089/thy.2011.0343.

Shames, Richard. Telephone interview by Mary Shomon, August 22, 2015.

Shomon, Mary J. 2005. *Living Well with Hypothyroidism: What Your Doctor Doesn't Tell You That You Need to Know*, 2nd ed. New York: HarperCollins.

Sipos, Jennifer. Telephone interview by Dana Trentini, August 28, 2015.

Slama, Remy, Oluf Hansen, Beatrice Ducot, Aline Bohet, Sebastien Bottagisi, Lyliane Rosetta, Niels Keiding, and Jean Bouyer. 2012. "Estimation of the Frequency of Involuntary Infertility on a Nation-Wide Basis." *Human Reproduction* 27 (5) (May): 1489–98. doi: 10.1093/humrep/des070.

Stagnaro-Green, Alex, Sheila H. Roman, Rhoda H. Cobin, Essam El-Harazy, Michael Alvarez-Marfany, and Terry F. Davies. 1990. "Detection of At-Risk Pregnancy by Means of Highly Sensitive Assays for Thyroid Autoantibodies." *Journal of American Medical Association* 264 (11) (September): 1422–25. http://www.ncbi.nlm.nih.gov /pubmed/2118190.

Stagnaro-Green, Alex, Emmerita Dogo-Isonaige, Elizabeth N. Pearce, Carole Spencer, and Nancy D. Gaba. 2015. "Marginal Iodine Status and High Rate of Subclinical Hypothyroidism in Washington DC Women Planning Conception." *Thyroid* 7 (August). http://www.ncbi.nlm.nih.gov/pubmed/26160595.

Stagnaro-Green, Alex, Scott Sullivan, and Elizabeth N. Pearce. 2012. "Iodine Supplementation During Pregnancy and Lactation." *Journal of American Medical Association* 308 (23) (December): 2463–64. doi: 10.1001/jama.2012.45423.

Stagnaro-Green, Alex, Marcos Abalovich, Erik Alexander, Fereidoun Azizi, Jorge Mestman, Roberto Negro, Angelita Nixon, Elizabeth N. Pearce, Offie P. Soldin, Scott Sullivan, and Wilmar Wiersinga. 2011. "Guidelines of the American Thyroid Association for the Diagnosis and Management of Thyroid Disease During Pregnancy and Postpartum." *Thyroid* 21 (10) (October): 1081–1125. doi: 10.1089/thy.2011.0087.

Stephen, E. H., and A. Chandra. 2006. "Declining Estimates of Infertility in the United States: 1982–2002." *Fertility and Sterility* 86 (3) (September): 516–23. http://www.ncbi.nlm.nih.gov/pubmed/16952500.

Tennant, Peter W. G., Rudy W. Bilous, Shamini Prathapan, and Ruth Bell. 2015. "Risk and Recurrence of Serious Adverse Outcomes in the First and Second Pregnancies of Women With Preexisting Diabetes." *Diabetes Care* 38 (4) (April): 610–19. doi: 10.2337/dc14–1888.

Thangaratinam, Shakila. 2011. "Association Between Thyroid Autoantibodies and Miscarriage and Preterm Birth: Meta-Analysis of Evidence." *BMJ* 342 (May). doi: http://dx.doi.org/10.1136/bmj.d2616.

Twig, Gilad, Avi Shina, Howard Amital, and Yehuda Shoenfeld. 2012. "Pathogenesis of Infertility and Recurrent Pregnancy Loss in Thyroid Autoimmunity." *Journal of Autoimmunity* 38 (2–3) (May): J275–J281. doi: 10.1016/j.jaut.2011.11.014.

UCSF Department of Radiology & Biomedical Imaging. "CT and MR Pregnancy Guidelines." http://www.radiology.ucsf.edu/patient-care/patient-safety/ct-mri-pregnancy.

Unfer, Vittorio, Emanuela Raffone, Piero Rizzo, and Silvia Buffo. 2011. "Effect of Supplementation with Myo-Inositol Plus Melatonin on Oocyte Quality in Women Who Failed to Conceive in Previous in Vitro Fertilization Cycles for Poor Oocyte Quality: A Prospective, Longitudinal, Cohort Study." *Gynecological Endocrinology* 27 (11) (November): 857–61. doi: 10.3109/09513590.2011.564687.

Wartofsky, Leonard, Daniel Glinoer, Barbara Solomon, Shigenobu Nagataki, Raphael Lagasse, Yuji Nagayama, and Motomori Izumi. 2009. "Differences and Similarities in the Diagnosis and Treatment of Graves' Disease in Europe, Japan, and the United States." *Thyroid* 1 (2): 129–35. http://online.liebertpub.com/doi/abs/10.1089/thy.1991.1.129.

Wentz, Izabella. E-mail to Dana Trentini, August 15, 2015.

Weschler, Toni. E-mail to Dana Trentini, August 12, 2015.

Woodruff, Tracey J., Ami R. Zota, and Jackie M. Schwartz. 2011. "Environmental Chemicals in Pregnant Women in the United States: NHANES 2003–2004." *Environmental Health Perspectives* 119 (6) (June): 878–85. doi: 10.1289/ehp.1002727.

World Health Organization. 1975. "The Epidemiology of Infertility. Report of a WHO Scientific Group." *World Health Organization Technical Report Series* 5 (82): 1–37.

Wright, Jonathan V. E-mail to Dana Trentini, August 15, 2015.

Yoshihara, Ai, Noh Jaeduk Yoshimura, Watanabe Natsuko, Mukasa Koji, Ohye Hidemi, Suzuki Miho, Matsumoto Masako, Kunii Yo, Suzuki Nami, Kameda Toshiaki, Iwaku Kenji, Kobayashi Sakiko, Sugino Kiminori, and Ito Koichi. 2015. "Substituting Potassium Iodide for Methimazole as the Treatment for Graves' Disease During the First Trimester May Reduce the Incidence of Congenital Anomalies: A Retrospective Study at a Single Medical Institution in Japan." *Thyroid* 28 (August). doi: 10.1089/thy.2014.0581.

Zhu, Qing, Li Wu, Bo Xu, Mei-Hong Hu, Xian-Hong Tong, Jing-Juan Ji, and Yu-Sheng Liu. 2013. "A Retrospective Study on IVF/ICSI Outcome in Patients with Anti-Nuclear Antibodies: The Effects of Prednisone Plus Low-Dose Aspirin Adjuvant Treatment. " *Reproductive Biology and Endocrinology* 11 (98) (October). doi: 10.1186/1477-7827-11-98.

Index